AF574500

Vestibular Disorders

Vestibular Disorders

HUGH O. BARBER, M.D., F.R.C.S.(C.)

Professor of Otolaryngology
University of Toronto
Department of Otolaryngology
Sunnybrook Medical Centre
University of Toronto Clinic
Toronto, Ontario, Canada

JAMES A. SHARPE, M.D., F.R.C.P.(C.)

Professor of Neurology
University of Toronto
Department of Medicine
The Toronto Hospital
Toronto, Ontario, Canada

YEAR BOOK MEDICAL PUBLISHERS, INC.

CHICAGO • LONDON • BOCA RATON

2 3 4 5 6 7 8 9 0 KC 92 91 90 89

Library of Congress Cataloging-in-Publication Data

Barber, Hugh O.

Vestibular disorders/Hugh O. Barber, James A. Sharpe.

p. cm.

Includes bibliographies and index.

ISBN 0-8151-0419-7

1. Vertigo. 2. Vestibular function tests. 3. Equilibrium (Physiology) I. Sharpe, James A. II. Title.

[DNLM: 1. Dizziness. 2. Eye Movements. 3. Reflex Vestibulo-Ocular. 4. Vestibular Function Tests—methods. WV 255 B234v]

RF260.B27 1988 87-34085

616.8′41—dc19 CIP

DNLM/DLC

for Library of Congress

Sponsoring Editor: David K. Marshall

Assistant Director, Manuscript Services: Frances M. Perveiler

Production Project Manager: Carol A. Reynolds

Proofroom Supervisor: Shirley E. Taylor

Contributors

ROBERT W. BALOH, M.D.
Professor of Neurology, UCLA School of Medicine, Los Angeles, California

HUGH O. BARBER, M.D., F.R.C.S.(C.)
Professor of Otolaryngology, University of Toronto; Department of Otolaryngology, Sunnybrook Medical Centre, University of Toronto Clinic, Toronto, Ontario, Canada

JACOB BLOOMBERG, B.Sc.
Aerospace Medical Research Unit, McGill University, Montreal, Quebec, Canada

LOUIS R. CAPLAN, M.D.
Professor and Chairman, Neurology, Tufts University; Neurologist-in-Chief, New England Medical Center, Boston, Massachusetts

JOSEPH M. R. FURMAN, M.D., Ph.D.
Assistant Professor, Departments of Otolaryngology and Neurology, University of Pittsburgh, Eye and Ear Hospital of Pittsburgh, Pittsburgh, Pennsylvania

VICENTE HONRUBIA, M.D., D.M.Sc.
Professor, Director of Research, Division of Head and Neck Surgery, UCLA School of Medicine, Los Angeles, California

KATHLEEN M. JACOBSON, B.A.
Staff Research Associate, Department of Neurology, UCLA School of Medicine, Los Angeles, California

GEOFFREY MELVILL JONES, M.D.
Hosmer Research Professor of Applied Physiology, Director, Aerospace Medical Research Unit, Department of Physiology, McGill University, Montreal, Quebec, Canada

DONALD B. KAMERER, M.D.
Associate Professor, Department of Otolaryngology, University of Pittsburgh School of Medicine; Chief, Division of Otology, Eye and Ear Hospital of Pittsburgh, Pittsburgh, Pennsylvania

ATHANASIOS KATSARKAS, M.D. F.R.C.S.(C.)
Associate Professor, Department of Otolaryngology, McGill University, Montreal, Quebec, Canada

R. JOHN LEIGH, M.D.
Associate Professor, Departments of Neurology, Otolaryngology, and Biomedical Engineering, Case Western Reserve University, Cleveland, Ohio

JOSEPH A. McCLURE, M.D.
Clinical Associate Professor, Department of Otolaryngology, The University of Western Ontario, London Ear Clinic, London, Ontario, Canada

MARK J. MORROW, M.D.
Fellow in Neuro-Ophthalmology, University of Toronto; Division of Neurology, Department of Medicine, The Toronto Hospital, Toronto, Ontario, Canada

JAMES E. OLSSON, M.D., F.A.C.S.
Clinical Associate Professor, Division of Otorhinology, The University of Texas Health Science Center at San Antonio, San Antonio, Texas

BARRY W. PETERSON, Ph.D.
Professor, Department of Physiology and Rehabilitative Medicine, Northwestern University Medical School, Chicago, Illinois

LEONARD R. PROCTOR, M.D.
Associate Professor, Department of Otolaryngology—Head and Neck Surgery, The Johns Hopkins University School of Medicine, Baltimore, Maryland

PAUL J. RANALLI, M.D., F.R.C.P.(C.)
Lecturer, Division of Neurology, Department of Medicine, University of Toronto; Research Fellow, Neuro-Ophthalmology Unit, Playfair Neuroscience Unit, The Toronto Hospital, Toronto, Ontario, Canada

BERNARD SEGAL, Ph.D.
Assistant Professor, Department of Otolaryngology, Sir Mortimer B. Davis Jewish General Hospital, McGill University, Montreal, Quebec, Canada

JAMES A. SHARPE, M.D., F.R.C.P.(C.)
Professor, Departments of Medicine, Ophthalmology, and Otolaryngology, Director, Neuro-Ophthalmology Unit, The Toronto Hospital and Playfair Neuroscience Unit, University of Toronto, Toronto, Ontario, Canada

CHARLES W. STOCKWELL, Ph.D.
Director of Vestibular Laboratory, Greater Detroit Otology Center, Farmington Hills, Michigan

R. DAVID TOMLINSON, Ph.D.
Associate Professor, Departments of Physiology and Otolaryngology, Playfair Neuroscience Unit, The Toronto Hospital, University of Toronto, Toronto, Ontario, Canada

CONRAD WALL, III, Ph.D.
Associate Professor of Otolaryngology, Director, Vestibular Laboratory, Massachusetts Eye and Ear Infirmary, Harvard Medical School, Boston, Massachusetts

DOUGLAS G. D. WATT, M.D., Ph.D.
Professor, Aerospace Medical Research Unit, Department of Physiology, McGill University, Montreal, Quebec, Canada

ROBERT D. YEE, M.D.
Professor and Chairman, Department of Ophthalmology, Indiana University School of Medicine, Indiana University Medical Center, Indianapolis, Indiana

DAVID S. ZEE, M.D.
Professor of Neurology, Department of Neurology, The Johns Hopkins Hospital, Baltimore, Maryland

Preface

In no area of neuroscience have recent advances in fundamental research had more profound impact on clinical research and practice than vestibular studies. *Vestibular Disorders* presents the latest viewpoints of both basic and clinical scientists on the disordered physiology of the vestibular system, with goals of understanding its disturbances and providing scientific bases for testing its functions, and for managing patients. The text is divided into four parts that deal with (1) the neurophysiology of orientation; (2) the comparative merits of different vestibular function tests; (3) smooth eye movement disorders; and (4) the diagnosis and management of dizziness. This book is directed at physicians and physiologists who are concerned with dizzy patients. The contents are not encyclopedic; the book is intended to be sufficiently broad to satisfy the needs of experienced otologists or neurologists and to provide a foundation for residents. We have selected topics by expert contributors to highlight recent important advances. Contributors have discussed those aspects of physiology most pertinent to understanding vestibular disorders.

Hugh O. Barber, M.D., F.R.C.S.(C.)
James A. Sharpe, M.D., F.R.C.P.(C.)

Contents

PART ONE

Recent Concepts of the Neurophysiology of Orientation

1

*Experiments on Vestibular Adaptation and Its Clinical Significance**

Geoffrey Melvill Jones, M.D.

Bernard Segal, Ph.D.

Athanasios Katsarkas, M.D.

Jacob Bloomberg, B.Sc.

It is well known to the neurotologist that the vestibular system as a whole exhibits a remarkable potential for clinical rehabilitation after pathologic lesions. Even after the extreme insult of unilateral ablation of the peripheral end organ and/or its peripheral innervation, there often is progressive recovery toward apparent behavioral normality, including return of the patient to the work force. Nevertheless, there remains much to learn about the fundamental underlying physiologic processes responsible for this kind of neurologic rehabilitation.

For example, although neurologic lesions can certainly generate central plastic reactions such as neural sprouting, reactive synaptoge-

*This research was supported by Canadian Medical Research Council grants MT-5630, MA-9715; the McGill Hosmer Foundation; and the Department of Otolaryngology, Sir Mortimer B. Davis Jewish General Hospital. B. Segal was supported by McGill Faculty of Medicine Fraser-Monat-McPherson bequest, and J. Bloomberg holds a graduate student fellowship of the Canadian National Sciences and Engineering Research Council of Canada.

nesis, and deafferentation supersensitivity,[7–9, 56, 57] the extent to which these processes need to be brought under behavioral control for full functional recovery remains debatable.[17, 34, 58, 61] Despite these uncertainties, at least some key factors are clear. Thus, even in the absence of any lesion, purely behavioral stimuli can readily be made to induce extensive adaptive plastic changes of reflex function.[2, 26, 33, 40] Moreover, these behaviorally induced changes of reflex function appear to be associated with correlated central neurophysiologic changes of a plastic nature.[18, 29, 43] However, the rehabilitative process is not restricted to these mechanisms. An additional feature is the organized recruitment of allied sensory-motor systems to "make good," or "substitute" for, lasting deficiencies incurred by the primary pathologic impairment.[28, 49] No doubt in practice any call for "action" initiates a multifactoral "search" for "best" solutions to a particular problem, drawing in idiosyncratic fashion from the available repertoire of these physiologic options.[1]

We review briefly first the experimental basis of behaviorally induced vestibular adaptation in normal subjects. Next we describe some recent studies which demonstrate the correction of vestibulo-ocular inadequacy by the synergistic contribution of complementary saccadic eye movements acting in the *compensatory* direction. Finally, we address the clinical relevance of these findings as reflected in the overall rehabilitation of a patient subjected to unilateral 8th nerve neuronectomy due to acoustic neuroma.

REVIEW OF ADAPTIVE PLASTICITY IN THE SLOW-PHASE COMPONENT OF THE VESTIBULO-OCULAR REFLEX (VOR)

Behavioral Experiments

In the Introduction, we questioned the extent to which a patient's plastic neural reactions to an internal lesion could be brought under behavioral control through an active working encounter with the external environment. At first it seemed difficult to conceive how the essentially internal phenomenon of central neural plasticity could, *of itself,* serve to reestablish a proper degree of sensory-motor correspondence[36] at the interface with the external physical world. Presumably for functionally meaningful recovery, the active process of internal neurologic rearrangement would have to be guided by some kind of adaptive informational feedback from the working brain-world interface.

Following these guidelines, it was argued that if such feedback could be activated in the *abnormal* subject by physical contact with our *normal* environment, then conversely it should surely be possible to induce analogous effects in the laboratory by exposing the *normal* human subject to an *abnormal* encounter with the external environment. It was essentially this "guess," together with the recognized need for active maintenance of even the normal "status quo" (neurologic homeostasis), which first triggered[14] an extended series of experimental studies designed to investigate the potential for purely behavioral induction of adaptive plasticity within the CNS.

Initial experiments utilized the VOR as a model sensory-motor system. Leaning on the outcome of psychologic studies of Kohler,[27] optically reversing prism goggles were used to "ask" the involuntary VOR to reverse itself. The prism goggles were arranged on the head so that when turning, say, to the right, the eyes would have to move smoothly *also to the right* if they were to "see" a stable image of the external world on the retina during head rotation, which is exactly opposite to normal VOR compensation. Short durations of exposure to this demanding situation resulted in relatively large degrees of attenuation in slow-phase gain of the dark-tested reflex (slow phase VOR gain = [compensatory eye velocity]/[head angular velocity]).[15]

Figure 1–1 summarizes results obtained from 7 human subjects. The lower curves show the mean daily reduction in (normalized) VOR gain resulting from two successive 8-minute exposures to mirror reversal of vision during sinusoidal whole body rotation, repeated on 3 successive days. On each day there was a highly significant VOR attenuation amounting to about 20% of the initial condition, albeit with almost (but not quite) complete recovery between days. The top row of control points demonstrates that this attenuation was not due to simple habituation, since exactly the same vestibular stimulus profile (⅙ Hz, 60°/sec amp) conducted *without* vision reversal produced no significant alterations in the dark-tested reflex, as has been confirmed for this stimulus frequency by other authors.[23]

Bearing in mind that Kohler's subjects needed weeks, not minutes, of continuous vision inversion to produce effective functional adaptation in locomotive and sportive activities, we similarly extended our experimental exposures in the reversed vision paradigm. As illustrated in Figure 1–2,A, after about 2 weeks ambulatory activity with continuous left-right vision reversal, the *dark-tested* VOR produced an adaptively altered pattern of ocular response in which both the slow and quick phases of resulting nystagmus became effectively the reverse of normal.[16, 32] This new condition was approached gradually through a combination of progressively reduced gain (upper

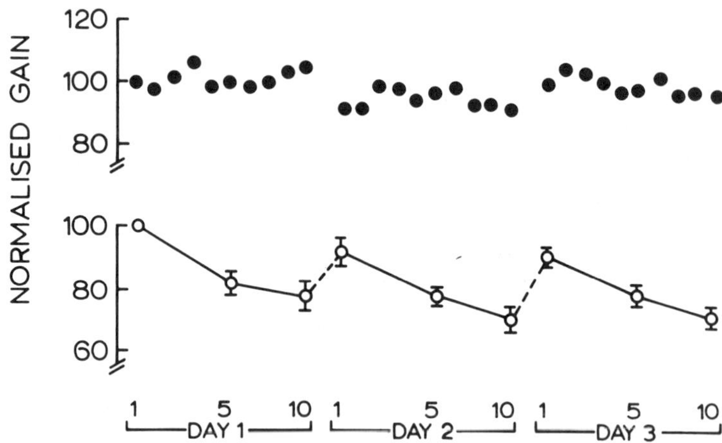

FIG 1–1.
Short-term adaptive changes in the human VOR. Upper control data points define the lack of habituation produced by repeated 2-min exposures to horizontal sinusoidal rotation with normal vision. Each point shows dark-tested VOR gain measured after each 2-min period of normal vestibular-visual interaction. Lower curves show progressive attenuation of dark-tested VOR, with 8 min of reversed visual-vestibular conflict between each point. Note restoration of VOR gain between consecutive daily tests, with a small but significant decline of initial test results on each of 3 consecutive days. (Data from Gonshor A, Melvill Jones, G: Short-term adaptive changes in the human vestibulo-ocular reflex arc. *J Physiol* 1976; 256:361–379.)

curves in each figure) coupled with changes of phase (lower curves) that had a trend toward a reversed response, which would ideally be represented in these figures by a 180° phase shift. Figure 1–2,B, shows similar patterns of change in the cat exposed to very long durations of continuous dove prism reversal of vision.[37] The inset in Figure 1–2 shows samples of original tracings of compensatory nystagmus from the human subject during sinusoidal whole body oscillation in the dark, (a) during a control test and (b) after 14 days of adaptation to the reversed visual-vestibular conflict. Notice the almost complete reversal of the adapted reflex response, although at somewhat reduced gain, denoted by the respective calibration bars.

Important in Figure 1–2 are the following three features: (1) effects were long-lasting; (2) observed changes were adaptive in that they improved the functional goal of retinal image stabilization during head rotation; (3) given adequate time (roughly equal to the duration of the preceding reversed vision experience) a return to normal vision completely restored the normal VOR, although in a somewhat complex

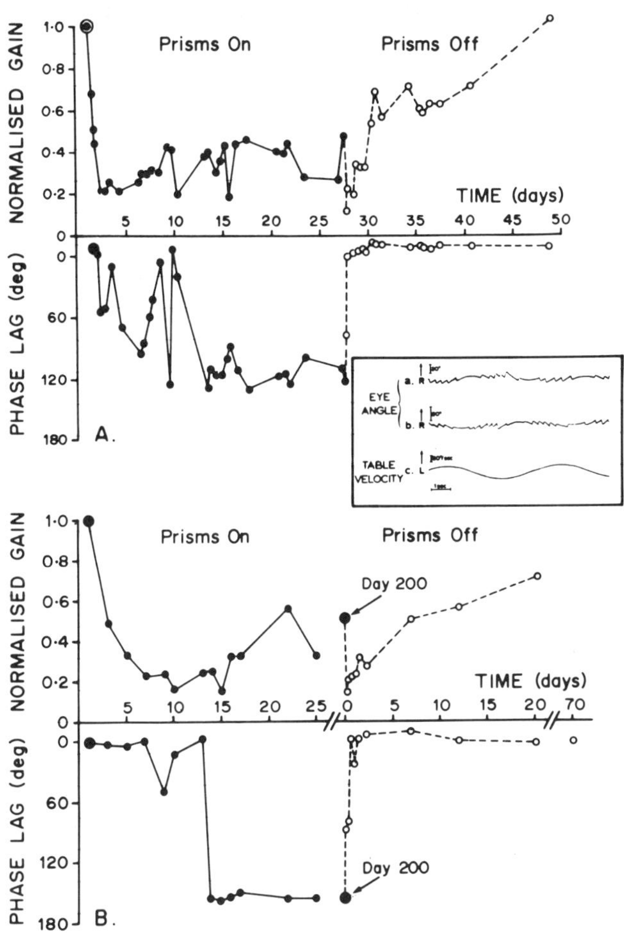

FIG 1–2.

Time course of long-term VOR adaptive changes in gain and phase during (●) and after (○) the wearing of horizontally reversing dove prisms. **A,** man, tested at 1/6 Hz, 60°/sec peak amplitude. **B,** cat, tested at 1/8 Hz, 5°/sec. The phase is registered relative to perfect normal compensation. All tests were conducted in darkness. *Inset* shows samples of normal *(upper)* and adapted ("reversed") nystagmus tested in the dark after 14 days of continuous vision reversal. (Adapted from Melvill Jones G: Plasticity in the adult vestibulo-ocular reflex arc. *Philos Trans R Soc Lond* [*Biol*] 1977; 278:319–334.)

manner.[39] These characteristics led us to adopt the term "adaptive plasticity" to describe the general features of this phenomenon.

Additional animal experiments both replicated and extended the findings of these early studies in the cat[31, 48]; in the rabbit[22]; in the monkey[42]; in the chicken[59]; and in the goldfish.[50]

For example, Figure 1–3 illustrates the systematic augmentation of VOR gain produced in monkeys who wore binocular spectacles which, instead of reversing the seen world, simply magnified it by a factor of 2.[42] After a week or so of wearing these binoculars, the monkey's dark-tested VOR had appropriately nearly doubled itself. This condition was approached approximately exponentially and tended to be retained indefinitely in the absence of further visual-vestibular interaction. However, as in the earlier human experiments, the VOR could be completely restored to normal by reexposure to normal vision and movement, albeit with a somewhat faster time course than the original adaptation. Moreover, reexposure of the same animal to the same adaptive stimuli repeatedly produced an identical time course of VOR gain change, emphasizing the almost "machine-like" nature of the adaptive process. In line with these findings, Miles and Eighmy[42] also showed that substituting miniaturizing lenses for the magnifying ones produced the appropriate effect of attenuating, rather than augmenting, slow-phase VOR gain.

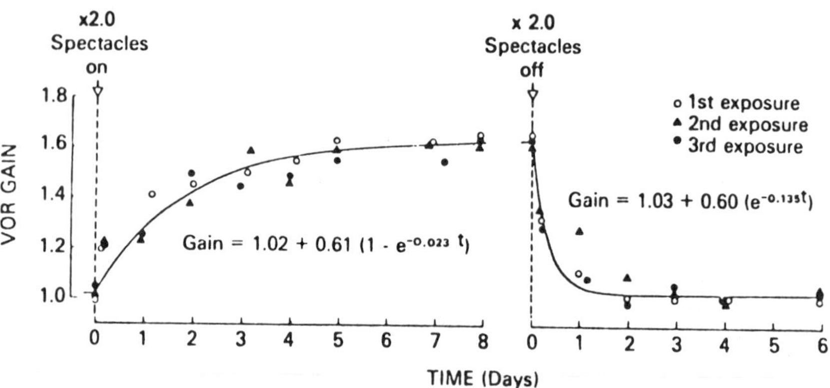

FIG 1–3.
Adaptive enhancement and recovery of VOR gain in a monkey exposed to continuous ×2 binocular vision. The different symbols represent data from the same animal obtained on different occasions. The similarity of the curves they depict emphasizes the "machine-like" characteristics of the adaptive process. (From Miles FA, Eighmy BB: Long-term adaptive changes in primate vestibuloocular reflex: I. Behavioral observations. *J Neurophysiol* 1980; 43:1406–1425. Used by permission.)

Numerous additional studies have now demonstrated the apparent universality of this kind of behaviorally induced central plasticity in the absence of a neurologic lesion. For example, artificial obstruction of fluid circulation in the lumen of one semicircular canal (without affecting its peripheral innervation) effectively halves slow-phase VOR output as an immediate consequence of the obstruction to endolymph circulation.[45–47] Yet following normal behavioral exposure to the normal visual world, vestibulo-ocular slow-phase output is progressively restored to near normal in the absence of recanalization of the peripheral end organ.

Even the direction of ocular response to a given peripheral vestibular stimulus can be adaptively changed by rotationally oscillating the normal animal in one plane (e.g., vertical) but artificially causing a coordinated movement of the visual scene in *another* plane (e.g., horizontal).[51] Nor is the phenomenon restricted to horizontal and sagittal vertical planes: the slow phase of torsional VOR (TVOR) in the frontal plane proves equally susceptible to adaptive modulation as illustrated in Figure 1–4.[3] Here the upper (dotted) traces show the oscillatory torsional eye rotation induced reflexly by oscillatory rotation of a human subject about a vertical axis, with the head tilted back 90° and the eyes looking (in darkness) vertically upward. Before adaptation, there was a brisk TVOR. After 3 weeks of wearing prisms which reversed the seen visual image movement in both torsional and horizontal planes, TVOR was much reduced. The analyzed data of the lower half of the figure show that roughly proportionate adaptive changes of gain occurred in these two affected planes.

Central Mechanisms

From these and related studies of visual-vestibular interactions,[35] the importance of active behavioral contact with the environment is well proven today. When the normal adult subject is exposed to an abnormal sensory-motor interface with the external world, there is an immensely powerful potential for bringing about appropriate (i.e., adaptive) remodeling in relevant central neural networks—notably, without the intrusion of an invasive lesion. What do we know about the nature of these central mechanisms? Are they compatible with the kind of central neural plasticity known to result from internal lesions?

To the latter question we may give a cautiously affirmative answer, although the nature and sites of induced plastic change remain unclear. Briefly, it seems certain that cerebellar function is intimately involved, since vestibular cerebellar ablation generally blocks adap-

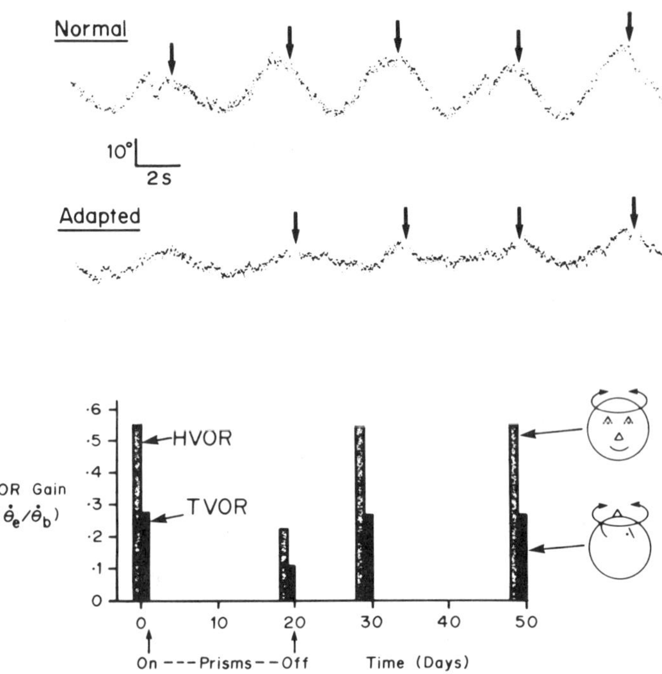

FIG 1–4.
Adaptive attenuation of torsional VOR in a human subject exposed to 3 weeks of dove prism vision, which reverses visual movement in both frontal and horizontal planes. **Upper traces,** original records obtained by frame-to-frame measurement (individual dots) of torsional eye movement by means of infrared cinephotography (stimulus amp 35°; 1/5 Hz). *Vertical arrows,* estimated moments of peak angular deviation of turntable. **Lower "bar" figure** compares adaptive changes of gain in horizontal *(HVOR)* and torsional *(TVOR)* planes in the same subject. Note that similar degrees of adaptive attenuation and recovery were attained in each plane. (Data from Berthoz A, Melvill Jones G, Bégué AE: Differential visual adaptation of vertical canal-dependent vestibulo-ocular reflexes. *Exp Brain Res* 1981; 44:19–26.)

tive plasticity of VOR gain.[21, 44, 48] However, whereas Ito and colleagues favor plastic changes located at a cellular level in the *cerebellar cortex itself* and induced by retinal image slippage,[18–20] Miles and associates[43, 44] point to the cerebellar cortex merely as an important "way station." They suggest that, instead of itself undergoing plastic change, the cortex rather serves to assemble a new neural signal; namely, a signal coded in cortical Purkinje cells and representing *error in gaze stabilization relative to space.* In turn, this internally generated error signal is presumed to bring about relevant changes of synaptic efficacy (the necessary cellular plastic change) within some target relay station located in the vestibular nuclei.[43] The resulting slow-phase VOR output would thereby be altered in a manner which reduces that error and hence improves reflex gaze stabilization during head rotation. Contemporary neurophysiologic findings of Lisberger and colleagues[29, 30] support the latter hypothesis as does the behavioral demonstration that purely mental suppression of the VOR leads to its adaptive attenuation *in the absence of any real visual conflict.*[41]

However, both views are in good accord with theoretical predictions of Galiana et al.[12] and Galiana,[11] reviewed in Galiana.[10] No doubt ultimately the two hypotheses will prove equally substantive in spelling out different components in a multifactoral process.

We turn next to entrainment of the saccadic oculomotor system as a complement to VOR slow-phase insufficiency in the automatic stabilization of visual gaze. Note that the term "gaze" is defined as the direction of regard relative to space (i.e., gaze = [eye position re: head] + [head position re: space]).

VOR-SACCADIC SYNERGY IN GAZE STABILIZATION

Normal Unadapted Human Subjects

It has frequently been noted that when, *with head still,* slow phase *visual* pursuit of a moving target proves inadequate, supplementary saccadic catch-up eye movements tend to make good the visual tracking error,[6] particularly when there is pathologic attenuation of slow-phase visual tracking capability.[38, 60] Recent studies in our laboratories showed that an analogous saccadic supplementation of the slow-phase VOR tends to occur in normal human subjects during head rotation in the dark.[4, 52–54] The *internal* nature of the phenomenon is emphasized by the fact that it occurs when the VOR is tested in complete darkness, while the subject tries to "look" at an (unseen) stationary (i.e., Earth-fixed) target that has just been viewed before extinguishing the lights.

Figure 1–5 illustrates an example of this kind of VOR-saccadic synergy. Eye movements from one subject during two turns in opposite directions are shown. In each case, the subject looked first at a small, stationary target in the light. Then the light was extinguished while he continued trying to "look" at the now-remembered target. Shortly thereafter, but at an unpredictable time, the subject was suddenly rotated through 20° to the right or left at a steady angular veloc-

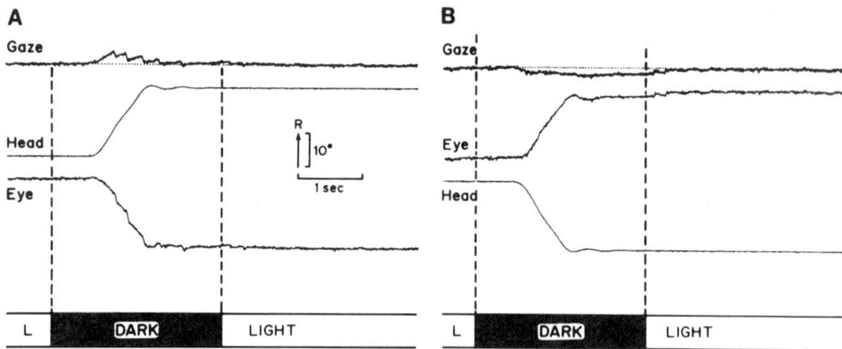

FIG 1–5.
Oculomotor response to transient rotation in total darkness while the subject tried to stabilize direction of gaze on an imagined, Earth-fixed target. **A,** when turned to right, the slow-phase VOR undercompensated, but undercompensation was successively corrected by clearly defined saccades in compensatory direction. Note that these supplementary saccades were "injected" during the head rotation in total darkness, with only minor corrective eye movement onto target when the lights were turned on. **B,** when turned left, the right-going slow-phase VOR almost completely compensated for head rotation without saccadic supplementation, as determined by minimal corrective eye movement after reilluminating target. Gaze trace computed by summation of eye and head movement traces after adjustment for equal calibrations. It clarifies the functional role of saccades in left-hand set of traces, since they repeatedly brought the direction of visual regard back toward the real (but unseen) target *(horizontal dotted line).*

ity of 40°/sec, the head being locked to the rotating turntable by means of a dental bite. After cessation of all movement and while still "looking" at the imagined target, the light was turned on again, and, if required, a corrective saccade was then made onto the original, now visible, target. The method is somewhat similar to that of Gauthier and Robinson.[13] As shown in the left-hand figure, when the head began rotating to the right, there was a virtually synchronous slow-phase compensatory eye movement of VOR origin. But part way through the turn, there were clear-cut saccadic eye movements, *in the same compensatory direction* as the slow phase, followed again by continuation of the slow-phase VOR as it corrected for the damped head oscillations associated with cessation of turntable rotation.

Both the presence and functional significance of these saccades are highlighted in the computed curve of gaze (summation of eye and head movement traces), which ideally should have been stabilized during head rotation, as indicated by the dotted horizontal line. Evidently each saccade appropriately moved the gaze direction toward the intended spatial target after deviation from it due to undercompensation of the VOR. Note particularly that these saccades took place in complete darkness and during the very brief head rotation. Further, after cessation of head rotation, as can be seen from the final very small corrective saccade in the light, the *net* ocular compensation was almost perfect, notably because of these interjected saccades. If their effects had been disregarded, as is customary when using cumulative slow-phase analysis of VOR, the presumed vestibular compensatory response (i.e., the cumulative slow-phase eye movement) would have been deemed to have undercompensated for the head movement with a gain of only 0.66. However, inclusion of the supplementary saccades leads to a new estimated *net* compensatory gain amounting to 0.98. The internal brain apparently "knew" where to place the gaze relative to space despite inadequacy of the slow-phase component of the VOR.

Another feature, to which we return later in a clinical context, is shown in the right-hand set of traces. When this subject was turned in the opposite direction, compensation was almost completely achieved by means of the VOR slow phase. This proved to be a consistent form of asymmetry in this subject, even to the point of his particular asymmetry's amounting to a readily recognized performance "signature."

The consistency of saccadic supplementation is well illustrated in the accumulated control data of Figure 1–6, shown in the left-hand pair of columns. Here we see results obtained from an experiment in which the subject of Figure 1–5 was repeatedly rotated to right or left for a total of 40 turns in the control phase of the experiment. Right and left turns were imposed in random order so that the subject could not predict the direction of the next turn. In this "bar" figure the ordinate is expressed as the degree of "stabilization," defined as the fraction of ideal compensation achieved respectively by slow phase alone (shaded areas) and saccadic supplements (clear areas). Net compensation is represented by the total height of the bar.

There was a general tendency to contribute saccadic supplements, with the special feature that in this subject there was a consistent directional asymmetry in VOR slow phase gain. Despite this marked asymmetry of VOR slow-phase gain, there was no significant difference between *net* compensation in the two directions, due to the organized "injection" of appropriate supplementary saccades, augmented in the VOR-deficient direction.

Bearing in mind that all test turns were conducted in the dark, the question arises, how does the *internal* neural system "know" how large a saccadic contribution to make? Certainly this contribution is not arbitrary, since the net response does achieve the intended goal to

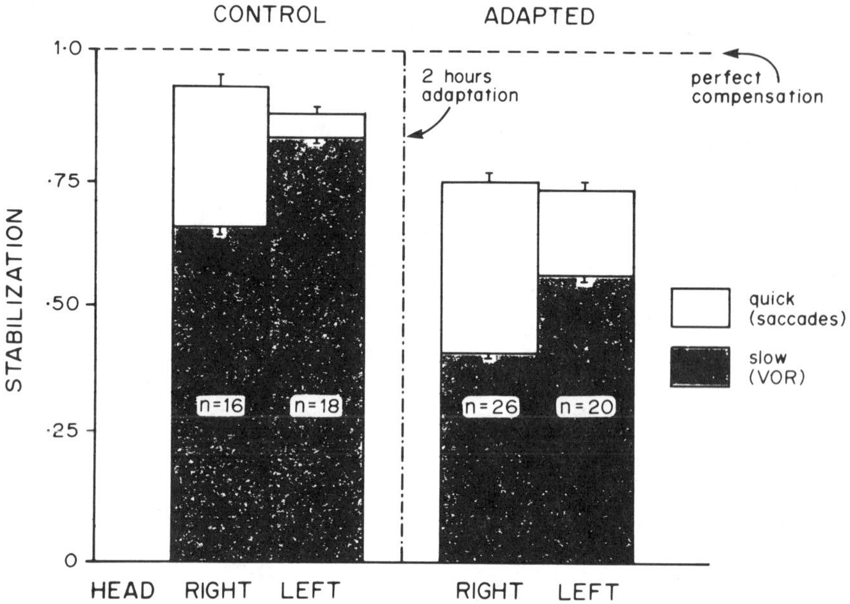

FIG 1–6.
Cumulative data from subject in Figure 1–5 showing average slow-phase and saccade contributions in *control* tests and similar tests conducted after 2 hr of an *adaptive* stimulus comprising visual suppression of VOR (see text and Fig 1–7). Note (1) asymmetric slow-phase VOR gain *(shaded bars)* elicited by turns of opposite direction; (2) restoration of compensatory gaze stabilization by enhanced saccadic contributions *(clear bars)* when turning in direction associated with low VOR gain; (3) inverse VOR and saccadic asymmetries were retained after 2-hr period of adaptive stimulus; (4) retention of directional symmetry in net gain of adapted response; (5) significantly lowered value of net gain after adaptation. (Selected data from Bloomberg, Melvill Jones G, Segal B: Quick and slow-phase interaction following adaptive attenuation of the human vestibulo-ocular reflex (VOR). *Can J Physiol Pharmacol* 1986; 64(4):Aiii.)

a good approximation, a conclusion which is clinched by a highly significant negative correlation between the respective magnitudes of slow phase and saccadic contributions during individual turns. In other words, low slow-phase gains are associated with high saccadic contributions and vice versa.[4, 53, 54]

Adaptive Phenomena

Given the fact that slow phase VOR gain can readily be adaptively modulated, what would be the relative roles of slow phase and saccadic elements in the adapted response? We chose to use the well-tried adaptive stimulus of synchronous rotation of the subject and the surrounding visual scene. The subject sat on a servo-driven turntable surrounded by an independently servo-driven "optokinetic" cylinder (Fig 1–7). When the two systems are rotationally oscillated with the same phase and amplitude, vision calls for cancellation of the VOR. There is progressive attenuation of slow phase VOR gain as tested in the dark. We used sinusoidal horizontal rotation of ⅙ Hz and 40°/sec peak angular velocity, extended over a total exposure of 2 hours, to produce adaptive attenuation of slow-phase VOR amounting to about 30%.

The outcome for the above subject is shown in the adapted segments of Figure 1–6 (the right-hand pair of columns). As expected, the slow-phase VOR gain, tested as in Figure 1–5, was systematically attenuated by about 30%. However, this led to retention of an asymmetric response in the absolute values of right and left slow-phase

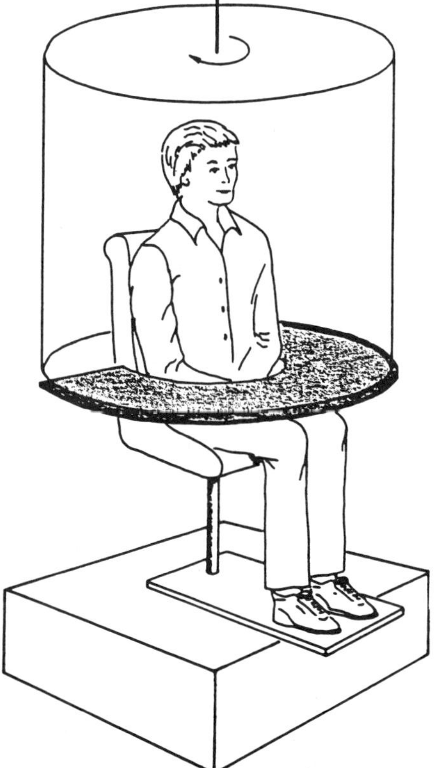

FIG 1–7.
Method for producing visual-vestibular conflict. Subject and surroundings were synchronously rotated in sinusoidal fashion for 2 hr at 1/6 Hz and peak velocity of 40°/sec with lights on. For clear vision, subject was obliged to suppress visually VOR over this period of conflict stimulus.

VOR gains. The question was how would the saccadic component respond to the adaptive stimulus? The answer is twofold. First, saccades successfully resolved the asymmetric condition by contributing larger compensatory elements during turns in the direction which produced smaller slow-phase VOR gains. Despite this, there remained a highly significant reduction of the *net* response relative to control conditions, even though there was some augmentation of the saccadic contribution per se. The *goal* of the whole synergistic system had been altered, and despite asymmetry in the adapted VOR, the modification of this goal appeared to remain independent of direction as reflected in the net overall achievement.

We conclude that (1) the saccadic elements served to carry the direction of gaze to an *internally perceived* location of the unseen target *independently of VOR performance*, and that (2) the perceived movement of that location relative to the head was adaptively attenuated approximately in line with adaptive attenuation of the brain stem slow-phase VOR. In other words, the phenomenon of sensory-motor correspondence[36] tends to be maintained at both reflex and cognitive levels, even after exposure to the adaptive stimulus.

A CLINICAL STUDY

How can these findings and emerging ideas be applied to clinical vestibular problems? Given a clinically defined vestibular asymmetry (e.g., peripheral unilateral vestibular afferent inactivation), could the rehabilitative process of clinical compensation include an asymmetric augmentation of the saccadic contribution to a permanently penalized slow-phase VOR? Kasai and Zee,[24] investigating the *cervico*-ocular reflex in a subject with complete absence of labyrinthine function, noted that he " . . . used quick phases to help stabilize gaze rather than to redirect the centre of visual attention." If quick phase supplementation of VOR occurs in a case of partial vestibular deficiency, then (1) such a phenomenon could mask an underlying VOR incompetence in a patient who had apparently reached a level of full behavioral recovery, and (2) conventional vestibular function tests, which quantify only the slow-phase component of the VOR, would fail to identify the more crucial functional level of recovery of the whole synergistic vestibular gaze control system.

Recent clinical investigations conducted by Segal and Katsarkas at the Sir Mortimer B. Davis-Jewish General Hospital[25, 55] examined patients with specifically unilateral vestibular pathology. Some early findings from one patient, obtained 3 months after complete right-sided 8th nerve neuronectomy for acoustic neuroma, are shown in Figure 1–8. The vertical columns are similar to those of Figure 1–6—their height represents the fraction of compensatory eye movement relative to ideal. However, unlike Figure 1–6, this patient was tested over a wide range of stimulus angular velocities (8°–170°/sec) on the grounds that response asymmetries might manifest themselves at high (but not low) velocities due to peripheral response cut-off in the unilateral sensory system. This was indeed the case. First, in response to test rotations contralateral to the neuronectomy (left-hand pair of col-

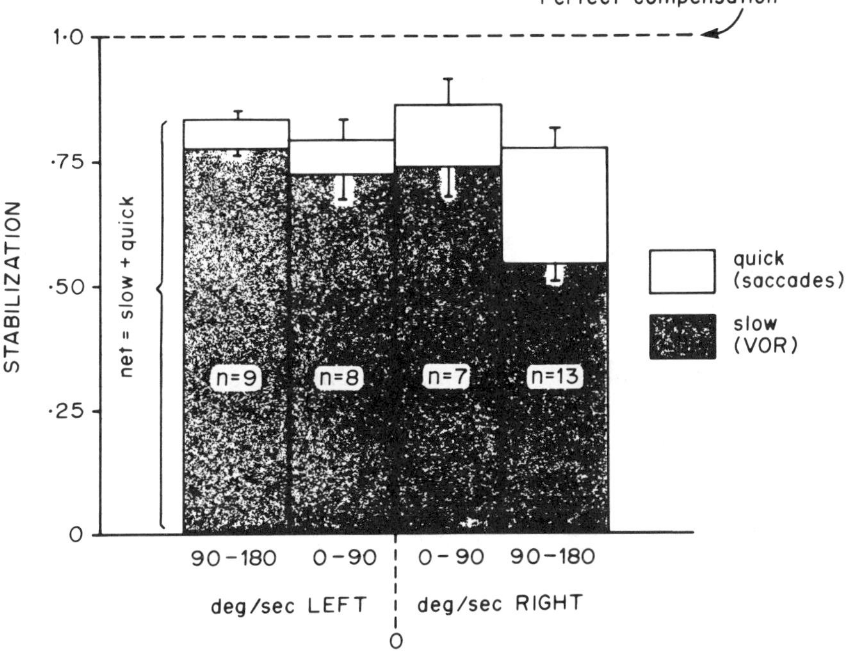

FIG 1–8.

Results obtained from clinical patient 3 months after right unilateral 8th nerve neuronectomy due to acoustic neuroma. On turning left (left pair of columns), there was good gaze compensation both below and above 90°/sec velocity stimuli. In contrast, during turns ipsilateral to the lesion (right pair of columns), there was attenuation of VOR in the higher velocity range. Note that this permanent pathologic VOR attenuation was effectively offset by enhanced saccadic contributions restoring symmetry in the automatic stabilization of gaze. (Selected data from Segal BN, Katsarkas A: Long-term deficits of goal-directed vestibulo-ocular function following total unilateral loss of peripheral vestibular function. *Acta Otolaryngol (Stockh)* 1988; in press.)

umns), both the slow-phase VOR and the supplementary saccadic contributions were independent of rotational velocity over the tested range. Moreover, in this direction the net response was consistently not far removed from the ideal value of unity, indicating that substantial adaptive rehabilitation of VOR gain had occurred. However, in contrast to this, when turning in the opposite direction (i.e., ipsilateral to the lesion and inhibitory to the remaining afferent input), there was a marked velocity dependence of VOR slow-phase gain (right-hand pair of columns). Although up to 90°/sec the mean VOR gain was 0.72 (± SE, 0.058), above this speed it fell to 0.53 (± 0.035), representing a significant drop of about 25%. The finding emphasizes the importance of extenuating the system by using high-velocity stimuli in clinical function testing.

Particularly relevant to this article is the additional finding that in this "rehabilitated" patient, a residual asymmetry in the slow-phase VOR was effectively rectified by the "injection" of larger saccadic compensatory elements (clear bar areas) when turning in the "bad" direction. To appreciate the implications of this observation, recall that these rotational tests were all conducted in complete darkness. The enhanced saccadic contribution could not have been visually generated: it must have derived from an internal central origin which had "learned" to improve the impaired gaze compensation at these high velocities by invoking enhanced corrective saccades *especially in the needed direction.*

We propose that this phenomenon represents a high hierarchical level of adaptive response, manifested as the informed choice of an altered motor strategy based on an internal (neurologic) comparison of estimated ocular slow-phase achievement (oculomotor efferent copy) with a multifactoral cognitive estimate[5] of the relative displacement of external space.

SUMMARY

A broad range of experiments of vestibular adaptation have definitively shown that active behavioral contact with the external environment can readily induce substantial changes in reflex sensory-motor relations, even in the normal adult organism. Our recent studies demonstrated a degree of correspondence in sensory-motor rearrangements so induced at both reflex and perceptual levels of neurologic function. In particular, it appears that "normal" deficits of the slow-phase VOR tend systematically to be corrected by the "injection" of supplementary saccadic eye movements acting in the same compensatory direction as the VOR. Furthermore, the goal to which these saccades direct the gaze can also be altered by an allied adaptive process. Initial results from clinical studies suggest that after unilateral vestibular ablation, the subsequent process of vestibular compensation comprises not only the partial restoration of slow-phase VOR asymmetry and gain, but also the introduction of an appropriately corrective saccadic contribution which permits both reacquisition of approximate symmetry and the restoration of near-normal net gain in the overall stabilization of gaze.

Acknowledgments

We appreciate the secretarial and technical support of Ms. E. Wong and Ms. H. Meyer, respectively.

REFERENCES

1. Berthoz A: Adaptive mechanisms in eye-head coordination, in Berthoz A, Melvill Jones G (eds): *Adaptive Mechanisms in Gaze Control, Reviews in Oculomotor Research.* Amsterdam, Elsevier, 1985, vol 1, pp 177–201.
2. Berthoz A, Melvill Jones G (eds): *Adaptive Mechanisms in Gaze Control: Reviews in Oculomotor Research.* Amsterdam, Elsevier, 1985, vol 1.
3. Berthoz A, Melvill Jones G, Bégué AE: Differential visual adaptation of vertical canal-dependent vestibulo-ocular reflexes. *Exp Brain Res* 1981; 44:19–26.
4. Bloomberg J, Melvill Jones G, Segal B: Quick and slow-phase interaction following adaptive attenuation of the human vestibulo-ocular reflex (VOR). *Physiol Canada* 1985; 16:50.
5. Bloomberg J, Melvill Jones G, Segal B: Vestibular-contingent voluntary saccades based on cognitive estimates of remembered vestibular information, in Pirodda E, Pompeiano O (eds): *Advances in Otorhinolaryngology.* Basel, S. Karger, 1987.
6. Collewijn H, Tamminga EP: Human smooth and saccadic eye movements during voluntary pursuit of different target motions on different backgrounds. *J Physiol* 1984; 351:217–250.
7. Dieringer N, Precht W: Mechanism of compensation for vestibular deficits in the frog: I. Modification of the excitatory commissural system. *Exp Brain Res* 1979; 36:311–328.
8. Dieringer N, Precht W: Mechanism of compensation for vestibular deficits in the frog: II. Modifications of the inhibitory pathways. *Exp Brain Res* 1979; 36:329–341.

9. Flohr H, Precht W (eds): *Lesion-Induced Neuronal Plasticity in Sensorimotor Systems*. Berlin, Springer, 1981.
10. Galiana HL: Commissural vestibular nuclear coupling: A powerful putative site for producing adaptive change, in Berthoz A, Melvill Jones G (eds): *Adaptive Mechanisms in Gaze Control: Reviews in Oculomotor Research*. Amsterdam, Elsevier, 1985, vol 1, pp 327–339.
11. Galiana HL: A new approach to understanding adaptive visual-vestibular interactions in the central nervous system. *J Neurophysiol* 1986, 55:349–374.
12. Galiana HL, Flohr H, Melvill Jones G: A reevaluation of intervestibular nuclear coupling: Its role in vestibular compensation. *J Neurophysiol* 1984; 51:242–259.
13. Gauthier GM, Robinson DA: Adaptation of the human vestibulo-ocular reflex to magnifying lenses. *Brain Res* 1975; 92:331–335.
14. Gonshor A, Melvill Jones G: Plasticity in the adult human vestibulo-ocular reflex arc. *Proc Can Fed Biol Soc* 1971; 14:11.
15. Gonshor A, Melvill Jones G: Short-term adaptive changes in the human vestibulo-ocular reflex arc. *J Physiol* 1976; 256:361–379.
16. Gonshor A, Melvill Jones G: Extreme vestibulo-ocular adaptation induced by prolonged optical reversal of vision. *J Physiol* 1976; 256:381–414.
17. Igarashi M, Alford BR, Kato Y, et al: Effect of physical exercise upon nystagmus and locomotor dysequilibrium after labyrinthectomy in experimental primates. *Acta Otolaryngol Stockh* 1975; 79:214–220.
18. Ito M: Cerebellar control of the vestibulo-ocular reflex: Around the flocculus hypothesis. *Annu Rev Neurosci* 1982; 5:275–296.
19. Ito M: *The Cerebellum and Neural Control*. New York, Raven Press, 1984.
20. Ito M: Synaptic plasticity in the cerebellar cortex that may underlie the vestibulo-ocular adaptation, in Berthoz A, Melvill Jones G (eds): *Adaptive Mechanisms in Gaze Control: Reviews in Oculomotor Research*. Amsterdam, Elsevier, 1985, vol 1, pp 213–221.
21. Ito M, Shiida T, Yagi N, et al: The cerebellar modification of rabbit's horizontal vestibulo-ocular reflex induced by sustained head rotation combined with visual stimulation. *Proc Jpn Acad* 1974; 50:85–89.
22. Ito M, Nisimaru N, Yamamoto M: Specific patterns of neuronal connexions involved in the control of the rabbit's vestibulo-ocular reflexes by the cerebellar flocculus. *J Physiol* 1977; 265:833–854.
23. Jäger J, Henn V: Habituation of the vestibulo-ocular reflex (VOR) in the monkey during sinusoidal rotation in the dark. *Exp Brain Res* 1981; 41:108–114.
24. Kasai T, Zee DS: Eye-head coordination in labyrinthine defective human beings. *Brain Res* 1978; 144:123–141.
25. Katsarkas A, Segal BN: Chronic gaze stabilization deficits following unilateral loss of peripheral vestibular function. *Soc Neurosci Abst* 1986; 12(2):1090.

26. Keller EL, Zee DS (eds): *Adaptive Processes in Visual and Oculomotor Systems: Advances in the Biosciences.* Oxford, Pergamon Press, 1986.
27. Kohler I: Experiments with goggles. *Sci Am* 1962; 206:62–86.
28. Lacour M: Contribution à l'étude de la restauration des fonctions posturo-cinétiques après labyrinthectomie chez le singe et le chat. Thèse de Docteur ès Sciences, L'Université d'Aix-Marseille I, Marseille, France, 1981.
29. Lisberger SG: Properties of pathways subserving long-term adaptive plasticity of the vestibulo-ocular reflex in monkeys, in Ruben RJ, Van De-Water TR, Rubel EW (eds): *The Biology of Change in Otolaryngology.* Amsterdam, Elsevier, 1986, pp 171–183.
30. Lisberger SG, Pavelko TA: A brain stem site of plasticity in the vestibulo-ocular reflex in monkeys. *Soc Neurosci Abstr* 1987; 13(2):1094.
31. Mandl G, Melvill Jones G, Cynader M: Adaptability of the vestibulo-ocular reflex to vision reversal in strobe reared cats. *Brain Res* 1981; 209:35–45.
32. Melvill Jones G; Plasticity in the adult vestibulo-ocular reflex arc. *Philos Trans R Soc Lond [Biol]* 1977; 278:319–334.
33. Melvill Jones G: Auto-adaptive control of central plasticity: Observations and speculations, in Basar E, Flohr H, Haken H, et. al (eds): *Synergetics of the Brain: Springer Series in Synergetics.* Berlin, Springer-Verlag, 1983, vol 23, pp 122–138.
34. Melvill Jones G: Behavioural control of central plasticity: Fact or fiction? in Igarashi M, Black FO (eds): *Vestibular and Visual Control on Posture and Locomotor Equilibrium.* 7th International Symposium of the International Society of Posturography, Houston, Texas, 1983. Basel, Karger, 1985, pp 9–13.
35. Melvill Jones G: Adaptive modulation of VOR parameters by vision, in Berthoz A, Melvill Jones G (eds): *Adaptive Mechanisms in Gaze Control: Reviews in Oculomotor Research.* Amsterdam, Elsevier, 1985, vol 1, pp 21–50.
36. Melvill Jones G: Cognitive management of sensory-motor correspondence in visual, vestibular and oculomotor systems, in Keller EL, Zee DS (eds): *Adaptive Processes in Visual and Oculomotor Systems.* New York, Pergamon Press, Oxford, 1986, pp 3–10.
37. Melvill Jones G, Davies P: Adaptation of cat vestibulo-ocular reflex to 200 days of optically reversed vision. *Brain Res* 1976; 103:551–554.
38. Melvill Jones G, DeJong JD: Visual tracking of sinusoidal target movement in Parkinson's disease. Canadian Defense Research Board, AMRU Research Reports, 1976, vol V, pp 271–288.
39. Melvill Jones G, Gonshor A: Oculomotor response to rapid head oscillation (0.5–5.0 Hz) after prolonged adaptation to vision-reversal: "simple" and "complex" effects. *Exp Brain Res* 1982; 45:45–58.
40. Melvill Jones G, Mandl G: Neurobionomics of adaptive plasticity: Integrating sensorimotor function with environmental demands, in Desmedt JE (ed): *Advances in Neurology, vol 39: Motor Control Mechanisms in Health and Disease.* New York, Raven Press, 1983, pp 1047–1071.

41. Melvill Jones G, Berthoz A, Segal B: Adaptive modification of the vestibulo-ocular reflex by mental effort in darkness. *Exp Brain Res* 1984; 56:149–153.
42. Miles FA, Eighmy BB: Long-term adaptive changes in primate vestibulo-ocular reflex: I. Behavioral observations. *J Neurophysiol* 1980; 43:1406–1425.
43. Miles FA, Lisberger SG: Plasticity in the vestibulo-ocular reflex: A new hypothesis. *Annu Rev Neurosci* 1981; 4:273–299.
44. Miles FA, Braitman DJ, Dow BM: Long term adaptive changes in primate vestibulo-ocular reflexes: IV. Electrophysiological observations in flocculus of adapted monkeys. *J. Neurophysiol* 1980; 43:1477–1493.
45. Paige GD: Vestibulo-ocular reflex and its interactions with visual following mechanisms in the squirrel monkey: I. Response characteristics in normal animals. *J Neurophysiol* 1983; 49:134–151.
46. Paige GD: Vestibulo-ocular reflex and its interactions with visual following mechanisms in the squirrel monkey: II. Response characteristics and plasticity following unilateral inactivation of horizontal canal. *J Neurophysiol* 1983; 49:152–168.
47. Paige GD: Plasticity in the vestibulo-ocular and optokinetic reflexes following modification of canal input, in Berthoz A, Melvill Jones G (eds): *Adaptive Mechanisms in Gaze Control: Reviews in Oculomotor Research.* Elsevier, Amsterdam, 1985, vol 1, pp 145–153.
48. Robinson DA: Adaptive gain control of vestibulo-ocular reflex by the cerebellum. *J Neurophysiol* 1976; 39:954–969.
49. Schaefer KP, Meyer DL: Compensation of vestibular lesions, in Kornhuber HH (ed.): *Vestibular System, Handbook of Sensory Physiology.* Berlin, Springer, 1974, Vol VI, part 2, pp 463–490.
50. Schairer JO, Bennett MVL: Changes in gain of the vestibulo-ocular reflex induced by combined visual and vestibular stimulation in goldfish. *Brain Res* 1986; 373:164–176.
51. Schultheis LW, Robinson DA: Directional plasticity of the vestibulo-ocular reflex in the cat. Ann NY Acad Sci 1981; 374:504–512.
52. Segal BN: Goal-directed vestibulo-ocular reflex produces compensatory quick phase eye movements. *Physiol Canada* 1985; 16:211.
53. Segal B, Katsarkas A: Quick-phase eye movements of goal-directed vestibulo-ocular reflex reduce gaze error. *Soc Neurosci Abstr* 1986; 12(2):1090.
54. Segal BN, Katsarkas A: Goal-directed vestibulo-ocular function in man: Gaze stabilization by slow-phase and saccadic eye movements. *Exp Brain Res* 1988; in press.
55. Segal BN, Katsarkas A: Long-term deficits of goal-directed vestibulo-ocular function following total unilateral loss of peripheral vestibular function. *Acta Otolaryngol (Stockh)* 1988; in press.
56. Teuber HL: Recovery of function after brain injury in man in *Outcome of severe damage to the CNS, Ciba Foundation Symposium 34 (new series).* Elsevier, Amsterdam, 1975, pp 159–186.

57. Tsukahara N: Synaptic plasticity in the mammalian central nervous system. *Annu Rev Neurosci* 1981; 4:351–379.
58. Tsukahara N, Fujito Y: Physiological evidence of formation of new synapses from cerebellum in the red nucleus neurons following cross-union of forelimb nerves. *Brain Res* 1976; 106:184–188.
59. Wallman J, Velez J, Weinstein B, et al: Avian vestibuloocular reflex: Adaptive plasticity and developmental changes. *J Neurophysiol* 1982; 48:952–967.
60. White OB: Saint-Cyr A, Tomlinson RD, et al: Oculomotor deficits in Parkinson's disease: II. Control of the saccadic and smooth pursuit systems. *Brain* 1983; 106:571–587.
61. Xerri C, Lacour M: Compensation des déficits posturaux et cinétiques après neurectomie vestibulaire unilatérale chez le chat. Rôle de l'activité sensori-motrice. *Acta Otolaryngol (Stockh)* 1980; 90:414–424.

2

*Modulation and Cancellation of the Vestibulo-ocular Reflex: Physiologic and Clinical Considerations**

Barry W. Peterson, Ph.D.

R. John Leigh, M.D.

VOR MODULATION: PHYSIOLOGIC CONSIDERATIONS

Vestibular physiologists have been aware for some time that humans and animals can modify or override the vestibulo-ocular reflex (VOR) when both they and the object that they are tracking are moving. The simplest explanation of this capability is that it merely represents addition of smooth pursuit and vestibulo-ocular eye movements with no intrinsic modification of the VOR. Recent physiologic studies support another explanation: that the brain contains a system that allows rapid, voluntary regulation of the amplitude of vestibulo-ocular eye movements. Evidence supporting both points of view will be discussed.

Quantification of Vestibulo-ocular and Pursuit Performance

Physiologists have adopted techniques developed by engineers to describe the functional properties of the VOR and smooth pursuit sys-

*Work in Dr. Peterson's laboratory is supported by National Institutes of Health grants EY 05049 and EY 06485. Dr. Leigh is supported by Public Health Service grant EY 06717, the Veterans Administration, and the Evenor Armington Fund.

tems.[1] The amplitude of the eye movements produced by these systems in response to head rotation or target motion is expressed as a gain, which is the ratio of the eye movement to the stimulus, both measured in degrees of rotation. Responses are frequently tested with periodic stimuli such as sinusoidal rotations, in which case one can also measure response phase. Phase is defined as the amount by which the eye movement response leads or lags the stimulus, measured as a fraction of the stimulus cycle. It is usually expressed in degrees, one cycle equaling 360°. By measuring gain and phase over a range of stimulus frequencies, one can construct a Bode plot that represents the response of the system in the frequency domain (Fig 2–1).

The frequency response of the VOR exhibits several characteristic features. At moderate frequencies of rotation (e.g., 0.1–0.5 Hz) in the dark, VOR gain is not 1.0, as one might expect, but varies from about 0.5 to 0.9 with a mean of approximately 0.7. This "baseline" gain depends on the mental state of the subject, falling drastically if the subject becomes drowsy. The value of 0.7 is obtained in fully alert subjects who are prevented from tracking imagined visual targets by an appropriate mental task. Performing mental arithmetic is not always suitable, since some subjects visualize the numbers they are manipulating and thereby suppress their VOR. We have subjects manipulate a joy-stick to indicate their speed of rotation.[2] Others have subjects recite place names or participate in a dialogue with the experimenter (J. Goldberg, personal communication).

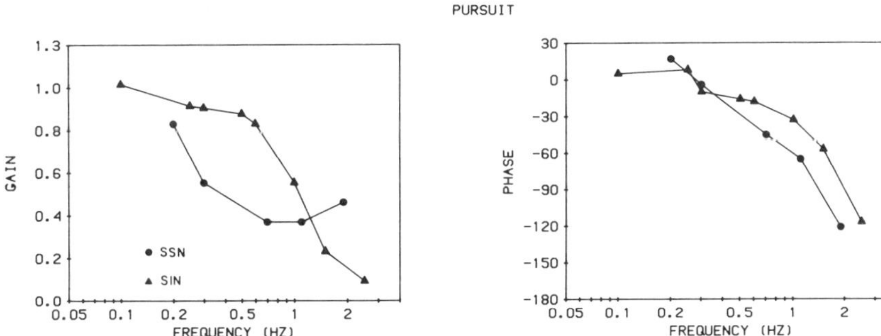

FIG 2–1.

Bode diagram showing gain and phase of slow phase pursuit eye movements in response to predictable, sinusoidal target motion *(circles)* and to pseudorandom, sum-of-sines target motion *(triangles)* at frequencies ranging from 0.1 to 2.5 Hz. (From McKinley PA, Peterson BW: Voluntary modulation of the vestibulo-ocular reflex by mental effort in darkness. *Exp Brain Res* 1985; 60:454–464. Used by permission.)

Another feature of the VOR is its low-frequency phase lead and gain decrease, which are seen at frequencies of 0.05 Hz and below. This behavior reflects the low-frequency time constant of the VOR, which is typically 15–20 sec in normal subjects. Although the high-pass filter behavior of the VOR arises from the basic mechanical properties of the semicircular canals, the time constant is lengthened by CNS mechanisms[1, 3] and therefore reflects the central processing of vestibular signals.

VOR performance is excellent at frequencies of 1–7 Hz, which represent the upper end of the head movement power spectrum.[4] Phase remains close to 0 over this range, and gain rises gradually, often reaching 1.0 or above between 1 and 2 Hz.

The performance of smooth pursuit is quite different from that of the VOR. At low frequencies, below 0.5 Hz, pursuit phase is near 0 and gain close to 1.0, unless the target moves at high velocity. At higher frequencies, however, pursuit gain falls rapidly, and a large phase lag develops.[5, 6] Over the entire frequency range pursuit is limited in the speed of target motion that can be followed. For humans the limit is often given as 100–150° sec, although Lisberger et al.[5] argued that the limiting value is the *acceleration* of the target, with the gain of human pursuit of periodic targets falling below 0.7 when acceleration exceeds 600–1800°/sec^2.

The parameters of pursuit performance given above apply when the target motion is predictable. When motion is unpredictable, tracking ability declines dramatically, as illustrated in Figure 2–1. Typically the performance decline occurs over most of the frequency range of the applied stimulus and depends on the high-frequency content of the signal.[6] When they used pseudorandom target motion, Lisberger et al.[5] found that the limiting target acceleration fell to 150–175°/sec^2.

Modulation of the VOR

Typically VOR modulation occurs when a subject attempts to fixate on a visual target while he is rotating. Fixating a stationary visual target results in a VOR gain that is close to 1.0 at all frequencies up to 5 Hz or more and a phase close to 0. More complex behavior occurs when the subject attempts to fixate on a target that rotates with him—the classic VOR cancellation situation (Fig 2–2). Here VOR gain is less than 0.1 up to about 0.5 Hz, above which it rises steadily toward 1.0.[2, 7] The frequency response of VOR cancellation during periodic rotations is thus similar to that of pursuit, which led Barnes et al.[7] to hypothesize that the pursuit system was responsible for cancellation.

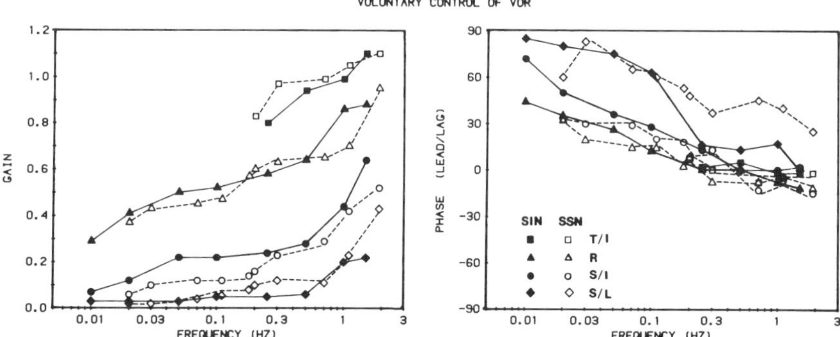

FIG 2–2.
Bode plots of VOR frequency responses under 4 instructional sets: track imagined target *(squares),* relax *(triangles),* suppress by tracking imagined target moving with chair *(circles),* suppress by tracking visible LED attached to chair *(diamonds). Filled symbols,* responses to predictable, sinusoidal rotation; *open symbols,* responses to an unpredictable, sum-of-sines rotation. Note essentially identical dynamics of responses to predictable and unpredictable stimuli when no visible target was present. Phase shifts seen with visible suppression target may be related to participation of smooth pursuit in this situation. (From McKinley PA, Peterson BW: Voluntary modulation of the vestibulo-ocular reflex by mental effort in darkness. *Exp Brain Res* 1985; 60:454–464. Used by permission.)

Their hypothesis received support from clinical observations that CNS lesions typically impaired pursuit and cancellation equally.[2, 8]

A challenge to the hypothesis that modulation of the VOR was executed by the pursuit system came from observations that humans could increase their VOR gain during rotation in the dark by attempting to track an imagined earth-fixed target or decrease their gain by attempting to track a target moving with them.[9] An example of this modulation is shown in Figure 2–3. It was argued that smooth pursuit could not be responsible, since it is only observed when a moving target is present. Those supporting the hypothesis argued, however, that pursuit may be able to utilize vestibular signals as its input in this special situation.

McKinley and Peterson[2] tested the hypothesis further by comparing the frequency responses of pursuit and VOR modulation when pseudorandom stimuli were used. As illustrated in Figure 2–1, the pseudorandom stimulus resulted in a large decrease in pursuit gain. In contrast, enhancement and suppression of the VOR by tracking imagined targets was the same for pseudorandom and predictable stimuli (see Fig 2–2). Another indication that pursuit was not involved in modifying the VOR came from the absence of a phase shift in the enhanced and suppressed VOR at high frequencies. As seen in

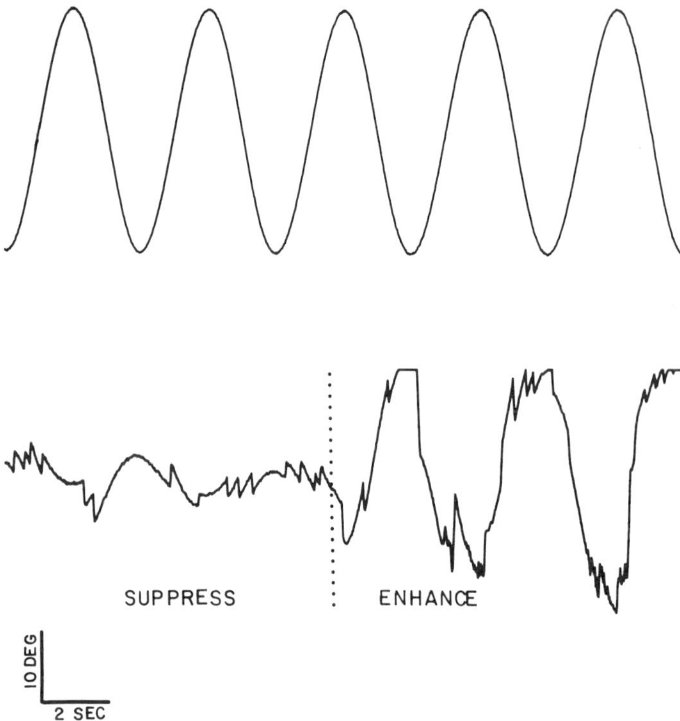

FIG 2–3.
Voluntary modulation of VOR using imagination. At beginning of record, subject was suppressing VOR by imagining that he was fixating on a target rotating with him. At point indicated by *dashed line,* he was asked to imagine that he was fixating on a target fixed on the wall. After approximately 0.3 sec, his VOR changed from suppression to enhancement, generating eye movements *(lower trace)* with slow phases nearly equal and opposite to the chair rotation shown in the *top trace.* (From McKinley PA, Peterson BW: Voluntary modulation of the vestibulo-ocular reflex by mental effort in darkness. *Exp Brain Res* 1985; 60:454–464. Used by permission.)

Figure 2–1, pursuit develops a large phase lag for frequencies above 0.5 Hz, and if pursuit signals were summing with the baseline VOR to generate the gain changes seen in Figure 2–2, the phase of the suppressed and enhanced VOR should exhibit significant phase leads and lags, respectively.

Other evidence against the hypothesis that VOR modulation is due to pursuit comes from electrophysiologic and clinical studies. Second-order vestibulo-ocular relay neurons carry a signal related to smooth pursuit.[1] Tomlinson and Robinson[10] observed that this signal is not present when monkeys suppress their VOR. Instead, a specific group of brain stem neurons appears to become active when the VOR is suppressed.[11] Also, clinical cases have now been reported where pursuit and VOR suppression were altered differentially.[12]

VOR Modulation as an Independent Brain Function

On the basis of the evidence presented above, it seems reasonable to conclude that the smooth pursuit system is not responsible for modulation of the VOR. Instead, this function is mediated by an independent pathway, presumably involving the neurons described by May and McCrea.[11] Although the system fails at high frequencies, as does pursuit, it does not depend on predictability of the stimulus or show the large phase lags associated with pursuit. When tested in the dark with imagined targets, the VOR suppression mechanism cannot completely suppress vestibulo-ocular eye movements. Thus, pursuit may in fact play a role in VOR cancellation by opposing the residual eye movements that remain after suppression has lowered the gain to 0.1–0.2. The standard cancellation test may therefore measure the action of the two systems working in concert. It is not correct to assume, however, that cancellation can be used as a test of the integrity of the pursuit system.

That there is an independent system capable of modulating the VOR is also of interest to the physician interested in helping patients to compensate for labyrinthine deficits. The important role of VOR modulation in the recovery of some unilateral labyrinthectomized patients is discussed in chapter 3. With proper exercises, it may be possible to train patients to develop their ability to modulate the VOR as a means of restoring gaze stability following labyrinthine lesions.

VOR CANCELLATION: CLINICAL CONSIDERATIONS

"VOR suppression," or "VOR cancellation,"[13] is routinely tested in vestibular laboratories during *passive* rotation of patients in a vestibular chair to which a fixation light is rigidly attached. In fact, this is an artificial situation which has no equivalent during natural activities. VOR cancellation normally occurs during *active* combined eye-head tracking. Since the purpose of such combined, eye-head tracking—like smooth pursuit with the head stationary—is to keep the image of the moving target close to the fovea, it makes sense to measure "tracking gain" (e.g., peak gaze velocity/peak target velocity). This is easily done if eye and head movements are measured using a magnetic search coil system, but most laboratories use electro-oculography; in the latter case, correction should be made for the different axes of rotation of the head and of the eyes in the head.[14]

Leigh et al.[15] recently compared tracking gain during smooth pursuit and active eye-head tracking in a group of 10 normal subjects and in 10 patients with deficient labyrinthine function. They found that in normal subjects, smooth pursuit and active eye-head tracking were *similar* for a variety of sinusoidal stimuli. In the labyrinthine-deficient patients, however, active eye-head tracking was *superior* to smooth pursuit (Fig 2–4). The latter result could mean that the labyrinthine-deficient patients had less VOR to cancel during eye-head tracking than did the normal subjects.

Do these results during active eye-head tracking differ from the more usual laboratory situation of "passive cancellation?" To answer this question directly, it would be necessary to compare tracking gain during smooth pursuit and during passive cancellation. This has not

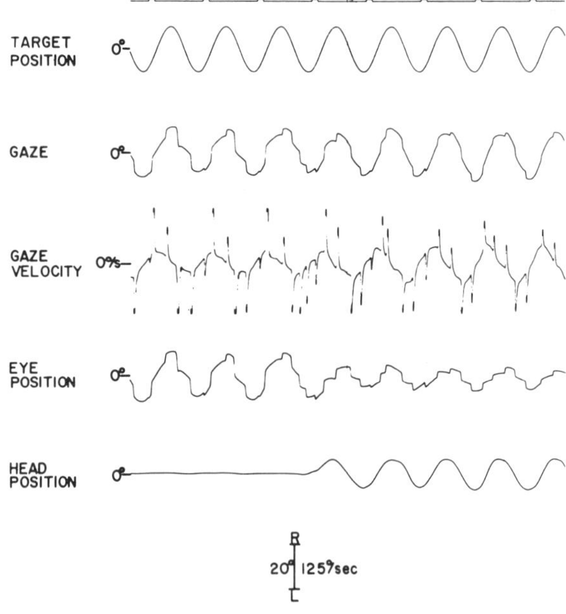

FIG 2–4.

Comparison of smooth pursuit *(left)* and combined eye-head tracking *(right)* in a patient with deficient labyrinthine function (magnetic search coil technique). Note how tracking gain *(gaze velocity)* increases when the patient starts to move his head.

often been done; however, Leigh et al.[15] made such a comparison and found that normal subjects have a higher tracking gain during passive cancellation than during smooth pursuit. McKinley and Peterson[2] reported similar results using nonpredictable stimuli.

Most commonly, tracking gain is not measured, but a cancellation gain is calculated. The purpose of the latter is to account for any inadequacies in the VOR and so come up with a cancellation gain value that can be directly related to smooth pursuit gain. This approach presents considerable problems, principally because of the way that VOR gain varies according to "mental set."

A Method for Measuring Passive VOR Cancellation

This may be calculated by making the following measurements. (1) Rotate the subject while he fixates on a target moving with the head. In the laboratory, the target may be either a light-emitting diode (LED) rigidly attached to the chair in which the patient is rotated or a laser spot projected onto a screen whose motion is coupled to that of the chair. Measure the maximum eye velocity during this cancellation test (E_C). (2) Rotate the subject using the same stimulus, but this time in darkness. Measure maximum eye velocity during this stimulation (E_V). It is then possible to calculate VOR cancelation gain from:

$$\frac{E_V - E_C}{E_V}$$

It is well-known that the gain of the VOR varies considerably with mental set, being highest if the subject imagines an earth-fixed target and lowest with imagination of a target moving with the subject's head; mental arithmetic produces intermediate gain values.[9] It is not clear what mental set governs the VOR gain during passive VOR cancellation. However, Koenig and colleagues[16] have recently shown that cancellation gain most closely approximated smooth pursuit gain when the VOR was evaluated as their subjects performed mental arithmetic. If subjects imagine a head-fixed target during VOR testing, cancellation gain is lower than smooth pursuit gain.[16] If subjects imagine an Earth-bound target, the calculated cancellation gain will be higher than for smooth pursuit.[15] Even with these general trends, it is likely that other factors will confound estimates of cancellation gain (for example, the effect of spectacle correction on VOR gain).[17]

Therefore, in deciding what is an abnormal VOR cancellation

gain, it is important that any measured value from the patient be compared with the normal range of VOR cancellation gain for normal subjects for that laboratory under specified conditions, and it is inappropriate to compare VOR cancellation gain with smooth pursuit gain in the same subject for the reasons discussed above. Although it has been reported that disorders of the CNS may selectively impair VOR cancellation,[18] much more work is required to determine exactly what disorders are responsible. Generally, abnormalities that impair smooth pursuit also cause impairment of VOR cancellation. Thus, disease affecting any part of the pursuit pathway will also impair VOR cancellation. For example, impaired VOR cancellation during rotation clockwise and smooth pursuit to the right will occur with right posterior cortical lesions, lesions of the right midbrain or pons, lesions of the right cerebellum, and perhaps with disorders affecting the vestibular nuclei. More commonly, VOR cancellation is impaired bilaterally and is then generally a nonspecific finding similar to bilateral impairment of smooth pursuit.

Bedside Testing of VOR Cancellation

It is easy and convenient to test VOR cancellation at the bedside. Conventionally, the subject is asked to fixate on the end of a pointer which is attached to the head. The subject is then either rotated passively or actively moves the head. Since it has been shown that active eye-head tracking has properties similar to those of smooth pursuit, it is probably best to ask the patient to generate his own head movements. One advantage of testing VOR cancellation in this situation over smooth pursuit is in individuals with nystagmus. By keeping the eye close to primary position or some other point where nystagmus is minimal, it is sometimes possible to estimate smooth tracking ability uncontaminated by the effect of moving the eye to an eccentric position in the orbit.

In summary, testing of cancellation of the VOR is a useful and sensitive screening test for visual-vestibular interaction. However, interpretation of findings requires caution because we are judging a response not to one but to two stimuli: visual and vestibular. During natural, combined eye-head tracking, it appears that VOR cancellation does have properties very similar to smooth pursuit. However, during passive rotation in a chair, VOR cancellation and smooth pursuit performance are often different. Finally, visual suppression of nystagmus induced by caloric stimulation is quite different from natural combined eye-head tracking and, because of the semiquantitative nature of the caloric stimulus, is the most difficult to interpret.

REFERENCES

1. Robinson DA: Control of eye movements, in Brooks VB (ed): *Handbook of Physiology, The Nervous System, II: Motor Control.* Baltimore, Williams and Wilkins, pp 1275–1320.
2. McKinley PA, Peterson BW: Voluntary modulation of the vestibuloocular reflex in humans and its relation to smooth pursuit. *Exp Brain Res* 1985; 60:454–464.
3. Skavenski AA, Robinson DA: Role of abducens neurons in vestibuloocular reflex. *J Neurophysiol* 1973; 36:724–728.
4. Donaghy M: The cat's vestibulo-ocular reflex. *J Physiol* 1980; 300:337–352.
5. Lisberger SG, Evinger C, Johanson GW, et al: Relationship between eye acceleration and retinal image velocity during foveal smooth pursuit in man and monkey. *J Neurophysiol* 1981; 46:229–249.
6. Yasui S, Young LR: On the predictive control of foveal eye tracking and slow phases of optokinetic and vestibular nystagmus. *J Physiol* 1984; 347:17–33.
7. Barnes GR, Benson AJ, Prior ARJ: Visual-vestibular interaction in the control of eye movement. *Aviat Space Environ Med* 1978; 49:557–564.
8. Baloh RW, Lyerly K, Yee RD, et al: Voluntary control of the human vestibulo-ocular reflex. *Acta Otolaryngol (Stockh)* 1984; 97:1–6.
9. Barr CC, Schultheis LW, Robinson DA: Voluntary, non-visual control of the human vestibulo-ocular reflex. *Acta Otolaryngol (Stockh)* 1976; 81:365–375.
10. Tomlinson RD, Robinson DA: Is the vestibulo-ocular reflex cancelled by smooth pursuit? in Fuchs A, Becker W (eds): *Progress in Oculomotor Research.* New York, Elsevier/North-Holland, 1981, pp 533–539.
11. May EF, McCrea RA: Physiological characteristics of neurons in the medial vestibular nucleus and reticular formation of the squirrel monkey involved in foveal cancellation of the horizontal vestibulo-ocular reflex. *Soc Neurosci Abstr* 1985; 11:1039.
12. Dell'Osso LF, Abel LA, Daroff RB, et al: Absence of VOR suppression in the presence of intact pursuit. *Invest Ophthalmol Vis Sci* 1981; 20(suppl):57.
13. Robinson DA: A model of cancellation of the vestibulo-ocular reflex, in Lennestrand G, Zee DS, Kelly EL (eds): *Functional Basis of Ocular Motility Disorders.* Oxford, Pergamon, 1982, pp 5–13.
14. Wist ER, Brandt TH, Krafczyk S: Oscillopsia and retinal slip. *Brain* 1983; 106:153–168.
15. Leigh RJ, Sharpe JA, Ranalli PJ, et al: Comparison of smooth pursuit and

combined eye-head tracking in normal subjects with deficient labyrinthine function. *Exp Brain Res* 1987; 66:458–464.

16. Koenig E, Dichgans J, Dengler W: Fixation suppression of the vestibulo-ocular reflex (VOR) during sinusoidal stimulation in humans as related to performance of the pursuit system. *Acta Otolaryngol (Stockh)* 1986; 102:423–431.
17. Cannon SC, Leigh RJ, Zee DS, et al: The effect of the rotational magnification of corrective spectacles on the quantitative evaluation of the VOR. *Acta Otolaryngol (Stockh)* 1985; 100:81–88.

3

Recovery From Peripheral Vestibular Defects: VOR and VSR

Douglas G.D. Watt, M.D., Ph.D.
Barry W. Peterson, Ph.D.

NORMAL FUNCTION OF VESTIBULAR REFLEXES

It is well known that if the head is caused to rotate, the eyes must compensate by moving in the opposite direction if normal visual acuity is to be maintained. Gaze stabilization in the face of perturbations that disturb head position can be attained in two ways: through movements of the eyes in the head that compensate for movement of the head in space or through reflex activation of muscles that act to maintain the head stable in space. Turning initially to the first alternative, three sensorimotor mechanisms can contribute to compensatory eye movements: the vestibulo-ocular reflex (VOR), the cervico-ocular reflex (COR), and visually guided eye movements produced by the smooth pursuit (SP) and optokinetic (OK) systems. The properties of these four systems have been extensively studied in normal subjects.[1] Predictive mechanisms can also contribute if the perturbing head movement is predictable.

The ocular stabilizing mechanisms listed above are limited in the amplitude of eye movements that they can produce. An important corollary is that if the head can be stabilized, control of gaze is greatly simplified. Unfortunately, the head is a very important platform supported by a very unstable body. Nevertheless, it can be seen to remain remarkably stable despite severe perturbations such as those encountered during locomotion.[2]

If the nervous system is to control where the head is by means of appropriate motor outputs, it must have a knowledge of its precise location at all times through sensory feedback. Information concerning head orientation and movement is obtained from at least four sources. These include efference copy (a knowledge of motor commands), vision, somatosensory inputs (proprioceptive, tactile), and the vestibular system. Of these, only the last is always available and has a fixed frame of reference (gravitoinertial space) under normal circumstances. All other sources of information have significant restrictions. Efference copy only tells the nervous system about intended movement, not what was actually accomplished. Vision is certainly of no help when the eyes are closed or the individual is in the dark. Tactile inputs can vary dramatically depending on surface texture or the type of clothing being worn. Finally, proprioception provides information as to the position of body parts relative to one another, not to the world. Thus, the vestibular system and vestibulospinal reflexes may play a particularly vital role in the moment-to-moment control of posture and locomotion.[3]

MOTOR EFFECTS OF VESTIBULAR DEFECTS

A sudden change in vestibular input, as after unilateral labyrinthine damage, leads to severe loss of ocular stability due to the unbalancing of tonic vestibular input from the two labyrinths. The obvious clinical sign is unidirectional vestibular nystagmus with slow phases toward the lesioned side and fast phases toward the normal side. To eliminate these inappropriate responses, the CNS must undergo adaptive changes that restore the balance of tonic activity in the vestibular nuclei on the two sides. In otherwise healthy individuals this adaptation occurs within a few days following the lesion. The underlying mechanisms are poorly understood but appear to involve both ascending and descending signals from other regions of the CNS, since lesions of many structures can lead to decompensation.[4]

A second consequence of peripheral vestibular lesions is reduction in VOR gain that is proportional to the loss of receptors. Thus, a 50% reduction in VOR gain is to be expected following unilateral labyrinthectomy; 100% loss with total bilateral lesions.

The importance of vestibulospinal reflex control is underscored by the obvious deficits which are seen if the function of one or both labyrinths is suddenly compromised. (The onset must be sudden, as compensatory mechanisms can modify or even hide a gradually developing deficit—e.g., during aging.) The effects of peripheral defects are reasonably similar across all vertebrates, and even though they are less severe in higher species, they are still significant in man.[5]

In quadrupeds, unilateral lesions result in asymmetric body postures, including a tendency to roll and yaw the head toward the damaged side, and ataxia. As noted above, maintained nystagmoid eye movements are also characteristic, and though this does not reflect altered vestibulospinal activity, it can indirectly influence postural control by compromising stability based on visual inputs. Bilateral defects result in head oscillation, hypotonia and ataxia. Subjectively, vestibular lesions cause instability of the visual world and incorrect perceptions of self-movement which further compromise postural and locomotor stability. Finally, if one labyrinth is destroyed and then the other, after a period of hours to days, the effects of unilateral damage reappear but in the opposite direction. This phenomenon is currently known as "Bechterew compensation,"[6] and reflects some degree of recovery of function of central vestibular pathways on the side of the original damage.

RESTORATION OF OCULAR STABILIZING REFLEXES

To maintain image stability during head movements, gaze stabilizing reflexes must generate compensatory eye movements that are equal and opposite to the movements of the head. Reflex performance can be measured in terms of its gain, which is the ratio of eye movement to head movement. For ideal stabilization, this gain should be -1.0. In normal subjects the baseline VOR, measured in the relaxed state in total darkness, has a gain of -0.6 to -0.8. When image stability is required, this gain can be brought to the required level of -1.0 by voluntary enhancement of the VOR and by adding visually elicited eye movements (due to smooth pursuit and optokinetic systems) to those produced by the VOR.

Total unilateral loss of vestibular input would be expected to reduce baseline VOR gain to half its normal value immediately after the lesion. The question is then how is this loss compensated for to restore gaze stability during head movements? Oculomotor research has suggested the following three mechanisms that might contribute to restoration of gaze stability.

Plastic, Adaptive Increase in Baseline VOR Gain

Studies in normal humans[7] and animals[8] exposed to reversing or magnifying lenses showed that altered visual feedback during head rotation can lead to a recalibration of VOR gain that tends to restore gaze stability. Reports vary concerning whether such a recalibration of VOR gain occurs after unilateral labyrinthine loss. Paige[9] reported full recovery of baseline VOR gain measured in the dark in squirrel monkeys following unilateral plugging of semicircular canals. On the other hand, unilateral labyrinthectomized rabbits show little gain recovery,[10] and only 50% of the cats followed up by Maioli et al.[11] for several months after a unilateral labyrinthectomy exhibited a significant increase in gain.

Our recent studies of patients following resection of an acoustic neuroma[12] revealed a similar variation in amount of recovery of baseline VOR gain that could be attributed to VOR plasticity. When tested in the relaxed state during rotation in the dark, some individuals, such as patient 1 in Figure 3–1, had VOR gains that were half the normal value (filled diamonds). Patient 3, on the other hand, had a baseline gain in the high normal range indicating that substantial plastic gain recovery had occurred. The typical case, exemplified by patient 2, fell between the two extremes. The question of why plastic readjustment does not occur in all individuals remains a mystery. Maioli and Precht[13] showed that their low gain cats could plastically increase their gains to normal levels when exposed to passive whole body rotation in a stationary, illuminated environment, so that the reason does not seem to be a loss of adaptive capacity but a change in the VOR gain set point or in gaze strategy.

Voluntary Enhancement of the VOR

Recent studies have shown that VOR gain can be controlled voluntarily by having subjects attempt to follow imagined targets fixed with respect to their body (voluntary suppression) or to the earth (voluntary enhancement).[14, 15] Such voluntary control could play a role in maintaining gaze stability in labyrinthectomized individuals. In fact, patient 1 in Figure 3–1 appears to utilize this mechanism effectively. When he attempted to fix his eyes on an imagined earth-fixed target

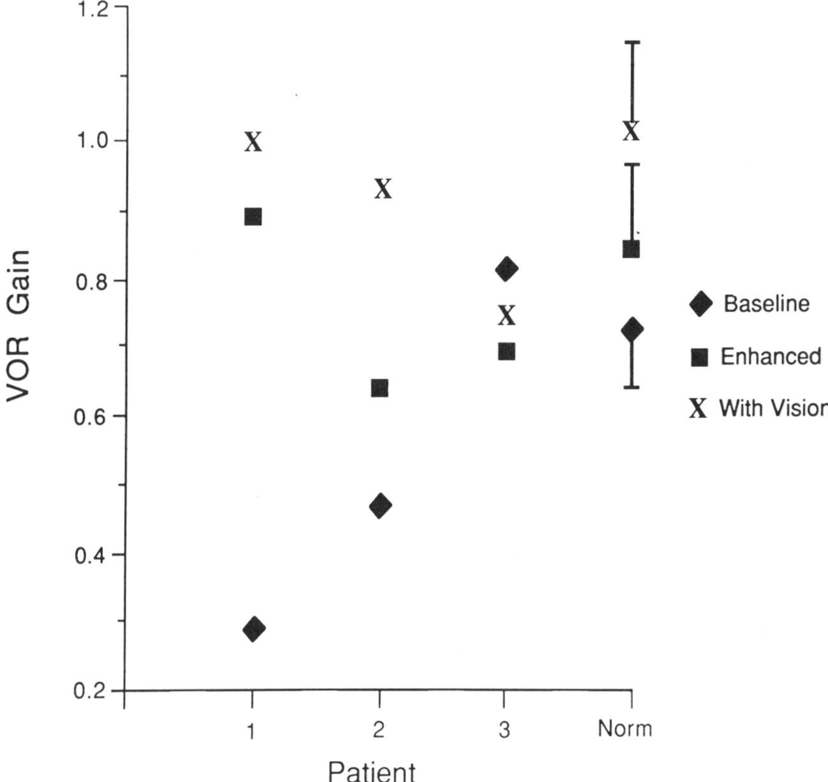

FIG 3–1.
Responses of three postsurgical acoustic neuroma patients in vestibulo-ocular (VOR) tests. Patients were tested 6–24 months after surgical resection of the tumor using three testing situations. In a baseline test, the patient was rotated in the dark while indicating the speed and direction of the rotation with a joystick. In an enhanced VOR test, the patient attempted to fixate on an imaginary, earth-fixed target while rotating. In a test with vision, the patient fixated on an earth-fixed LED target while rotating. All rotations were 80°/sec peak velocity sinusoids at a frequency of 0.25 Hz. VOR gain is the ratio of smooth-phase eye velocity to chair velocity. Columns *1, 2, 3,* the three patients; *Norm,* mean and SD of responses of seven normal subjects to the same tests.

during rotation in total darkness, his VOR gain rose from 0.25 to 0.97 (filled square). He thus appears to rely primarily on voluntary modulation of the VOR to obtain good gaze stabilization. Patient 3 is quite different. While her baseline VOR gain during relaxed rotation in the dark was above normal (0.8), her ability to override the VOR voluntarily was very poor: attempting to raise the gain by tracking an imagined earth-fixed target actually resulted in a gain reduction! Patient 2 had some ability to improve VOR gain voluntarily but could not attain the fully compensatory gaze performance shown by patient 1.

Increased Reliance on Visually Guided Image Stabilization

Smooth pursuit and optokinetic eye movements can help keep the eyes directed toward a target of interest provided that the target does not move too rapidly.[16] The contribution of smooth pursuit to gaze stabilization in the three patients in Figure 3–1 was tested by giving them an Earth-fixed light to fixate on during body rotation ("Xs" in Figure). The gain of patient 2 increased dramatically in this condition, indicating that he was utilizing visual pursuit to help stabilize his gaze. Gain in patient 1 did not change, since it was already brought to the required value by voluntary enhancement of the VOR. Patient 3 did not do well when given the visual target reference. She appears to rely solely on a plastic, adaptive increase in VOR gain to approach gaze stability.

Data from 4 other patients confirmed the patterns illustrated in Figure 3–1. Only 2 of 7 patients had baseline VOR gains in the normal range, indicating effective plastic recalibration of gain. Two patients exhibited large increases in gain when they attempted to track an imagined target. They appear to rely primarily on voluntary modulation of the VOR to obtain good gaze stabilization. The remaining 3 patients were like patient 2. They had only a modest gain recovery due to plastic, adaptive mechanisms and were not especially adept at increasing this gain by fixating on an imagined target. When given a visible target to track, however, they could attain gains approaching 1.0. They therefore appear to rely primarily on visual tracking mechanisms to stabilize gaze.

These findings leave two key questions to be answered. First, we must discover why there is so much variation in the recovery strategies adopted by different individuals. In particular it is unclear why plastic adaptation does not raise the VOR gain to normal levels in all individuals. Perhaps the answer is that alternative gaze stabilization mechanisms adopted early in the recovery period preempt the recovery process and prevent plastic adaptive changes from occurring.

The second question concerns whether one strategy or combination of strategies is better than another. If so, we would want to determine whether patients can be guided to adopt the optimal strategy. Such an approach offers the possibility of providing the physician with means of improving the recovery of his patients from loss of labyrinthine function.

RESTORATION OF POSTURAL AND LOCOMOTOR CONTROL

As in the case of the gaze stabilizing reflexes, the neurophysiologic changes underlying recovery of the vestibulospinal system are both widely distributed[17] and poorly understood.[18] The vestibular nuclei do appear to play a prominent role, however. They are well established as a major site for integration of vestibular, proprioceptive, and visual information. They appear to be necessary for a complete and normal recovery to occur.[19] Finally, their metabolic and unit activity reflect the recovery course seen at a behavioral level.[20]

While many investigators have recognized that the process of recovery occurs in stages,[21–23] the various classification schemes proposed are not always compatible. This is not surprising, since they were derived from measurements of a variety of parameters in different species. In the case of vestibulospinal reflexes in particular, it may not even be possible to define phases of recovery which can be applied in a uniform way to bipeds, quadrupeds, and inherently stable animals such as frogs, since the normal function of those reflexes could vary dramatically.

Nevertheless, recovery from vestibular defects does occur in several steps, probably reflecting different underlying mechanisms. These may be seen quite clearly in a unique "patient"—the returning astronaut. This otherwise healthy individual is suddenly confronted with a vestibular system which, having adapted to a weightless environment, can no longer provide appropriate information for use in postural and locomotor control. Of course, unlike patients with more permanent defects, he has the potential for completely normal function.

For the first few minutes on the ground, standing upright is a very demanding task, made even more difficult by varying amounts of postural hypotension. Voluntary head movements can result in apparent displacement of the external world and false sensations of self-motion. These severe initial symptoms pass quickly, however, apparently compensated for by means of very rapid recalibrations or adjustments of relevant reflex pathways, and by the adoption of more appropriate motor strategies. The latter phenomenon is responsible for the typical broad-based stance of the crew member emerging from the space shuttle.

Subjectively, postural and locomotor stability seem close to normal within 6–8 hours of landing, much of the recovery occurring in the first hour or two. Nevertheless, any situation which restricts vision can reverse this rapidly acquired compensation immediately. Several astronauts have discovered on their first night home that it is not appropriate to turn off the light and then walk to the bed. Apparently, visual inputs are substituting for vestibular sensation at this point. This has been confirmed by objective measurements of visual dependence of returning crew members.[24, 25]

Completely normal postural and locomotor control is restored within two weeks of returning to the ground.[26] At that point, it is presumed that long-term plastic adaptive phenomena have remodeled the nervous system so that the normal preflight balance of reflex and other mechanisms is reestablished. Certainly, all tests of these systems are normal, and, in particular, the measures of visual-vestibular interactions mentioned above are back to control values.

While it was not practical to detect the initial very rapid phase of compensation described above, the latter two stages (sensory substitution followed by long-term remodeling of reflexes) have been seen in baboons subjected to section of the 8th nerve.[27] In these experiments, electromyographic (EMG) activity was recorded from the splenius muscle during sudden falls, in some cases in the presence of normal vision (NV) and in others with stabilized vision (SV). The size of the postural reaction was normalized and plotted as a function of time after unilateral (UN) or bilateral (BN), 8th nerve section. These data have been redrawn in Figure 3–2,A. For the initial two weeks, recovery of the response in both UN and BN monkeys required normal vision during the falls. By three weeks, however, the situation was different, vision having little influence. At that point, the presence of the remaining labyrinth became the most important factor in determining the degree of recovery.

While the mechanisms which restore function following peripheral vestibular lesions can be remarkably effective, complete recovery from bilateral or even unilateral defects may not be possible. Since the substituted sensory inputs and neural pathways may not have been optimized by evolution for their new role, a sufficiently demanding situation may cause a limit to be exceeded. Thus, baboons show less than perfect performance when tested with sudden falls long after unilateral 8th nerve sections, especially in the presence of stabilized vision,[27] and unilaterally labyrinthectomized cats regain a significant degree of head tilt many days after they appear compensated if re-

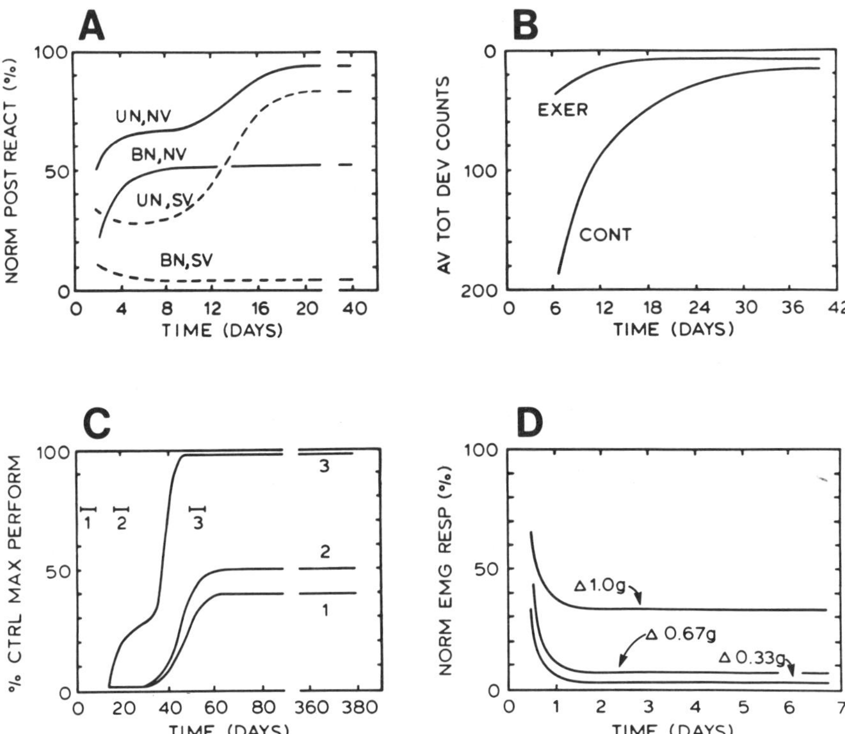

FIG 3–2.
Recovery from peripheral vestibular defects. **A,** two phases of recovery: sensory substitution followed by plastic adaptation. **B,** recovery occurs more rapidly through the use of a forced exercise program. **C,** early sensorimotor restriction can delay or even prevent full recovery. **D,** otolith-spinal reflex function is altered by going into weightlessness, and, with continued exposure, is lost almost completely.

turned to a dark environment.[28] These "hidden" deficits could pose a risk to the labyrinth-defective patient who steps off a curb unexpectedly or who is forced to walk in complete darkness.

THE ROLE OF SELF-GENERATED MOVEMENT IN THE RECOVERY PROCESS

There is now a substantial body of evidence which demonstrates a clear relationship between the rate and completeness of recovery from peripheral vestibular lesions and the amount of active behavior on the part of the experimental animal. For example, Igarashi et al.[29] measured locomotor performance in two groups of squirrel monkeys after unilateral labyrinthectomy. Five were exposed to 2.5 hours of exercise per day postoperatively, while another five received no special exercise. When the number of missteps which occurred during testing was plotted as a function of time after surgical intervention, the exercise group returned to the preoperative level of performance in significantly less time than was required by the nonexercised animals. These data have been redrawn in Figure 3–2,B.

Taking the opposite approach, Lacour and Xerri[27] studied the effects of deliberate sensorimotor restriction (SMR) on recovery of locomotor equilibrium following unilateral vestibular neurectomy in the cat. Selected animals were placed in a small cage (30 × 15 × 20 cm) for 7 consecutive days, in the 1st, 3rd, or 8th postoperative week. Performance on a rotating beam was measured repeatedly, except during the week of SMR, and plotted as a function of time after surgery. These data have been redrawn in Figure 3–2,C. The most striking effects were seen in those animals exposed to SMR early after surgery (curves 1 and 2), in which locomotor equilibrium never recovered fully, at least for more than one year. SMR applied after recovery had occurred (curve 3) had no effect.

Under normal circumstances, it would not be possible to conduct an experiment equivalent to that of Lacour and Xerri[27] on human subjects. However, a closely analogous situation may occur each time an astronaut enters the weightless condition of space. In the absence of the normal gravitational vector, most head movements produce patterns of vestibular afferent activity which differ from those experienced when the same head movements are performed on the ground. This is in many ways equivalent to suffering an instantaneous bilateral vestibular lesion. The nervous system then has the goal of compensating for this altered sensorimotor relationship, which would disrupt normal vestibulospinal reflex function. However, postural and locomotor control are completely abnormal in weightlessness, with stability in the upright position no longer relevant, so no meaningful exercise occurs at all. Under these conditions of ultimate sensorimotor restriction, vestibulospinal reflexes might not recover. (This is different from the case of the returning astronaut, who is exposed to normal, self-generated postural and locomotor activity almost immediately.)

This prediction has been tested by experiments conducted during the flight of *Spacelab-1*.[30] Astronaut subjects were exposed to sudden, unexpected falls, using a harness and elastic cords to provide an accelerating force. Electromyographic activity in response to this vestibular stimulus was recorded from gastrocnemius soleus. The earliest component of this response, which is considered to be an otolith-spinal reflex, was measured, normalized with respect to preflight controls, and plotted as a function of time in weightlessness (Figure 3–2,D). In contrast to the ground-based situation (Figure 3–2,A–C), there was no apparent recovery. In fact, with all but the strongest acceleration stimulus, no otolith-spinal reflex was detectable after mission day 1 (after 48 hours in space). Apparently, this is the proper, goal-directed adaptation to the unique biomechanical environment of space. Certainly, it is not simply the loss of a reflex as a result of disuse or irrelevancy. The VOR, for example, remains essentially normal in adult cats deprived of vision for over 4 months.[31]

The implications of these studies seem clear. Following a peripheral vestibular lesion, recovery of postural and locomotor control involves both sensory substitution and plastic adaptation occurring within the CNS. These processes require appropriate, actively generated motor activity with resulting sensory feedback to be effective. This activity must occur throughout the adaptive period, but it is most critical during the first few days. Therefore, active behavior must be encouraged as soon as possible following the onset of a peripheral vestibular defect, even though it will almost certainly aggravate accompanying symptoms of motion sickness, which will probably not be fully controllable pharmacologically. The potential consequences of restricting movement, however, far outweigh the short-term discomfort experienced by the patient.

The studies of the ocular component of gaze stability also indicate that it may be important to shape the applied stimuli or appropriately instruct the patient so that he develops an optimal combination of compensatory strategies. Whether this is also the case for the vestibulospinal component remains to be determined.

REFERENCES

1. Robinson DA: Control of eye movements, in Brooks VB (ed): *Handbook of Physiology, The Nervous System: III. Motor Control*. Bethesda, Md, American Physiological Society, 1980, pp 1275–1320.
2. Roberts TDM: *Neurophysiology of Postural Mechanisms*, ed 2. London, Butterworths, 1978, pp 182–192.
3. Nashner LM, Black FO, Wall C III: Adaptation to altered support and visual conditions during stance: Patients with vestibular deficits. *J Neurosci* 1982; 2:536–544.

4. Precht W, Maioli C, Dieringer N, et al: Mechanisms of compensation of the vestibulo-ocular reflex after vestibular neurotomy, in Flohr H, Precht W (eds): *Lesion-induced Neuronal Plasticity in Sensorimotor Systems.* New York, Springer-Verlag, 1981, pp 221–230.
5. Schaefer KP, Meyer DL: Compensation of vestibular lesions, in Kornhuber HH (ed): *Handbook of Sensory Physiology, Volume VI/2.* Berlin, Springer-Verlag, 1974.
6. Bechterew W von: Ergebnisse der durchschneidung des n. acusticus, nebst erorterung der bedeutung der semicircularen canale fur das korpergleichgewicht. *Pflugers Arch* 1883; 30:312–347.
7. Gonshor A, Melvill Jones G: Extreme vestibulo-ocular adaptation induced by prolonged optical reversal of vision. *J Physiol (Lond)* 1976; 256:381–414.
8. Miles FA, Eighmy BB: Long-term adaptive changes in primate vestibulo-ocular reflex: I. Behavioral observations. *J Neurophysiol* 1980; 43:1406–1425.
9. Paige GD: Vestibuloocular reflex and its interaction with visual following mechanisms in the squirrel monkey: II. Response characteristics and plasticity following unilateral inactivation of horizontal canal. *J Neurophysiol* 1983; 49:152–168.
10. Baarsma EA, Collewijn H: Changes in compensatory eye movements after unilateral labyrinthectomy in the rabbit. *Arch Otorhinolaryngol* 1975; 211:219–230.
11. Maioli C, Precht W, Ried S: Short- and long-term modifications of vestibulo-ocular response dynamics following unilateral vestibular nerve lesions in the cat. *Exp Brain Res* 1983; 50:259–274.
12. Hart CW, McKinley PA, Peterson BW: Compensation following acute unilateral total loss of peripheral vestibular function, in Graham MD, Kemink JL (eds): *The Vestibular System: Neurophysiologic and Clinical Research.* New York, Raven Press, 1987.
13. Maioli C, Precht W: On the role of vestibulo-ocular reflex plasticity in recovery after unilateral peripheral vestibular lesions. *Exp Brain Res* 1985;59:267–272.
14. Barr CC, Schultheis LW, Robinson DA: Voluntary, non-visual control of the human vestibulo-ocular reflex. *Acta Otolaryngol (Stockh)* 1976; 81:365–375.
15. McKinley PA, Peterson BW: Voluntary modulation of the vestibuloocular reflex in humans and its relation to smooth pursuit. *Exp Brain Res* 1985; 60:454–464.
16. Lisberger SG, Evinger C, Johanson GW, et al: Relationship between eye acceleration and retinal image velocity during foveal smooth pursuit in man and monkey. *J Neurophysiol* 1981; 46:229–249.
17. Llinas R, Walton K: Vestibular compensation: A distributed property of the central nervous system, in Asanuma H, Wilson VJ (eds): *Integration in the Nervous System.* Tokyo, Igaku-Shoin, 1979.
18. Xerri C, Gianni S, Manzoni D, et al: Central compensation of vestibular

deficits: I. Response characteristics of lateral vestibular neurones to roll tilt after ipsilateral labyrinth deafferentation. *J Neurophysiol* 1983; 50:428–448.

19. Igarashi M, Levy JK, Reschke MF, et al: Locomotor dysfunction after surgical lesions in the unilateral vestibular nuclei region in squirrel monkeys. *Arch Otorhinolaryngol* 1978; 221:89–95.
20. Flohr H, Bienhold H, Abeln W, et al: Concepts of vestibular compensation, in Flohr H, Precht W (eds): *Lesion-induced Neuronal Plasticity in Sensorimotor Systems*. Berlin, Springer-Verlag, 1981.
21. Ryu JH, McCabe BF: Central vestibular compensation. *Arch Otolaryngol* 1976;102:71–76.
22. Lacour M, Xerri C, Hugon M: Compensation of postural reactions to fall in the vestibular neurectomized monkey: Role of the remaining labyrinthine afferences. *Exp Brain Res* 1979; 37:563–580.
23. Pfaltz CR: Vestibular compensation: Physiological and clinical aspects. *Acta Otolaryngol (Stockh)* 1983; 95:402–406.
24. Young LR, Shelhamer M, Modestino S: MIT/Canadian vestibular experiments in Spacelab-1: 2. Visual vestibular tilt interaction in weightlessness. *Exp Brain Res* 1986; 64:299–307.
25. Benson A, Baumgarten R von, Berthoz A, et al: Some results of the European vestibular experiments in the Spacelab-1 mission, in *Results of Space Experiments in Physiology and Medicine and Informal Briefings by the F-16 Medical Working Group, AGARD-CP-377*. Neuilly sur Seine, France, AGARD, 1984.
26. Homick JF, Reschke MF, Miller EF II: Effects of prolonged exposure to weightlessness on postural equilibrium, in Johnston RS, Deitlein LF (eds): *Biomedical Results from Skylab, NASA SP-377*. Washington, DC, US Government Printing Office, 1977.
27. Lacour M, Xerri C: Vestibular compensation: New perspectives, in Flohr H, Precht W (eds): *Lesion-induced Neuronal Plasticity in Sensorimotor Systems*. Berlin, Springer-Verlag, 1981.
28. Putkonen PTS, Courjon JH, Jeannerod M: Compensation of postural effects of hemilabyrinthectomy in the cat: A sensory substitution process? *Exp Brain Res* 1977; 28:249–257.
29. Igarashi M, Levy JK, O-Uchi T, et al: Further study of physical exercise and locomotor balance compensation after unilateral labyrinthectomy in squirrel monkeys. *Acta Otolaryngol (Stockh)* 1981; 92:101–105.
30. Watt DGD, Money KE, Tomi LM: MIT/Canadian vestibular experiments on Spacelab-1: 3. Effects of prolonged weightlessness on a human otolith-spinal reflex. *Exp Brain Res* 1986; 64:308–315.
31. Harris LR, Cynader M: The eye movements of the dark-reared cat. *Exp Brain Res* 1981; 44:41–56.

4

Gaze Shifts and the Vestibulo-ocular Reflex

R. David Tomlinson, B.Sc., M.Sc., Ph.D.

To understand the questions involved in eye-head coordination, it is first necessary to understand something of the function of the eye movement systems involved. The first part of this chapter is aimed at providing the necessary background.

THE VESTIBULO-OCULAR REFLEX

The basic function of the VOR is to generate compensatory eye movements which are equal in amplitude but opposite in direction to the head movements which cause them. Thus, if one defines "gaze" direction as the direction of the visual axis in space (that is, eye-in-head + head-in-space), the VOR can be thought of as a system which stabilizes gaze during head movements. The reflex is based on a three-neuron arc (Fig 4–1). The head velocity signal, $\dot{H}$, derived from the semicircular canals, is linked through to the ocular motoneurons with the minimum amount of processing to provide the signal to drive the eyes at the same velocity.

The performance of the VOR is most commonly defined in terms of its gain: (eye velocity)/(head velocity). Thus, for the reflex to be compensatory and to stabilize images on the retina during head movements, the gain must be close to unity, as is found when the measurement is made at frequencies close to those experienced during natural head movements (>0.5 Hz). Experiments in humans by Pulaski et al.[1] have shown that the human VOR saturates with head velocities above 350°/sec. As a result of this saturation, when the head velocity is below 350°/sec, the gain is close to unity but decreases progressively as head velocity continues to increase. Thus, the VOR generates compen-

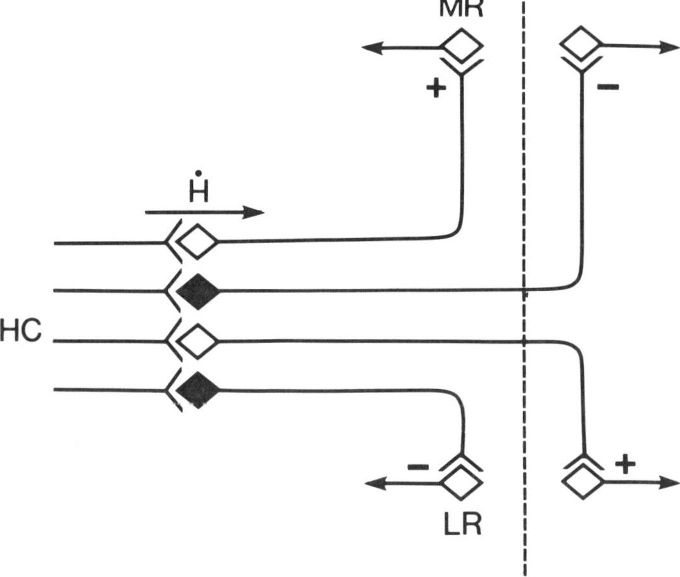

FIG 4–1.
Three-neuron arc on which VOR is based. Signal carried by these neurons is *H,* head velocity. In consequence of this arrangement, head movements result in (approximately) equal and opposite eye movements. *HC,* horizontal semicircular canal afferents; *LR,* lateral rectus motoneurons; *MR,* medial rectus motoneurons; neurons *(filled symbols)* are inhibitory.

satory eye movements in response to head movements within a wide range of head velocities and frequencies and, under normal circumstances, does not appear to depend on any other sensory systems besides the vestibular labyrinth.

THE SACCADIC SYSTEM

The saccadic system functions to move the fovea from one target of interest to another as quickly as possible. Recordings from ocular motoneurons indicate that the signal required to drive the eye consists of a pulse or burst of firing which moves the eye to the new position, along with a step change in firing rate to hold the eye at that new position. Stated somewhat differently, the burst is a velocity command and the step a position command.

All eye movement systems are believed to be organized in the same basic fashion. A control network generates a velocity command which is sent both to the eye muscles and to an integrator, which, since position is the integral of velocity, has an output which encodes eye position and supplies the necessary position command to the ocular motoneurons.

Both neuronal recordings and lesion studies indicate that the horizontal and vertical components of saccades are separately controlled by centers in the pontine[2, 3] and mesencephalic[4, 5] reticular formation, respectively. Most current models of saccadic control are variations of the original "bang-bang" controller proposed by Zee et al.[6]

A simplified version of the model is illustrated in Figure 4–2. Simply stated, an internal copy of eye position, E′, is compared to target position, T, the difference between the two being the desired movement, or motor error, e. This signal is used to drive the burst neuron, BN, which provides the drive to the motor neuron needed to overcome the viscoelastic drags and to move the eye to its new position. Note that the BN fires rapidly during saccades and is otherwise completely silent. The same BN signal is fed through an integrator to generate the eye position signal necessary to hold the eye in the new position. Between saccades, the burst neuron is inhibited by the pause neuron (PN), which in turn is inhibited by the burst neuron. Thus, to initiate a saccade, the pause neuron is first turned off by a trigger signal, allowing the burst neuron to respond to its motor error input. Once a saccade has been initiated in this fashion, it will continue until the motor error is reduced to zero, or at least below some threshold value.

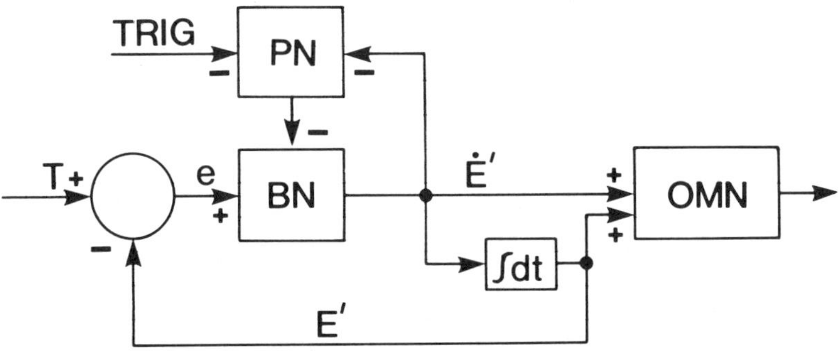

FIG 4–2.
Simplified version of "bang-bang" controller believed to be responsible for control of saccadic eye movements. Operation of this model is described in the text. *E'*, internal copy of eye position; *T*, target position; $e = T - E'$, motor error; *BN*, burst neuron; *PN*, pause neuron; *TRIG*, saccadic trigger signal; *OMN*, ocular motoneurons; *dt*, oculomotor integrator which generates an eye position signal by integrating velocity command produced by burst neurons.

It is important to remember that under natural conditions, all moderately sized saccades are accompanied by a head movement that keeps the eye reasonably centered in the orbit and thus prepared to make another movement.

EYE-HEAD COORDINATION

Even casual observations of either humans or animals show that eye and head movements are tightly linked. This coupling has been strikingly demonstrated at the neuronal level by the observation that the burst neurons which drive saccadic eye movements also project to the cervical spinal cord.[7] Indeed, in both cat and monkey, when the head is restrained, neck muscle EMG is seen to be clearly related to eye position in the orbit.[8, 9] In spite of this, most studies of the oculomotor system have been done in humans or in animals with fixed (immobile) heads, thereby avoiding the question of eye-head coordination. Recently, however, several groups have begun to investigate eye-head coordination in more detail.

Since the late 1960s the mechanism responsible for eye-head coordination has been widely accepted to be the VOR. It was believed that when a saccadic eye movement was executed in conjunction with a head movement, the vestibular and saccadic commands were summed linearly (presumably at the motoneuron).[10, 12] Thus, since the

VOR generates compensatory eye movements which are (approximately) equal and opposite to the head movement, any head movement which occurred during the course of a saccade would be automatically subtracted from the saccadic command, so that the change in gaze angle (gaze = eye-in-head + head-in-space and thus represents the direction of the visual axis relative to the world) would still be equal to the programmed saccade. This concept is illustrated in Figure 4–3, where the head is seen to move about 15° during the course of a 50° gaze saccade. The result of the head movement is that the saccade amplitude is reduced by this same 15°, so that gaze falls on target as desired. Thus, assuming a VOR gain of close to unity, the velocity-amplitude characteristics of saccadic gaze shifts should be the same whether the head moves or not.

Problems, however, exist with the addition hypothesis. Specifically, recordings in the vestibular nuclei[13, 14] and in the medial longitudinal fasciculus[15, 16] have shown that the secondary vestibular neuron on which the VOR is based pauses during all saccades. The result of this pause in firing is that the semicircular canals are functionally disconnected from the the ocular motoneurons (see Fig 4–1) during saccades. This observation alone seems to argue strongly against linear addition, as it implies that the VOR should be switched off during saccades. In addition, since the VOR generates compensatory eye movements in response to head movements, the head cannot contribute to changes in gaze. That is, whatever amount the head

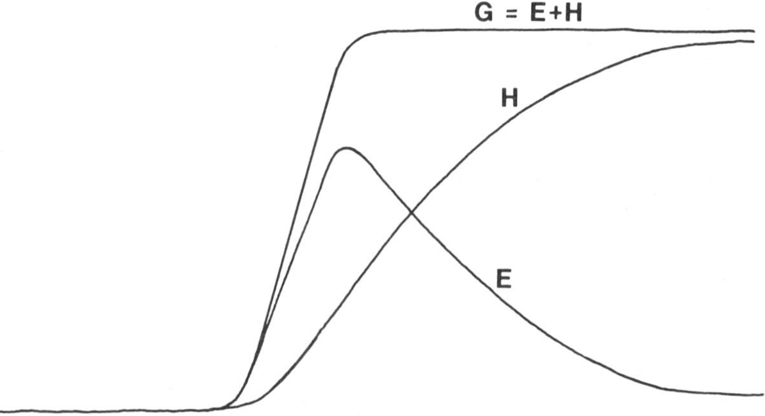

FIG 4–3.
Eye *(E)*, head *(H)*, and gaze *(G = E+H)* trajectories typically seen during a combined eye-head gaze shift. Note that saccadic eye movement amplitude is reduced by an amount equal to head movement, so that gaze arrives on target even though head moves.

moves, according to linear addition the VOR should subtract an equal amount. If this were true, gaze shifts should be limited to lie within the normal range of eye movements, about ± 45° in humans. This implies that targets far out in the peripheral visual field often could be foveated only through the use of multiple saccades, an approach which is clearly inefficient.

The results of recent experiments, however, have shown that the addition hypothesis is not entirely correct. Instead, Tomlinson and Bahra,[17, 19] working in rhesus monkeys, demonstrated that during small-amplitude saccades (<20°), the VOR is functional, and linear addition is obeyed. During large saccades, however, this does not happen. Instead, the VOR is disconnected so that linear addition does not occur. Similar observations have been made in human subjects by several groups.[20, 21]

In addition to the above findings, Laurutis and Robinson[21] also demonstrated that gaze saccades are highly accurate, even though the VOR is not functioning. Furthermore, gaze saccades were shown to be accurate even when the head movement was suddenly and unexpectedly altered by an externally applied perturbation. These observations have been confirmed by other groups[19, 20] (Fig 4–4). In view of the accuracy of gaze saccades, even in the face of externally applied perturbations, some other as yet unknown mechanism must be replacing the VOR and must be responsible for coordinating the eye and head during large gaze saccades.

To explain these observations, several new models have been proposed, all having the common feature of assuming that saccades are controlled based on gaze (rather than eye) coordinates (Fig 4–5). The important aspect of this model is that an internal copy of gaze position, G′, is generated by adding a copy of eye position to an internal estimate of head position. If the head does not move, gaze position and eye position are the same, so this model reduces to the old saccade model. When the head moves, however, the head's contribution to the change in gaze angle will be reflected in the internal estimate of gaze position, so that saccades will remain accurate, as the saccade will continue until the gaze (rather than the eye) is on target. An important property of this model is that it predicts that gaze saccade accuracy should be achieved even when the head is perturbed. Furthermore, the compensation for the perturbation should be achieved by changing the duration of the saccadic movement. Thus, gaze saccades would be predicted to continue as long as necessary to achieve the desired change in gaze angle. This is precisely what has been observed in the experiments to date.[19–21]

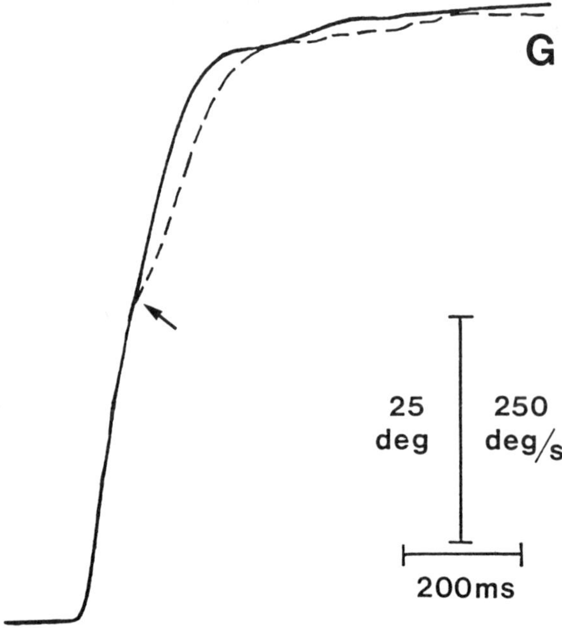

FIG 4–4.
Illustration of two superimposed combined eye-head gaze saccades made to visual targets. In one saccade *(dashed line),* the head was unexpectedly perturbed *(arrow)* during the movement, while in the other saccade *(solid line)* it was not. Note two saccades are of equal amplitude despite perturbation.

The above observations have considerable potential clinical relevance. They imply that it may be possible for certain neurologic conditions to disrupt gaze saccades while sparing eye saccades and the VOR. This could come about by damaging the pathway which carries the internal copy of head position, H′ (see Fig 4–5). The result of such damage can be simply understood by considering the effect on the internal copy of gaze G′, which is subtracted from desired gaze, Gd, in order to obtain the motor error signal. Specifically, if G′ were too small, the computed motor error would be too big, while if G′ were too large, the motor error would be too small. These mistakes would only be made, of course, when the head actually moved during the course of the saccade. If the head does not move, as is the case when the saccadic system is tested with the head fixed, then G′ = E′, and the system behaves normally. Thus, damage of the type described here would result in a condition wherein eye saccades would still be accurate, but combined eye-head gaze saccades would not be. Further,

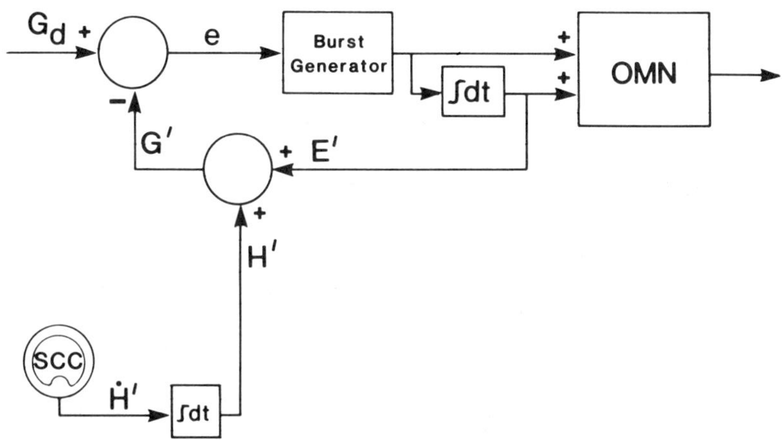

FIG 4–5.
Model of saccadic control system based on gaze (rather than eye) coordinates. Operation of this model is described in the text. *E′*, internal copy of eye position; *H′* and *Ḣ′*, internal copies of head velocity and position, respectively; *G′*, internal copy of gaze position; *e*, motor error.

if the lesion occurred after the integrator which generates the internal copy of head position, conventional vestibular testing might yield normal results. Indeed, we have evidence for such a dissociation in parkinsonian patients,[22] who exhibit grossly inaccurate and inappropriate gaze-changing behavior even though their VOR is only mildly abnormal.

The expected consequence of disruption of the gaze saccade system in isolation is simply this—the patient would make inaccurate gaze saccades, even though conventional tests of vestibular and saccadic function would be normal. Since large head movements are normally made only during gaze saccades, and since those saccades might be very inaccurate, patients could report that they became disoriented during head movements. This is one possible explanation for patients who become disoriented during head movements but have normal vestibular function test results.

Of course, this is only a theory for which we have limited clinical evidence. Nonetheless, the results of the physiologic experiments are highly suggestive. Since testing of the gaze saccade mechanism is relatively easy and can be done without any equipment beyond that found in any clinical vestibular testing laboratory, it would certainly be a worthwhile test, particularly for patients who report disorientation but have aparently normal vestibular function.

TESTING GAZE SACCADES

As mentioned previously, large-amplitude gaze saccades are under normal circumstances highly accurate, particularly when they are self-paced and are directed toward unchanging, clearly visible targets. A testing technique suggests itself immediately. It is necessary only to have the patient make large-amplitude gaze saccade between two targets which subtend a sufficiently large angle; e.g., 100°. The patient should be encouraged to make the refixation as rapidly as possible. Although we do not now have sufficient data to specify the normal range with confidence, most people seem to be able to make saccades that are within 5° of the target under these conditions. It is not necessary to measure the amplitude of the primary saccade (which might well exceed the linear range of the extra-ocular muscles) or of the

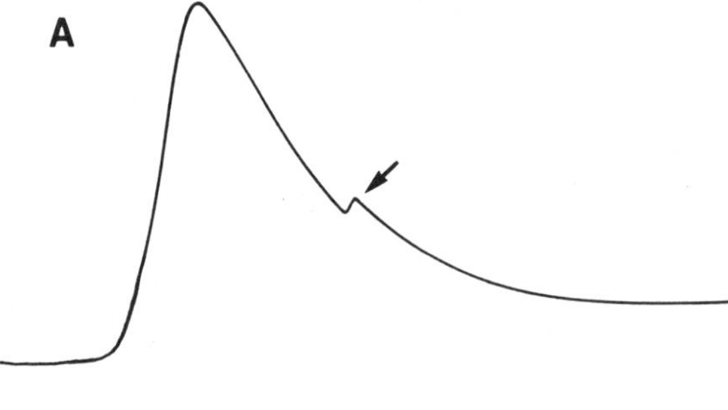

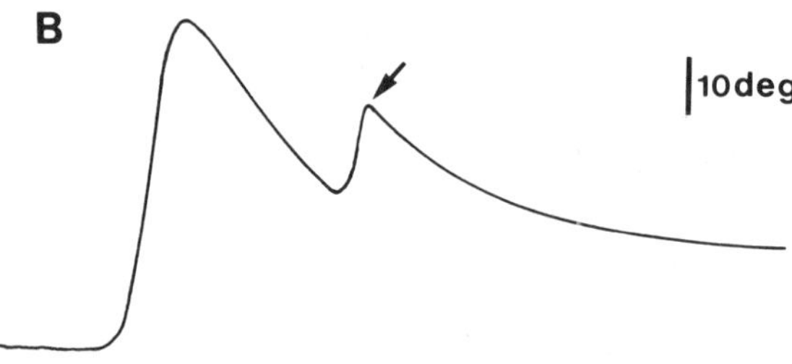

FIG 4–6.
Typical eye trajectories during 100° gaze saccades showing **(A)** example with normal accuracy (small [or absent] correction saccade, *arrow*); and **(B)** example with reduced accuracy (large 17° correction saccade, *arrow*).

head movement. Instead, if the amplitude of the correction saccade (normally less than 5°) is measured, it will immediately provide a measure of the accuracy within which the system is operating (Fig 4–6). Any failure of the gaze saccade mechanism will result in abnormally large correction saccades.

Recent demonstrations of the failure of linear addition of saccadic and vestibular signals during coordinated eye-head gaze saccades demonstrated that some mechanism for coordinating eye and head movements other than the VOR must exist. The functional integrity of this system can be tested by measuring the amplitude of the corrective saccade following a large amplitude gaze saccade.

REFERENCES

1. Pulaski PD, Zee DS, Robinson DA: The behaviour of the vestibulo-ocular reflex at high velocities of head rotation. *Brain Res* 1981; 222:159–165.
2. Henn V, Cohen B: Coding of information about rapid eye movements in the pontine reticular formation of alert monkeys. *Brain Res* 1976; 108:307–325.
3. Henn V, Lang W, Hepp K, et al: Horizontal or global gaze palsy induced by kanic acid lesions in the pons of the monkey. *Soc Neurosci Abstr* 1982; 8:157.
4. King WM, Fuchs AF, Magnin M: Vertical eye movement related responses of neurons in the midbrain near the interstitial nucleus of Cajal. *J Neurophysiol* 1981; 46:549–562.
5. Henn V, Schnyder H, Hepp K, et al: Loss of vertical rapid eye movements after kanic acid lesions in rostral mesencephalon in rhesus monkey. *Soc Neurosci Abstr* 1983; 9:749.
6. Zee DS, Optican LM, Cook JD, et al: Slow saccades in spinocerebellar degeneration. *Arch Neurol* 1976; 33:243–251.
7. Grantyn R, Baker R, Grantyn A: Morphological and physiological excitatory pontine reticular neurons projecting to the cat abducens nucleus and spinal cord. *Brain Res* 1980; 198:221–228.
8. Vidal PP, Roucoux A, Berthoz A: Horizontal eye position related activity in neck muscles of the alert cat. *Exp Brain Res* 1982; 46:448–453.
9. Lestienne E, Vidal PP, Berthoz A: Gaze changing behaviour in head restrained monkey. *Exp Brain Res* 53:349–356.
10. Bizzi E, Kalil RE, Tagliasco V: Eye-head coordination in monkeys: Evidence for centrally patterned organization. *Science* 1971; 173:452–454.
11. Dichgans J, Bizzi E, Morasso P, et al: Mechanisms underlying recovery of eye-head coordination following bilateral labyrinthectomy in monkeys. *Exp Brain Res* 1973; 18:548-562.
12. Whittington DA, Lestienne F, Bizzi E: Behaviour of preoculomotor burst neurons during eye-head coordination. *Exp Brain Res* 1984; 55:215–222.

13. Tomlinson RD, Robinson DA: Responses of vestibular nuclei cells during vertical vestibular and pursuit eye movements. *Soc Neurosci Abstr* 1980; 6:477.
14. Tomlinson RD, Robinson DA: Signals in vestibular nucleus mediating vertical eye movements in the monkey. *J Neurophysiol* 1984; 51:1121–1136.
15. King WM, Lisberger SG, Fuchs AF: Responses of fibres in medial longitudinal fasciculus (MLF) of alert monkeys during horizontal and vertical conjugate eye movements evoked by vestibular or visual stimuli. *J Neurophysiol* 1976; 39:1135–1149.
16. Pola J, Robinson DA: Oculomotor signals in medial longitudinal fasciculus of the monkey. *J Neurophysiol* 1978; 41:245–259.
17. Tomlinson RD, Bahra PS: Interactions of the vestibulo-ocular reflex with the saccadic system during combined eye-head gaze shifts in the monkey. *Soc Neurosci Abstr* 1984; 10:389.
18. Tomlinson RD, Bahra PS: Combined eye-head gaze shifts in the primate; I. Metrics. *J Neurophysiol* 1986; 56:1542–1557.
19. Tomlinson RD, Bahra PS: Combined eye-head gaze shifts in the primate: II. Interactions between saccades and the vestibulo-ocular reflex. *J Neurophysiol* 1986; 56:1558–1570.
20. Guitton D, Volle M: Gaze control in humans: Eye-head coordination during orienting movements to targets within and beyond the oculomotor range. *J Neurophysiol* 1987; 58:427–459.
21. Laurutis VP, Robinson DA: The vestibulo-ocular reflex during human saccadic eye movements. *J Physiol (Lond)* 1986; 373:209–233.
22. White OB, St Cyr J, Tomlinson RD, et al: Ocular motor deficits in Parkinson's disease: III. Coordination of eye and head movements. *Brain* In press.

PART TWO

Vestibular Function Testing

5

Conventional Bithermal Caloric Tests

Charles W. Stockwell, Ph.D.

The bithermal caloric test has been the mainstay of vestibular function testing for the past 30 years. This chapter is a brief review of the principles of bithermal caloric testing. It provides a background for the following discussions of alternative methods.

In 1942, Fitzgerald and Hallpike[1] first described the clinical use of the bithermal caloric test. They irrigated each ear twice—once with water at 30° C for 40 sec and once with water at 44° C for 40 sec—and watched the patient's eyes to determine the duration of the nystagmus response. In 1956 Aschan et al.[2] described the use of electronystagmography to monitor the nystagmus response with eyes closed. Today we require the patient to perform a mental task to maintain alertness while his nystagmus is being recorded, and we use peak slow-phase eye velocity rather than duration of nystagmus as the index of caloric response strength. Otherwise, we perform the bithermal caloric test exactly as Aschan et al. described it.

MECHANISM OF CALORIC STIMULATION

Caloric stimulation produces nystagmus by modulating the firing rates of the afferent nerves of the horizontal semicircular canals. For many years it was assumed that the mechanism of stimulation was endolymph convection, first described by Barany[3] in 1906, in which the thermal stimulus causes convection currents within the endolymph of the horizontal canal that deflect the cupula and thus modulate the firing rates of the afferents. When the patient is in the standard nose-up caloric test position, warm stimuli increase the firing rates and cool stimuli decrease them. In 1967 Coats and Smith[4] showed that endolymph convection is not the only mechanism of stimulation. They found that the caloric response was greater when the patient was in the nose-up position than when he was in the nose-down position and concluded that the caloric response is provoked by two mechanisms—endolymph convection, which depends on head position relative to gravity and accounts for approximately 80% of the response, and a direct thermal effect, which is independent of head position and accounts for approximately 20% of the response. However, the entire endolymph convection hypothesis was recently called into question by the report of Scherer and Clarke[5] that caloric responses in space were as strong as those on earth. Endolymph convection could not have produced caloric responses in space, because convection depends on the presence of gravity. Scherer and Clarke offered an alternative hypothesis in which the thermal stimulus produces a local change in the volume of the endolymph that, in turn, leads to a pressure gradient around the semicircular canal, which causes deflection of the cupula. A definitive answer to the question of the mechanism of caloric stimulation awaits resolution of this issue.

CURRENT CLINICAL USE OF CALORIC TESTING

Whatever the exact mechanism of stimulation, the conventional bithermal caloric test has proved highly sensitive to unilateral peripheral vestibular lesions, i.e., to lesions of the labyrinth or vestibular nerve, because it permits the examiner to stimulate each ear separately. Other test procedures, such as rotation testing and posturography, necessarily involve stimulation of both ears together and therefore permit masking of abnormal responses arising from the damaged labyrinth by normal responses arising from the opposite ear. For this reason, the caloric test has been widely used over the years and is not likely to be soon replaced, despite its well-recognized shortcomings.

The caloric test is specifically a test of the horizontal semicircular canals, although inferences about the condition of the other receptors often are made on the basis of caloric test results. In theory, it should be possible to stimulate the vertical canals after appropriately positioning the head, but, in practice, vertical canal stimulation does not seem to work well. The vertical canals are deeply imbedded in the temporal bone far from the caloric stimulus. Furthermore the eye movements produced by vertical canal stimulation are primarily vertical-rotary and difficult to monitor by the electronystagmographic method.

The caloric stimuli used today by most examiners consist of 250 ml of water irrigated into the external ear canal within 30 sec. The temperature of the water is 30° C for the cool irrigation and 44° C for the warm irrigation. Some examiners use air (8 L at 24° C and 50° C within 60 sec) instead of water as caloric stimuli. Others use a "closed-loop" system, in which water continuously circulates within a water-tight system which includes a small balloon that inflates in the external ear canal during the irrigation. All three irrigating methods—water, air and "closed-loop"—yield approximately equivalent stimuli.

NORMAL CALORIC RESPONSES

Standard caloric stimuli produce nystagmus responses in normal individuals like those shown in Figure 5–1. The responses begin approximately 20 sec after the onset of the irrigation, reach peak intensity approximately 40 sec later, thereafter decline, and finally disappear after about 3 min. The cool irrigations provoke nystagmus with slow phases toward the irrigated ear, and the warm irrigations provoke nystagmus with slow phases away from the irrigated ear. The responses to warm and cool stimuli are mirror images of one another. The difference between the peak intensity of the cool response and the peak intensity of the warm response is commonly used as the index of caloric response strength of a particular ear. The basic assumption of the caloric test is that both ears receive equal caloric stimuli, and, if both ears are normal, they should produce equally strong caloric responses.

UNILATERAL WEAKNESS

To quantify the difference in caloric response strength of the two ears, most examiners use the formula proposed by Jongkees and Philipszoon,[6] which is as follows:

$$\frac{(RW + RC) - (LW + LC)}{RW + RC + LW + LC} \times 100 = \text{unilateral weakness,}$$

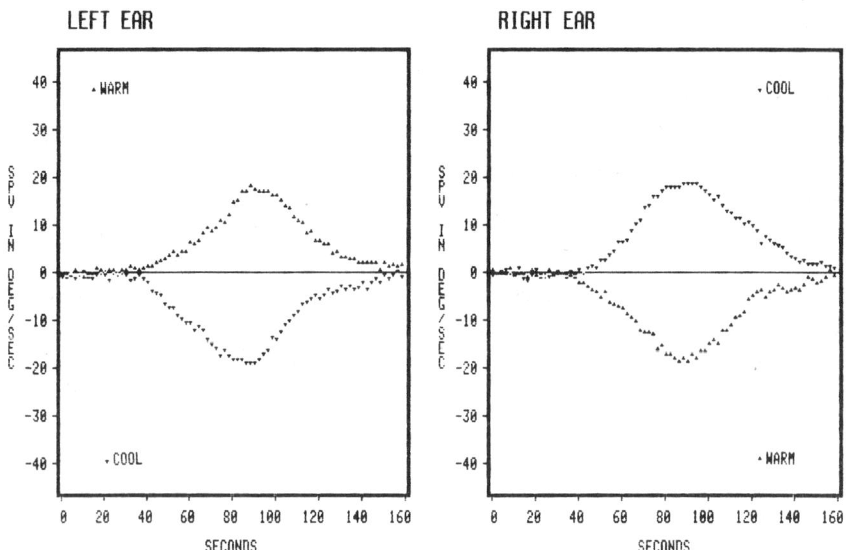

FIG 5–1.
Caloric responses of normal individual. Slow-phase velocity on vertical axis (positive values indicate rightward velocities; negative values indicate leftward velocities); time on horizontal axis.

where RW, RC, LW, and LC are peak slow-phase velocities for the responses to right warm, right cool, left warm, and left cool irrigations, respectively. The normal limit of 20%–25% is widely accepted.[7, 8]

Figure 5–2 shows the caloric responses of a patient who has a left peripheral vestibular lesion. Responses of the left ear are clearly weaker than those of the right ear, and calculation of unilateral weakness by the formula of Jongkees and Philipszoon[6] yields

$$\frac{(20 + 20) - (5 + 5)}{20 + 20 + 5 + 5} \times 100 = 60\%$$

which is well outside the normal limit.

DIRECTIONAL PREPONDERANCE

If all patients who underwent caloric testing displayed only normal responses or unilateral weaknesses, it would not be necessary to

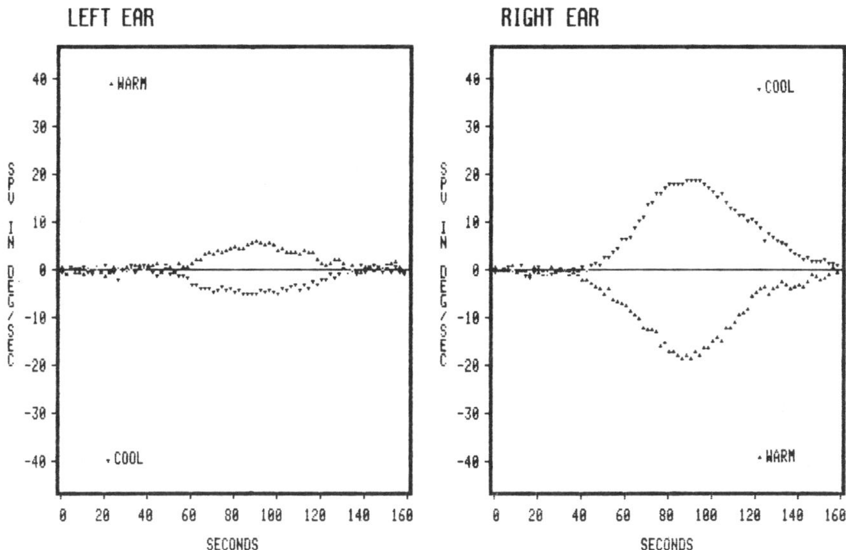

FIG 5–2.
Caloric responses of patient with long-standing left peripheral vestibular lesion. Axis labels are the same as in Figure 5–1.

irrigate each ear twice. One irrigation of each ear, either warm or cool, would suffice. However, some patients have a directional preponderance of caloric responses, i.e., their responses in one direction are stronger than their responses in the other direction.

A directional preponderance is the inevitable consequence of a sudden unilateral peripheral vestibular lesion. The lesion causes a reduction in the resting input coming from the damaged ear, producing an asymmetry of resting inputs coming from the two ears. This asymmetry mimics the asymmetry that would be produced by head acceleration away from the side of the lesion, and the result is tonic, or "spontaneous," nystagmus that would be appropriate for such acceleration, i.e., nystagmus with slow phases toward the side of the damaged ear. Figure 5–3 shows the caloric responses of a patient with a history characteristic of a sudden unilateral peripheral vestibular lesion—abrupt onset of vertigo with nausea and vomiting followed by gradual improvement. The caloric test was performed 3 days after the onset of symptoms. The responses clearly show a left unilateral weakness. Calculation of unilateral weakness by the formula of Jongkees and Philipszoon[6] yields

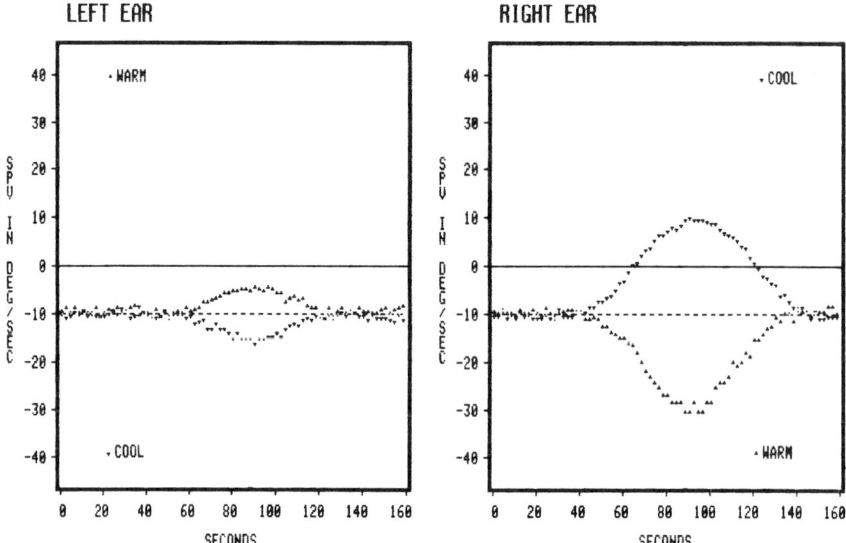

FIG 5–3.
Caloric responses of a patient with a recent left peripheral vestibular lesion. Axis labels are the same as in Figure 5–1; *horizontal dashed lines* indicate slow-phase velocity of subject's spontaneous nystagmus in darkness.

$$\frac{(30 + 10) - (-5 + 15)}{30 + 10 + -5 + 15} \times 100 = 60\%$$

which is outside the normal limit. (Note that the peak slow-phase velocity of the left warm response is entered into the formula as a negative value, since it is opposite the expected direction.)

The patient also has spontaneous nystagmus with leftward slow phases at velocities of 10°/sec, and the caloric responses are symmetric about a new baseline corresponding to the slow-phase velocities of this nystagmus. If the peak slow-phase velocities of the caloric responses are calculated with respect to zero velocity, the nystagmus responses with leftward slow phases—the responses to right warm and left cool irrigations—turn out to be stronger than responses with rightward slow phases—the responses to right cool and left warm irrigations.

To quantify directional preponderance, most examiners use the formula proposed by Jongkees and Philipszoon[6] as follows:

$$\frac{(RW + LC) - (LW + RC)}{RW + LC + LW + RC} \times 100 = \text{directional preponderance,}$$

where RW, LC, LW, and RC are the same as in the formula for unilateral weakness. The normal limit of 30% is widely accepted.[7, 8] Calculation of directional preponderance for the caloric responses shown in Figure 5–3 using this formula yields

$$\frac{(30 + 15) - (-5 + 10)}{30 + 15 + -5 + 10} \times 100 = 80\%$$

which is well outside the normal limit.

The directional preponderance in this case can be attributed to the left peripheral vestibular lesion, which created the asymmetry. Over time, it is expected that the process of vestibular compensation will rebalance the asymmetry and that the directional preponderance will disappear. Then, if the lesion resolves, subsequent testing is likely to show normal responses, like those shown in Figure 5–1. If the lesion does not resolve, subsequent testing would be expected to show a unilateral weakness without a directional preponderance, like that shown in Figure 5–2.

Figure 5–4 shows the caloric responses of a patient who has a directional preponderance without concomitant unilateral weakness.

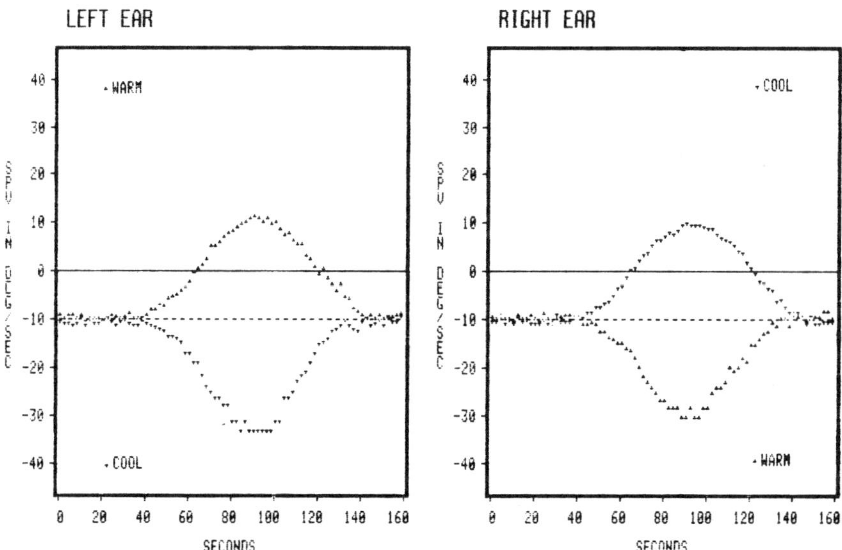

FIG 5–4.

Caloric responses of patient with nonlocalizing directional preponderance. Axis labels are the same as in Figure 5–1; *horizontal dashed lines* indicate slow-phase velocity of subject's spontaneous nystagmus in darkness.

Like the patient whose responses are shown in Figure 5–3, he has spontaneous nystagmus with leftward slow phases at 10°/sec, which creates a new baseline on which his caloric responses are superimposed. Calculation of directional preponderance by the formula of Jongkees and Philipszoon[6] yields

$$\frac{(30 + 30) - (10 + 10)}{30 + 30 + 10 + 10} \times 100 = 50\%$$

which is outside the normal limit.

The preponderance in this case cannot be attributed to a recent peripheral vestibular lesion, since the caloric responses of the two ears are equal. Calculation of unilateral weakness yields

$$\frac{(30 + 10) - (10 + 30)}{30 + 10 + 10 + 30} \times 100 = 0\%$$

This preponderance could have been caused by a lesion within the central vestibular pathways, but other explanations, such as recovery of a previously compensated peripheral lesion, are also possible. Therefore, a directional preponderance that cannot be attributed to a recent peripheral vestibular lesion generally must be regarded as nonlocalizing.

BILATERAL WEAKNESS

Whereas the bithermal caloric test is highly sensitive to unilateral peripheral vestibular lesions, it is relatively insensitive to bilateral lesions. The reason is that the caloric stimulus is uncalibrated. Even though the stimulus at the entrance to the external ear canal is the same for everyone, the amount of stimulus reaching the inner ear varies widely across individuals due to differences in the size and shape of the ear canal and middle ear structures. Therefore, normal limits for absolute response intensity are extremely wide, and bilateral caloric weaknesses must be severe to fall below them. The usual rule of thumb is that a bilateral weakness exists if caloric responses of both ears fall below 12°–15°/sec.[7] An example of caloric responses of a patient with a bilateral weakness is shown in Figure 5–5.

A bilateral weakness usually indicates bilateral peripheral vestibular lesions. Central nervous system disorders also produce bilateral

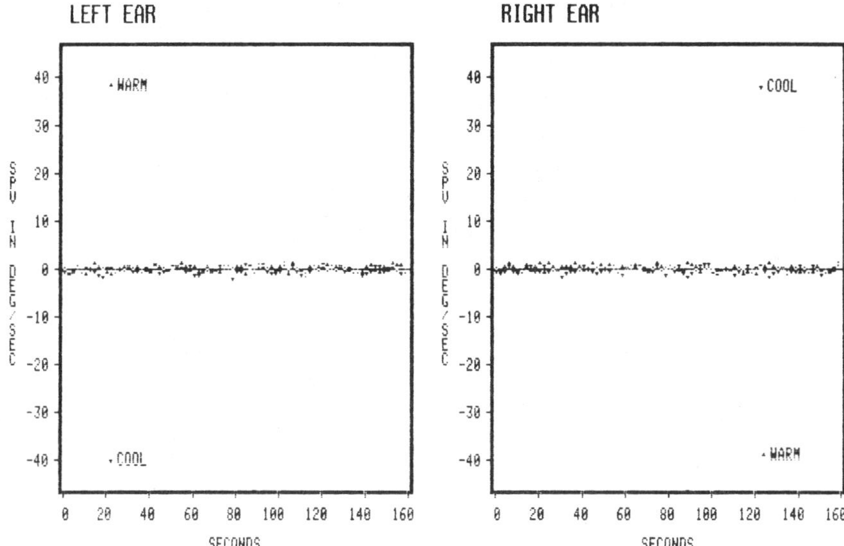

FIG 5–5.
Caloric responses of patient with bilateral weakness. Axis labels are the same as in Figure 5–1.

weaknesses, but bilateral weaknesses of CNS origin usually are accompanied by other signs of CNS dysfunction.[9]

REFERENCES

1. Fitzgerald G, Hallpike CS: Studies in human vestibular function: I. Observations on the directional preponderances, nystagmusbereitschaft, of caloric nystagmus resulting from cerebral lesions. *Brain* 1942; 65:115.
2. Aschan G, Bergstedt M, Stahle J: Nystagmography: Recording of nystagmus in clinical neuro-otological examinations. *Acta Otolaryngol (Stockh) [suppl 129]* 1956.
3. Barany R: Untersuchungen uber den vom Vertibularapparat ded Ohres reflektorisch ausgelosten rhythmischen Nystagmus und seine Begleiterscheinungen. *Monatsschr Ohrenheilk Laryngorhinol* 1906; 40:193.
4. Coats AC, Smith SY: Body position and the intensity of caloric nystagmus. *Acta Otolaryngol (Stockh)* 1967; 63:515.
5. Scherer H, Clarke AH: The caloric vestibular reaction in space. *Acta Otolaryngol (Stockh)* 1985; 100:328.
6. Jongkees LBW, Philipszoon AJ: Electronystagmography. *Acta Otolaryngol (Stockh) [suppl 189]* 1964.

7. Barber HO, Stockwell CW: *Manual of Electronystagmography*. St Louis, CV Mosby, 1980.
8. Coats AC: Electronystagmography, in Bradford LJ (ed): *Physiologic Measures of the Audio-Vestibular System*. New York, Academic Press, 1975, pp 37–85.
9. Simmons FB: Patients with bilateral loss of caloric response. *Ann Otol Rhinol Laryngol* 1973; 82:175.

6

*The Simultaneous Binaural Bithermal Caloric Test: An Evaluation Using Receiver-Operator Characteristic Methodology**

Joseph M.R. Furman, M.D., Ph.D.

Conrad Wall, III, Ph.D.

Donald B. Kamerer, M.D.

The simultaneous binaural bithermal caloric test, heretofore called the simultaneous test, has been advocated as a valuable adjunct to conventional, that is, alternate binaural bithermal caloric, testing.[1–4] This study was intended to: (1) compare the results from the alternate and the simultaneous tests; and (2) to compare their ability to distinguish between a healthy and patient population. Also, our goal was to determine whether combining the results from the alternate and simultaneous tests improved the ability to distinguish between a healthy and a patient population.

To perform our comparison of the simultaneous and the alternate tests, we used caloric test results from both populations. We were thereby able to compute the agreement and disagreement between the

*This work was supported by NIH grant NS00921 to Dr. Furman.

two tests. However, to compare directly the ability of each test to distinguish between healthy subjects and patients, we chose receiver-operator characteristic (ROC) methodology.[5, 6] This statistical technique provides a quantitative means of describing the ability of a test to separate two populations. ROC methods were developed for radar and then found application in psychology. Recently, ROC methods have been used to assess the diagnostic efficacy of several clinical tests, especially in the field of radiology. ROC methods have also been used for evaluating otologic tests.[7–10] An advantage of the ROC method is that the abilities of different diagnostic tests to distinguish between two populations can be compared to one another independent of the specific scoring criterion used to determine the normality of the test result. That is, the ROC method is independent of how strict or lax a criterion is used to determine normality. Thus, the intrinsic ability of a test to distinguish a healthy population from a patient population can be assessed.

An inherent difficulty in evaluating any vestibular test—and the caloric test is no exception—is the lack of a so-called gold standard. There is no means of determining absolutely which persons are truly normal and which patients are truly abnormal. Thus, the actual diagnostic efficacy of a new vestibular test cannot be determined, because there is no absolute standard against which to compare the results. This inherent limitation in the ability to evaluate a vestibular test is of less importance when comparing one test to another compared with determining the absolute efficacy of a single test.

METHODS

Patient Population

The patient population consisted of 652 persons between the ages of 5 and 91 years (mean, 50.3). The patients were an unselected group of persons referred to the Vestibular Laboratory at the Eye and Ear Hospital of Pittsburgh during a 2-year period. No attempt was made to identify a particular subgroup of these individuals.

Healthy Subjects

Forty asymptomatic persons between the ages of 16 and 69 years (mean, 27.0) were tested with both alternate and simultaneous testing. Healthy subjects were defined as persons who had no history of otologic or neurologic disease. In addition, each subject had to have normal oculomotor, positional, rotational, and posturography testing based on our laboratory's criteria. This group of healthy subjects can be considered to be a "supernormal" group. Again, with no gold standard, the absolute normality of our healthy subjects could not be determined. Using such a population, we expected fewer persons with abnormalities than would have been expected in a population of more average individuals. As a result of using such a highly selected population, false positive rates may have been underestimated for both the simultaneous and the alternate tests.

Testing Techniques

All caloric tests were performed using a closed-loop caloric irrigator (Grams/Brookler). All patients and normal subjects were tested with both simultaneous and alternate stimuli. Simultaneous testing consisted of irrigating both ears simultaneously with either warm or cool water. All persons first received a simultaneous cold irrigation, then cold irrigation of each ear separately. About half of the subjects had the left ear irrigated prior to testing the right. The others had the right ear tested prior to the left ear. We waited for 4 minutes between each of these three cold irrigations. Warm irrigations were performed 5 minutes following cold irrigations, starting with the simultaneous irrigation. Irrigation temperatures were 28° and 44° C, as these are the test temperatures recommended by the manufacturer of the closed-loop irrigator. Irrigations lasted for 40 seconds. During caloric testing, eye movements were monitored with electro-oculography (EOG) using silver-silver chloride electrodes affixed bitemporally. EOG electrodes were also placed above and below the right eye to record eye-blink artifacts. The EOG signal was amplified using dc coupling with a high-frequency filter of 40 Hz and recorded on chart paper. The EOG tracing was calibrated by instructing the subject to fixate on a target at ± 10°, horizontally.

Scoring of Caloric Responses

For alternate testing, the peak slow component velocity was determined by averaging the slow-component velocity of three beats at the peak of the response, which typically occurred between 60 and 90 seconds following the onset of irrigation. This peak slow-component velocity measure for each of the four alternate irrigations was then used to compute a percent reduced vestibular response (RVR) and percent directional preponderance (DP) using Jongkee's formula:[11, 12]

$$\% \text{ RVR} = \frac{(R30 + R44) - (L30 + L44)}{R30 + R44 + L30 + L44} \times 100$$

and

$$\% \text{ DP} = \frac{(R44 + L30) - (L44 + R30)}{R44 + L30 + L44 + R30} \times 100$$

Where R44 is the peak slow-component velocity measured following warm irrigation of the right ear; R30 is the peak slow component velocity following cool irrigation of the right ear; L44 is the peak slow-component velocity measured following warm irrigation of the left ear; and L30 is the peak slow-component velocity measured following cool irrigation of the left ear.

The RVR and DP values were used to assess the presence or absence of an RVR or DP by using threshold criteria.

Using the conventional technique of Brookler,[1, 2] simultaneous responses were characterized as type I, II, III, or IV depending on the presence and direction of the induced nystagmus. Type I responses were those with no nystagmus elicited by either simultaneous warm or simultaneous cool irrigations. Type II responses were those in which a right beating nystagmus was elicited with simultaneous warm irrigations and a left beating nystagmus elicited with simultaneous cool irrigations or those in which left beating nystagmus was elicited with simultaneous warm irrigations and right beating nystagmus was elicited with simultaneous cool irrigations. Type III responses were those in which the elicited nystagmus was either right beating or left beating with both simultaneous warm and simultaneous cool irrigations. Type IV responses were those in which either right or left beating nystagmus was elicited with either simultaneous warm or simultaneous cool irrigations, and no nystagmus was elicited with the other simultaneous irrigations. An example of a type IV response is the elicitation of right beating nystagmus with simultaneous warm irrigations and no nystagmus with simultaneous cool irrigations. It has been suggested that these response types may correspond to: type I equals normal, or bilaterally reduced, or bilaterally hyperactive; type II equals a reduced vestibular response, that is, an RVR; type III equals a directional preponderance, that is, a DP; and type IV equals a nonspecific abnormality.[1–3]

The response to simultaneous irrigations was evaluated by searching for the presence of nystagmus between 30 and 90 seconds after the onset of irrigation. Typically, nystagmus was considered present if there were at least five beats whose slow-component velocity exceeded 3°/sec. As described below, we also evaluated the simultaneous test responses with other techniques suitable for our statistical methods.

ROC Methods

To compare the ability of the alternate and the simultaneous tests to distinguish between our healthy and patient populations, we used ROC methodology.[5, 6] The ROC was generated by plotting sensitivity-specificity pairs for each test. We use the term "sensitivity" (and "hit rate") to mean that proportion of the patient population that was determined to have an abnormal test result, i.e., "true positives" (Fig 6–1). We use the term "specificity" (which equals 1 minus the false positive rate) to mean that proportion of the healthy population that was

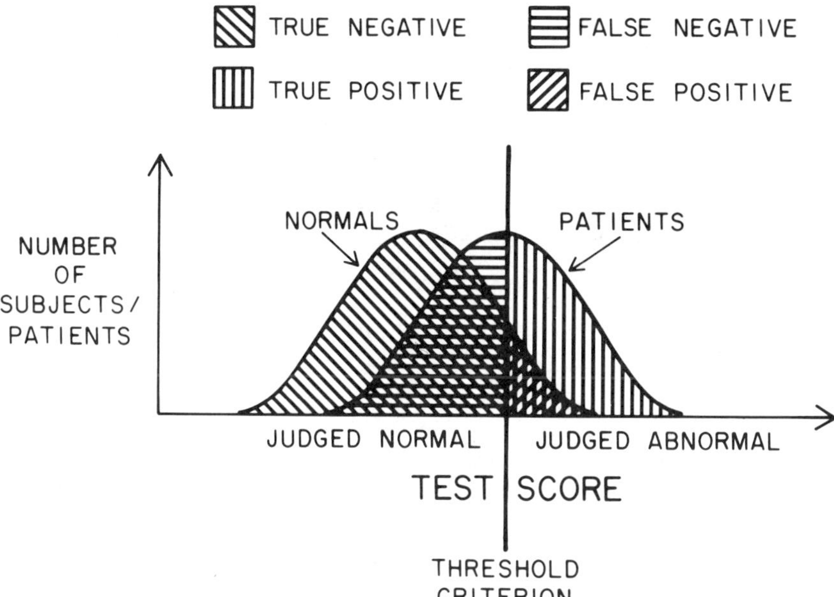

FIG 6–1.
Fictitious distributions of two populations with regard to number of persons having a particular score on a laboratory test. **Left,** supposed normal subjects; **right,** supposed patients. The threshold criterion determines the proportions of persons judged to be normal and abnormal.

determined to have a normal test result, that is, the proportion of "true negatives" (see Fig 6–1).

Again, without a gold standard to determine absolutely which persons are truly normal and which persons are truly abnormal, the proportion of true positives is in reality that portion of our patient population judged to be abnormal. Given the unselected nature of our patient population, this true positive rate is likely to be lower than the true positive rate that would be found if the patient population were instead a selected group of persons with known vestibular abnormalities. Thus, the sensitivity (and hit rate) for the alternate and the simultaneous test using our patient population is probably underestimated. The lack of a gold standard also influences the specificity measure, because we have no way of absolutely determining the normality of the healthy population. However, given the highly selected nature of this group, it is likely that the true negative rate (the specificity) of both the alternate and simultaneous tests is overestimated.

It can be seen in Figure 6–1 that by varying the location of the threshold criterion, the proportions of true positive, false positive, true negative, and false negative can be varied. Thus, the sensitivity and specificity of a given test can be varied. For instance, if the threshold criterion is increased (moved to the right in Fig 6–1), fewer normal subjects will be incorrectly judged to be abnormal, decreasing the false positive rate and increasing the specificity of the test. However, this increase in the threshold criterion will also increase the false negative rate and thereby decrease the true positive rate. The sensitivity of the test will, therefore, decrease as well. Thus, there is a trade-off between sensitivity and specificity as the value of the threshold criterion is changed.

By altering the threshold criterion in a systematic way, so that various sensitivity-specificity pairs can be generated, an ROC can be drawn. Shown in Figure 6–2 are ROCs, or plots of sensitivity-specificity pairs, for three hypothetical tests. The ability of a test to distinguish two populations can be evaluated using the ROC by computing its curvature. The diagonal line in Figure 6–2 represents the ROC of an ineffective test whose result is the same as that of chance alone. That is, the sensitivity and one minus the specificity are identical. An excellent test would have an ROC curve which is more like the dotted curve shown in Figure 6–2, wherein relatively high hit rates and thus high sensitivities are associated with relatively low false positive rates, thus, high specificities. Statistically, the curvature of the ROC reflects the ability of a test to distinguish between two populations, for example, those shown in Figure 6–1. Typically, the two popula-

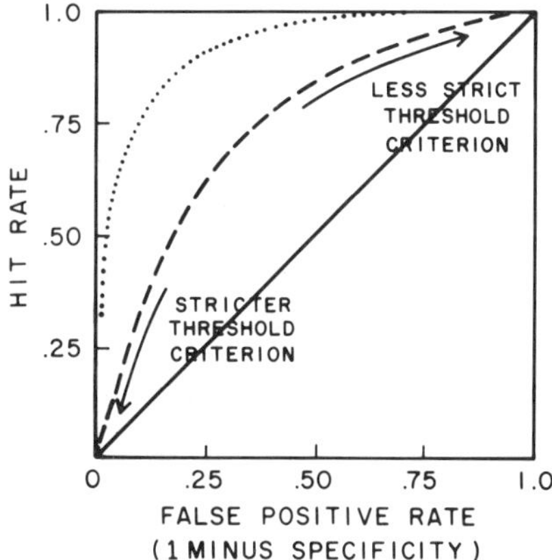

FIG 6–2.
Fictitious receiver-operator characteristics (ROC) for 3 different laboratory tests. Abscissa is false positive rate and ordinate is hit rate, or true positive rate. *Diagonal line,* ROC for completely ineffective test whose results are those expected by chance alone. *Dotted line,* ROC for a laboratory test good at distinguishing normal from diseased populations. *Dashed line,* ROC for a test not as good as that of the dotted line. Operating point on ROC can be changed by altering threshold criterion used to judge normality. Curvature of ROC, and thus efficacy of a test, is independent of the particular threshold criterion used. Points on ROC in **lower left** hit rate/false positive rate combinations generated by using a strict normality criterion, points on ROC in **upper right corner** are hit rate/false positive rate combinations generated by using a lax normality criterion.

tions used to determine an ROC are a normal and a diseased population. The classification of persons into one of the two groups requires a gold standard, or an absolute measure. For this study, we have no gold standard, and as a result we can only assess the ability of the caloric test to distinguish between our presumed normal and presumed diseased populations.

To generate an ROC, sensitivity-specificity pairs need to be generated by varying the threshold criteria used to determine normality. To alter the criteria for the alternate test, we varied the percent RVR or DP value from Jongkee's formula which was considered to be abnormal. However, for the simultaneous test, using the conventional method of Brookler, no quantitative value was available which could be used to alter the severity or laxity of the normality criteria. Therefore, we developed two nonconventional methods for evaluating the simultaneous test in a quantitative fashion so that normality criteria could be changed. We were then able to alter the sensitivity and specificity of the simultaneous test, generate sensitivity-specificity pairs, and thus generate an ROC.

Each of the nonconventional methods for quantifying the simultaneous test response required measuring the peak slow-component velocity attained. Peak slow-component velocity was measured using techniques similar to those described for scoring the alternate test. The first of the nonconventional methods for scoring the simultaneous test response considered the nystagmus elicited by a simultaneous stimulation to be insignificant if the peak slow-component velocity following irrigation did not exceed a particular threshold. For example, a person was judged to have a type II response on simultaneous testing only when right beating nystagmus whose peak slow-component velocity exceeded a threshold value was seen following simultaneous warm irrigations and left beating nystagmus whose peak slow-component velocity exceeded that same threshold value was seen following simultaneous cool irrigations. By increasing the value of this threshold, a larger proportion of persons was judged to have normal responses, and fewer persons were judged to have abnormal responses. The simultaneous test could thus be made more or less sensitive and, commensurately, less or more specific.

A second nonconventional method of quantifying the response to simultaneous testing (so that an ROC could be generated) was also used. We computed the difference between and the average of the peak slow-component velocity generated during simultaneous warm and that generated during simultaneous cold irrigations. As seen in Table 6–1, the presumed effect of an RVR is to increase the difference between the peak slow component velocities during simultaneous cold and during simultaneous warm. The presumed effect of a DP, however, is to cause no change in the difference between the cold and warm responses, but rather to alter the average of the cold and warm responses. These two values, the difference between and the average

TABLE 6–1.

Presumed Effects of RVR and DP on Simultaneous Calorics*

Abnormality	SC	SW	Difference (SC-SW)	Average (SC + SW/2)
Right RVR	↑	↓	↑	–
Left RVR	↓	↑	↓	–
Right DP	↑	↑	–	↑
Left DP	↓	↓	–	↓

*SC = simultaneous cold response; SW = simultaneous warm response; RVR = reduced vestibular response; DP = directional preponderance; ↑ = the effect of increasing the slow component velocity of a right beating nystagmus; ↓ = the effect of increasing the slow component velocity of a left beating nystagmus; – = no effect.

of the simultaneous responses, provide quantitative measures allowing the criteria for normality of the simultaneous test to be changed and thus an ROC to be generated.

We also wished to address the question of whether the ability to distinguish between our healthy and patient populations could be improved by performing both the alternate and the simultaneous tests. We generated an ROC for the combined use of the two tests. To do this, an algorithm was developed which combined the results from the simultaneous and alternate test so that a normality criterion could be applied and thus sensitivity-specificity pairs generated. Using this algorithm, persons were judged to have an RVR if their percent RVR from Jongkee's formula exceeded a particular threshold value; or if the person's percent RVR from Jongkee's formula was below that particular threshold, but between that threshold and the threshold minus 10 percentage points, the result from simultaneous testing, using the conventional criteria of Brookler, served as an additional measure. If the simultaneous test revealed a type II RVR in the same direction as the alternate test, only then was the person judged to have an RVR. For example, if the threshold for RVR on alternate testing was set at 25% and a patient had a 20% RVR as determined by Jongkee's formula, the patient would be judged as abnormal only if simultaneous testing showed a type II RVR in the same direction.

RESULTS

Of our patient population, 2.9% (19 cases) showed absent responses on both alternate and simultaneous testing. These persons' responses were not used in further evaluation of the data.

To compare the results of alternate and simultaneous testing, we determined the agreement between the results of the two tests in our patient population. For alternate testing we used normality criteria of 25% for RVR and 30% for DP, using Jongkee's formula. For simultaneous testing, we used the conventional criteria of Brookler to establish the type of the response. Shown in Table 6–2 are the agreement and disagreement data for the simultaneous and alternate tests. In general, the agreement between the simultaneous and alternate test results was low. Of note is that 17 cases, or 2.7%, of our patient population, showed an RVR on simultaneous and alternate tests which disagreed regarding the side of reduction. Frequently, the simultaneous test showed either an RVR or DP that was not shown on the alternate test and vice versa.

TABLE 6–2.
Agreement Between Alternate and Simultaneous Caloric Tests

Simultaneous Type	Alternate					
	Normal	RVR		DP		Both RVR and DP
I (50)	58.0% (29)	32.0% (16)		16.0% (8)		6.0% (3)
		Agree	Disagree			
II (276)	51.1% (141)	35.5% (98)	6.2% (17)	17.0% (47)		9.8% (27)
				Agree	Disagree	
III (106)	53.8% (57)	34.9% (37)		14.2% (15)	7.6% (8)	10.4% (11)
IV (201)	66.7% (134)	25.4% (51)		13.9% (28)		6.0% (12)

Alternate Abnormality	Simultaneous Type					
	Type I	Type II		Type III		Type IV
RVR		Agree	Disagree			
(219)	7.3% (16)	44.7% (98)	7.8 (17)	16.9% (37)		23.3% (51)
DP						
(106)	7.5% (8)	44.3% (47)		14.2% (15)	7.6% (8)	26.4% (28)

Using a criterion of 25% for RVR, the alternate test had a sensitivity of 33.5% and a specificity of 92.5%. Using the conventional criteria of Brookler for type II responses, the simultaneous test had a sensitivity of 44% and a specificity of 62.5%. Thus, the alternate test is more specific, while the simultaneous test is more sensitive.

Figure 6–3,A, illustrates the likelihood of finding a type II RVR on simultaneous testing as a function of the percent RVR on alternate testing. Figure 6–3,B, shows the likelihood of finding a type III DP on simultaneous testing as a function of the percent DP on alternate testing. It can be seen that persons with an RVR of less than 30% on alternate testing have approximately a one in four chance of showing a type II RVR on simultaneous testing. With an RVR on alternate testing greater than 30%, the likelihood of a type II RVR on simultaneous testing is about 50%. Also, with a large DP on alternate testing, the likelihood of a type III response on simultaneous testing is small. These findings are in agreement with the data in Table 6–2, which indicate a relatively poor agreement between the simultaneous and alternate caloric tests.

ROC Analysis

The results of ROC analysis for RVR on alternate caloric testing is shown in Figure 6–4,A. Highlighted is the operating point on the ROC

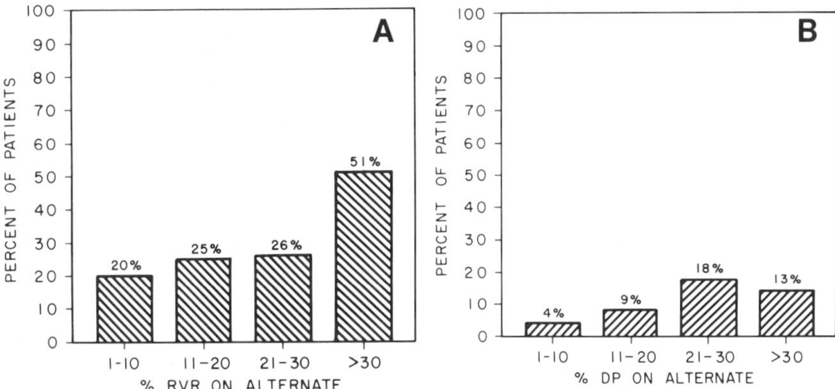

FIG 6–3.
Bar graphs of likelihood of finding a type II or type III response on simultaneous testing given % RVR or DP on alternate testing. **A,** likelihood of a type II given % RVR on alternate. **B,** likelihood of a type III given % DP on alternate.

when using a threshold criterion of 25% RVR. This operating point results in a sensitivity of 33.5% and a specificity of 92.5%. By making the threshold for normality less strict—for example, by using 20% RVR as the threshold for normality,—the sensitivity would increase to 41.2%, but the specificity would decrease to 85%. Figure 6–4,B and C, depict the ROCs generated by using the two techniques described in Methods for evaluating the response to simultaneous testing; namely, the variable threshold technique and the difference/average technique. Highlighted on Figure 6–4,B, is the operating point on the ROC when using the conventional scoring technique of Brookler. Figure 6–5 shows a comparison of the ROC from simultaneous and alternate testing for DP. The ability of the simultaneous test to distinguish between our healthy and our patient populations using RVR or DP is low. In fact, the simultaneous test gives results which are nearly those of what would be expected by chance alone. Figure 6–4,D, depicts the superimposition of the alternate and simultaneous ROCs. For a given specificity (i.e., the proportion of healthy subjects judged to be normal), the alternate caloric test has a higher sensitivity (i.e., the proportion of patients judged abnormal) than the simultaneous caloric test; and for a given sensitivity, the alternate caloric test has a higher specificity. Thus, despite the fact that the simultaneous test has a higher sensitivity (using the conventional criteria of Brookler for scoring), ROC analysis indicates that the false positive rate is so high (and thus the specificity so low) that the test is not well suited to distin-

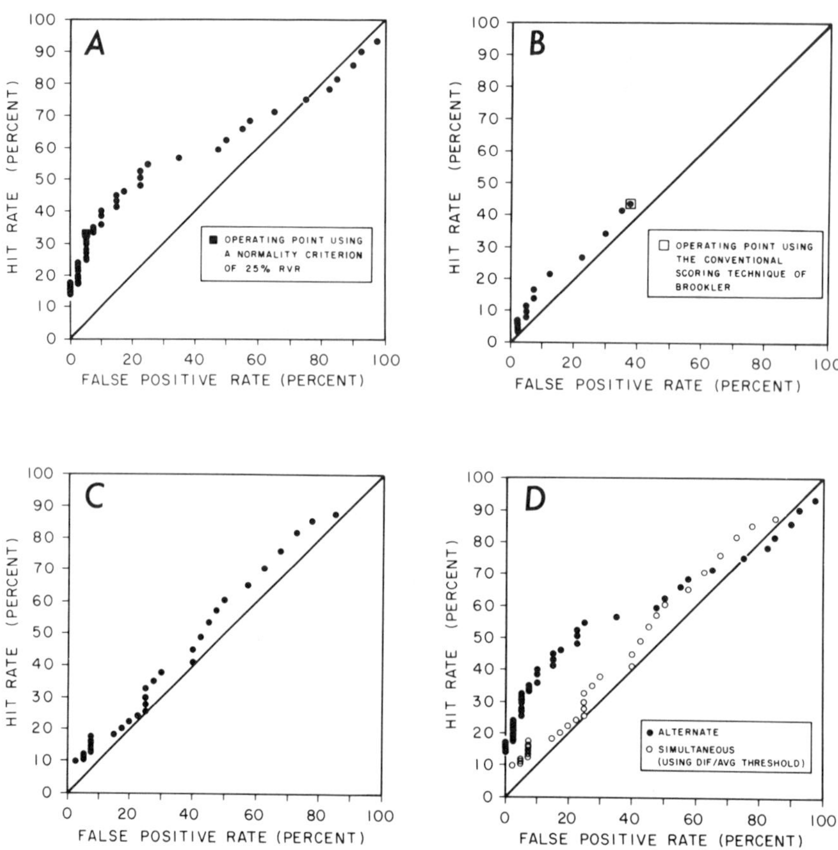

FIG 6–4.
Receiver-operater characteristics for caloric testing. Abscissa represents false positive rate based on evaluation of 40 healthy asymptomatic subjects. Ordinate represents hit rate, proportion of patients judged to have RVR. Each point on graph represents sensitivity-specificity pair. Data points toward the lower left corner represent the application of strict normality threshold criterion, while data points toward the upper right corner represent the application of lax normality threshold criterion. *Diagonal line,* ROC expected by chance alone. **A,** ROC for alternate testing for the determination of RVR; **B,** ROC for simultaneous testing for determination of RVR. Data points were generated by varying-threshold value for determination of type II responses. **C,** ROC for simultaneous testing for determination of RVR using difference between simultaneous cold and simultaneous warm responses. **D,** superimposition of ROCs for alternate and simultaneous testing (using difference method) for RVR.

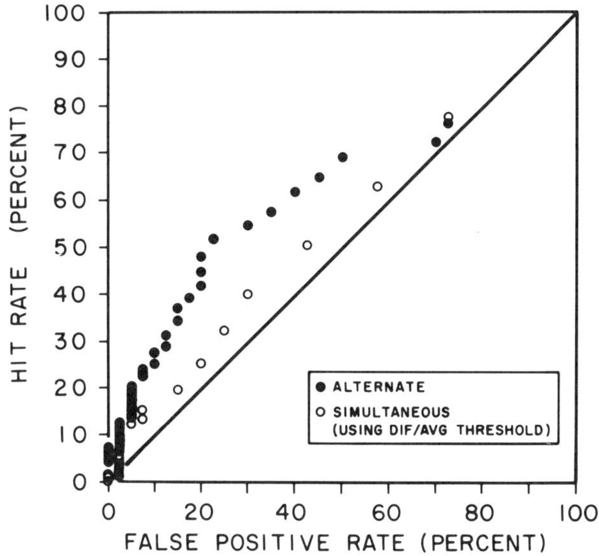

FIG 6–5.
Superimposition of ROCs for DP for alternate and simultaneous testing using a difference/average method. Ordinate and abscissa as in Figure 6–4.

guish our healthy population from our patient population. Moreover, if the threshold criterion for the alternate test is changed so that the alternate test has the same high sensitivity as the simultaneous test, the alternate test is still more specific.

Figure 6–6 shows the superimposition of the ROC for the alternate test and the ROC for the combination of results from alternate and simultaneous testing using the algorithm described in Methods. It is evident, using our algorithm, that there appears to be no change in the ability to distinguish our healthy from our patient population using the results from both tests as compared to using the result from the alternate test alone.

DISCUSSION

This study compared the results from simultaneous binaural bithermal and alternate binaural bithermal caloric testing of an unselected patient population. Our data indicate a poor agreement between the simultaneous and alternate tests. The reasons for such a

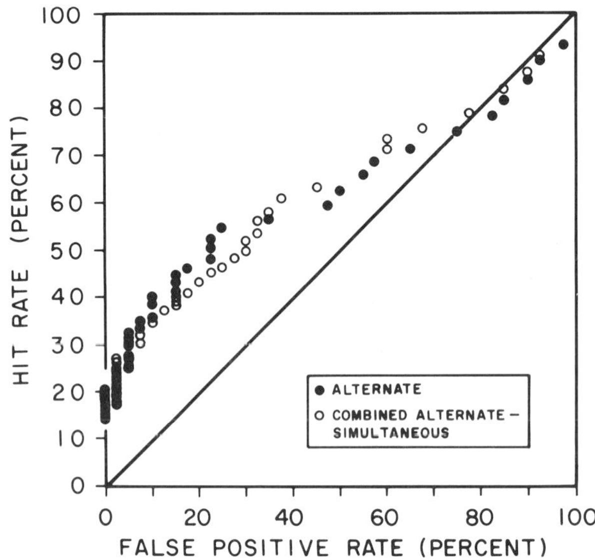

FIG 6–6.
Superimposition of ROCs for RVR for alternate testing and for the results of an algorithm which combines the results from simultaneous and alternate testing. Ordinate and abscissa as in Figure 6–4.

poor agreement may include the inherent variability of caloric testing due to variations in thermal conductivity of the temporal bone. Also, the simultaneous test is difficult to perform because both ears are irrigated at the same time. Further, the simultaneous caloric is a fundamentally different test than the alternate caloric. Where the alternate creates a difference in activity between the right and left horizontal ampullary nerves, the simultaneous excites or inhibits both the right and the left simultaneously. The effect of such simultaneous stimulation of the labyrinth and thus of the brainstem is not known, as no physiologic stimulus excites both ampullae simultaneously, and CNS recordings from animals are not available during simultaneous caloric testing. Thus, the relative influence of the vestibular periphery, the 8th nerve, the vestibular nuclei, and commissural pathways is not known. Although the results of simultaneous testing can be denoted as RVR (type II) and DP (type III), our data suggest that these categories may not be directly comparable to the RVR and DP as determined by alternate testing.

This study also compared the abilities of the simultaneous and the alternate caloric tests to distinguish between populations of healthy subjects and unselected patients. Because of the lack of a gold standard for any vestibular test, our study could compare the alternate and simultaneous tests only with regard to their ability to distinguish between our healthy population and our patient population, rather than assessing the ability of these tests to distinguish truly normal from truly abnormal persons. Using ROC analysis, the simultaneous test appears inferior to that of the alternate test in its ability to distinguish between our two populations. Also, there appeared to be no improvement when using an algorithm to combine the results from the two tests. Our algorithm is a simple and logical method; however, other algorithms for combining the simultaneous and alternate test results might yield a different conclusion. Our choice of an unselected patient population yields worst-case ROCs, thereby underestimating the ability of both the simultaneous and the alternate tests to distinguish healthy from patient populations.

Aside from their difference in ability to distinguish our healthy from our patient populations, the alternate and the simultaneous tests have several other differences: (1) The alternate test can identify both an RVR and a DP, while the simultaneous test can identify only an RVR or a DP. (2) The simultaneous test may give ambiguous results when the nystagmus response is of very low amplitude. In these cases, one interpreter might judge the response to be absent and another judge the response to be either right or left beating, thus changing the classification of response type. (3) If the time course of the thermal response of the two ears is different, nystagmus following simultaneous testing may be right beating at one time in the course of the response and left beating shortly thereafter, making response classification difficult. This was observed in 10% of normal subjects. (4) With alternate testing, there is the opportunity to repeat one or more of the irrigations if a discrepancy is noted between the response to a single irrigation and the response to the other irrigations. In our laboratory, approximately 20% of patients have at least one alternate irrigation repeated. With simultaneous testing, however, there is no opportunity for such a judgment to be made regarding repeated irrigation.

Prior to performing this study, our clinical impression was that the simultaneous test not infrequently identified a reduced vestibular response on the same side as that of the patient's complaints. Our data suggest that this impression may be an artifact because of the low specificity of the simultaneous test. Our data also suggest that if the threshold criteria for the alternate test were reduced to 19%, the alternate test would have the same high sensitivity as the simultaneous test (albeit with a higher specificity).

Acknowledgment

The authors wish to thank Vivian VanKirk for her assistance with data analysis.

REFERENCES

1. Brookler KH: Simultaneous bilateral bithermal caloric stimulations in electronystagmography. *Laryngoscope* 1971; 81:1014–1019.
2. Brookler KH: The simultaneous binaural bithermal: A caloric test utilizing electronystamography. *Laryngoscope* 1976; 86:1241–1250.
3. Hoffman RA, Brookler KH: The accuracy of the simultaneous binaural bithermal test in the diagnosis of acoustic neuroma. *Laryngoscope* 1979; 89:1046–1052.
4. Brookler KH: The use of the simultaneous binaural bithermal stimulus in neurootologic diagnosis, in Claussen CF, Kirtane MV (eds): *Optokinetic Tests*. Hamburg, Verlag, 1983, pp 160–166.
5. Metz CE: Basic principles of ROC analysis. *Semin Nucl Med* 1978; 8(4):283–298.
6. Metz CE: ROC methodology in radiologic imaging. *Invest Radiol* 1986; 21:720–733.
7. Mangham CA: Decision analysis of auditory brainstem responses and rotational vestibular tests in acoustic tumor diagnosis. *Otolaryngol Head Neck Surg* 1987; 96(1):22–29.
8. Turner RG, Frazer GJ, Shepard NT: Formulating and evaluating audiological test protocols. *Ear Hearing* 1984; 5(6):321–330.
9. Turner RG, Nielsen DW: Application of clinical decision analysis to audiological tests. *Ear Hearing* 1984; 5(3):125–133.
10. Turner RG, Shepard NT, Frazer GJ: Clinical performance of audiological and related diagnostic tests. *Ear Hearing* 1984; 5(4):187–194.
11. Baloh RW, Honrubia V: *Clinical Neurophysiology of the Vestibular System*. Philadelphia, FA Davis Co, 1979.
12. Barber HO, Stockwell CW: *Manual of Electronystagmography*. St Louis, CV Mosby Co, 1980.

7

Clinical Experience With a Short-Acting, Adjustable Caloric Stimulation*

Leonard R. Proctor, M.D.

Experimental studies have shown that the conventional caloric irrigation produces a labyrinthine stimulus that dissipates very slowly (Fig 7–1), with some degree of residual stimulation persisting for over 10 minutes.[1, 2] (Nystagmus stops after about two minutes because of a per-stimulatory adaptation.[2, 3]) Such a prolonged stimulation is objectionable, because patients often become uncomfortable and fatigued during the test session, and because a long waiting period is required between irrigations. Another problem is that the conventional method provides only one level of labyrinthine stimulation, which is often too strong and distressing in some patients but too weak for others. Kubo et al.[4] found that nearly half of 111 normal volunteers given conventional 40-sec irrigations complained of autonomic responses such as nausea and cold sweating.

Because of these difficulties clinical caloric testing is usually lim-

*United States patents have been obtained under the auspices of the National Institutes of Health to encourage commercial development: (1) U.S. Patent No. 4106493: Biphasic otoscopic air stimulator for performing clinical caloric tests, by L. R. Proctor and R. G. Byrnes; and (2) U.S. Patent No. 41064961: Method and apparatus for air caloric testing for the evaluation of aural vestibular disorders, by L. R. Proctor, R. C. Dix, and W. A. Metz.

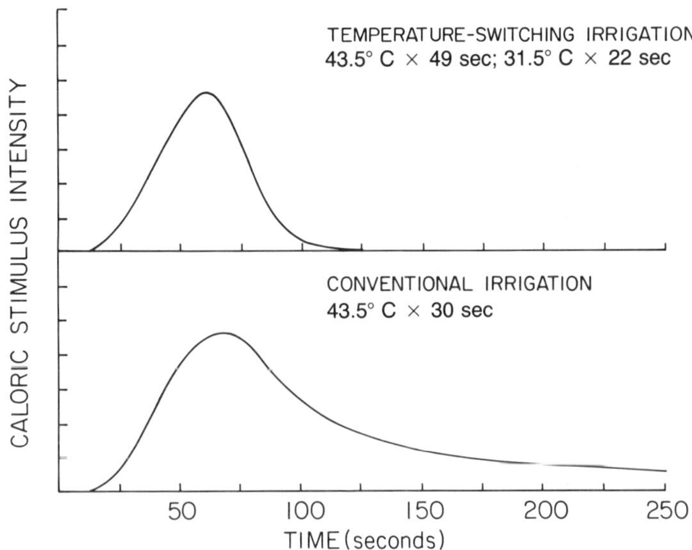

FIG 7–1.
Upper curve, time course of predicted caloric stimulus magnitude produced by temperature-switching aural irrigation (43.5° C × 49 sec; 30.5° C × 22 sec). **Lower curve,** time course of predicted caloric stimulus magnitude from conventional aural irrigation (43.5° C × 30 sec). Note that following conventional irrigation, a significant labyrinthine stimulus is still present beyond 250 sec.

ited to just four irrigations, even when responses are uncertain.[4–9] Further, the four irrigations cannot always be completed in patients who are experiencing nausea or other distress. Finally, there does not appear to be any useful purpose in maintaining thermal stimulation beyond the time when maximum nystagmus intensity is expected, since it has been shown that vestibular responsiveness is more precisely represented by the maximum slow-phase eye speed than by the duration of the nystagmus.[10]

The prolonged, often excessive stimulation of the conventional caloric test can be avoided through the use of a new irrigation technique that provides an easily adjustable, short-acting labyrinthine stimulus (Figs 7–1 and 7–2). In the new method, the temperature of a continuous aural irrigation is switched between hot and cold values at precisely specified times, based on a mathematical model of heat transmission in the labyrinth area.[11–15] Since the forces acting on the cupula-endolymph system are nearly proportional to the temperature difference across the semicircular canal, the magnitude of the caloric

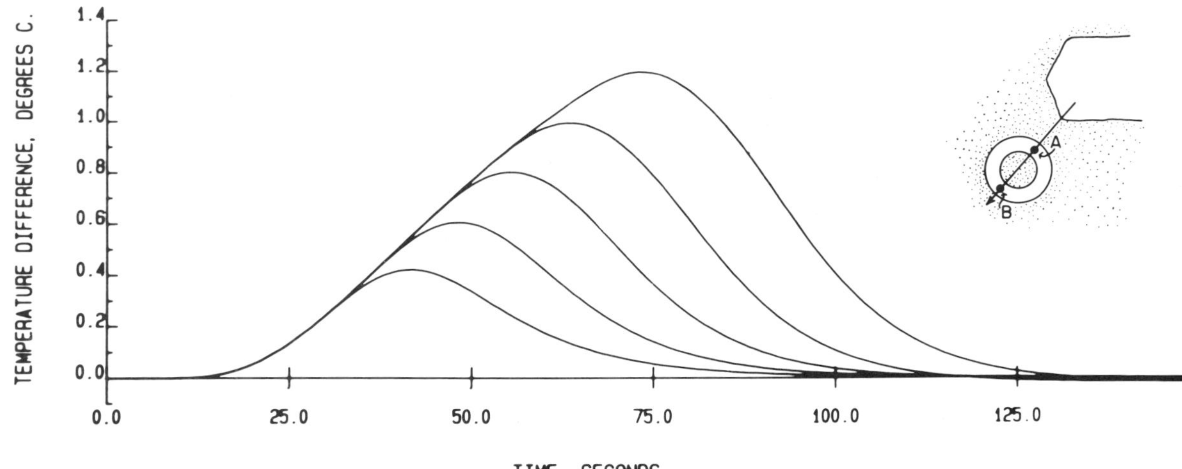

FIG 7–2.
Predicted temperature differences across the lateral semicircular canal *(A – B)* resulting from hot/cold water irrigations. Stimulus profiles shown are predicted from hot/cold pulses of 62/24, 49/22, 39/20, 29/17, and 21/14 sec (see Table 7–1). Similar stimulus profiles are produced by temperature-switching air irrigations using appropriate durations (see Figs 7–3 and 7–4).

stimulation is expressed as a (predicted) temperature difference in degrees centigrade. The temperature-switching caloric (TSC) method terminates the stimulus promptly and allows for convenient adjustment of the stimulus intensity through a range of predetermined values simply by changing the duration of irrigation pulses.

The relationship between the duration of various irrigation pulses and the resulting time profiles of caloric stimulations can be appreciated by comparing Table 7–1 and Figure 7–2. For example, Table 7–1 indicates that a water irrigation of 43.5°C for 49 sec, switched immediately to 30.5°C for 22 sec, will produce a peak temperature difference across the lateral semicircular canal of approximately 1.0°C. The time course of this stimulus is shown as the second highest curve in Figure 7–2 and the upper curve in Figure 7–1. The weakest stimulus that has been of practical use in our laboratory is 0.2°C.

Originally, a biphasic sinusoidal stimulus was employed.[8, 11–14] However, monophasic stimulations of the type shown in the upper curve of Figure 7–1 and in Figure 7–2 have been found to be more acceptable to patients and more practical for clinical testing.

The monophasic TSC method has been used to test over 6,000 patients at the Johns Hopkins Otological Vestibular Laboratory since January 1979 and has also been evaluated in several studies of normal subjects. The following is an overview of our clinical and experimental results.

TABLE 7–1.

Predicted Stimulation Levels (Peak Temperature Difference Across Lateral Semicircular Canal, °C) From Various Water Irrigations at 6.5°C Above or Below Body Temperature.*

Irrigation Duration (sec)		Predicted Stimulation Level†	
First Pulse	Second Pulse	Approximate	Actual
30	None*‡	1.0	1.06
62	24	1.2	1.19
49	22	1.0	.99
39	20	0.8	.80
29	17	0.6	.59
21	14	0.4	.39
13	10	0.2	.20

*Temperature-switching irrigation may be either hot/cold or cold/hot.
†Predicted from mathematical model.[11, 12]
‡Conventional test.

CLINICAL AND EXPERIMENTAL OBSERVATIONS

Our studies have shown that nystagmic responses rise to a peak and then fall promptly in close agreement with the time course and intensity of the predicted labyrinthine stimulus, both for the biphasic[8, 11–14] and monophasic[13, 15] stimulations. Because the stimulus is eliminated quickly, a waiting period of only 3 minutes is needed between the beginning of successive monophasic irrigations, instead of the 6–9 minutes recommended for the conventional method. Test results are comparable to the conventional caloric test and can be interpreted using standard formulas for right-left difference and directional preponderance.

Several studies were carried out using air as the irrigation fluid for the TSC instead of water. The combination of two air-water heat exchangers with electrically operated valves and timers[13, 16] provided the means for rapid switching of the air stream temperature between 51°C and 23°C at appropriate times. We found that appropriate irrigation pulse durations could still be calculated from the physical parameters determined by Young,[17] provided the heat transfer coefficient was reduced by 30%.[14] An example of the nystagmus response to a monophasic stimulus profile, using air irrigation (51°C × 58 sec/23°C × 45 sec) is shown in Figure 7–3. A plot of slow-phase eye speed averaged during successive 5-sec periods of this response is shown in Figure 7–4. The peak of the reaction occurred between 60 and 90 sec, and a moderate reversal of nystagmus began at 130 sec. Such a nystagmus reversal is observed commonly following either air or water TSC irrigations in both normal subjects and patients. The reversal nystagmus is sometimes intense and prolonged.

The reversal nystagmus is probably related to (1) the second irrigation pulse, which is intended to bring the labyrinthine stimulus back to 0,[15] and (2) adaptation effects that produce some degree of "secondary" nystagmus, even following conventional caloric irrigations.[3] We have not determined whether the reversal nystagmus associated with the new TSC irrigation method has any specific pathologic significance.

It has been reported by several authors that an incremental series of caloric stimulations may prove useful in clinical diagnosis of vestibular disorders.[19–22]. For example, Torok[20] found that some patients demonstrated a failure of caloric-induced nystagmus to increase appropriately in intensity with increased caloric stimulation. He termed

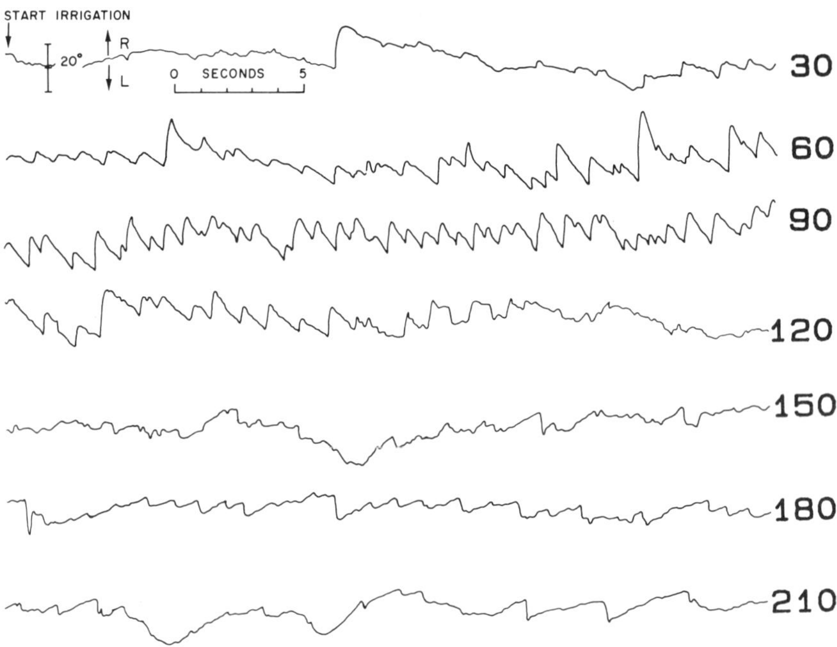

FIG 7–3.
Response of normal subject to monophasic air caloric test: 51° C × 58 sec/23° C × 45 sec. This irrigation sequence was predicted to produce a peak temperature difference across the lateral semicircular canal of 1.25° C at 82 sec. Numbers *(right margin)* are time in sec since onset of irrigation.

this "vestibular decruitment" and stated that this type of response profile was characteristic of central rather than peripheral vestibular disorders. To study this question, the growth of nystagmus intensity in response to incremental TSC caloric stimulations ("growth function" of the vestibulo-ocular reflex[22]) was measured in normal subjects[14, 22–25] and patients.[14, 22] Several studies indicated that small changes in TSC irrigation pulse durations produce consistent changes in the intensity of the induced labyrinthine stimulus.[14, 22–25] For example, the difference in average nystagmus response scores among 30 subjects tested at both 1.0°C and 0.8°C caloric stimulation levels was shown to be highly significant ($p<0.0001$).[25] (The mean scores were 22.66°/sec and 18.95°/sec, respectively.) However, some caution must be exercised when attempting to interpret the relative steepness or flatness of the growth function as an indication of vestibular system disorder: our analysis indicates that the slope of the growth function may be affected by variations in local anatomy and/or thermal diffu-

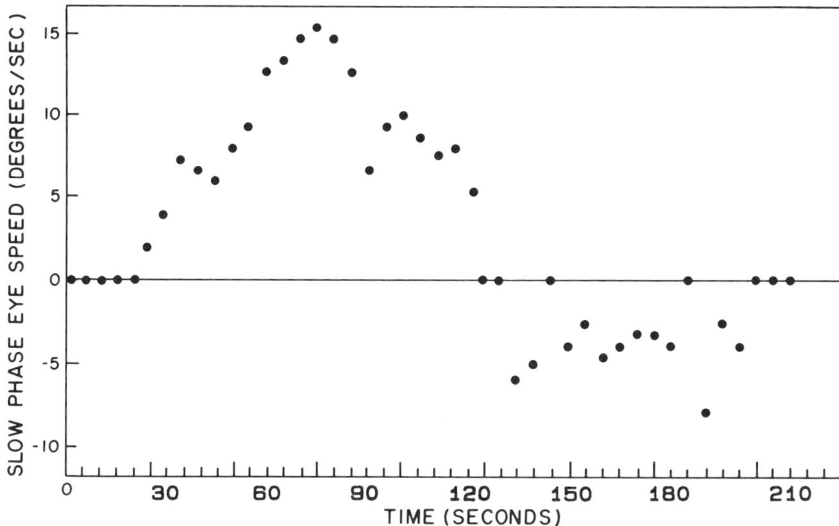

FIG 7–4.
Plot of average slow-phase eye speed during each 5 sec of response shown in Figure 7–3. Positive values indicate nystagmus fast phases directed toward the irrigated ear.

sivity in some cases.[23, 24] Further studies are needed to clarify this issue.

Despite the above reservations, we found interesting growth function patterns when patients were tested in this way.[14, 22] A careful study by Gursky[22] has shown that patients with central vestibular disorders exhibited growth functions that were significantly different from those observed in control subjects. Further, there were statistically significant differences in growth function scores between three categories of central lesion: (1) vestibular nerve only, (2) nerve and brain stem, (3) brain stem and cerebellum sparing the nerve.

Reference values for serial vestibular testing were determined by analyzing data from a study of 30 normal subjects who were participating in a study of aminoglycoside ototoxicity.[26] All subjects were tested on three successive days before drug administration was begun. Ten of the subjects, serving as controls, were tested on 11 subsequent occasions over a 7-week period. Intrasubject variability in test scores was significantly lower than that reported for conventional irrigations. Thus, individual TSC caloric test scores generally did not exceed a range of 55%–170% of their initial value, and there was very little evidence of vestibular habituation, either during the 3-day period (N = 30) or during the 7-week period (N = 10) of observation. For this group of 30 healthy young adult males, the "normal limits" of a drop in caloric test scores were determined to be 40% for individual scores (hot right or left; cold right or left) and 30% for averaged scores (hot plus cold). The upper normal limits of test-retest variation in scores for right-left difference and directional preponderance of caloric responses were 24% and 22%, respectively.

Clinical experience with the TSC test was described from a statistical analysis of anamnestic and diagnostic results in 100 consecutive patients.[18] The TSC procedure was well tolerated. Even though a number of patients were already dizzy or nauseated before the caloric irrigations were begun, a full set of four basic stimulations was completed in all but one patient. In 43 of the patients, additional tests beyond the four basic caloric irrigations were found to be useful, because the extra tests ensured a more reliable assessment of vestibular function. A review of our records since January 1979 indicates that only about one patient in 1,000 has experienced emesis as a result of TSC testing.

DISCUSSION

Similar favorable results with the TSC test have been described by Norre[27] in a study of 60 normal subjects and 90 patients. This author reported that the TSC method required a much shorter examination time, was more comfortable for patients, and provided a greater sensitivity than the conventional method.

As explained above, the TSC irrigation method produces a labyrinthine stimulus that is both of shortened duration and also conveniently adjustable through a range of preselected intensities. This provides the clinician with important options: for patients who are feeling anxious or distressed, or where a sensitivity to vestibular stimulation is expected, a weak stimulus can be chosen to begin the test session. If results are uncertain, the test can be repeated, perhaps with a stronger stimulus, without waiting an inordinate time. Either air or water can be used to apply the TSC irrigation. Test results are interpreted using standard formulas for right-left difference and directional preponderance.

Our investigations have demonstrated that the time course and intensity of the nystagmus response conform to the predicted TSC stimulus profile. A prominent secondary nystagmus often appears following the primary TSC reaction in both patients and normal subjects. Further studies are needed to determine the clinical implications of this phenomenon.

Small adjustments in irrigation pulse durations have been shown to produce the intended changes in the intensity of the nystagmus response. A series of incremental TSC irrigations, used to test the vestibulo-ocular growth function, have proved practical and well tolerated by patients and have demonstrated clinically useful results.

Serial TSC testing of normal subjects has demonstrated a lower degree of intrasubject variability and less "habituation" than is associated with conventional irrigations. The new method is well tolerated by patients and unpleasant reactions are rare, even though additional tests beyond the basic four are often employed.

Our experimental studies and clinical experience with the TSC test have indicated that this method is more acceptable to patients, easier to administer, and more comprehensive and reliable than the conventional method of caloric testing.

REFERENCES

1. Kleinfeldt D, Dahl D: Temperaturemessungen am menschlichen Bogengang nach thermisher Reizung. *Acta Otolaryngol (Stockh)* 1969; 61:411–419.
2. Hood JD: Persistence of response in the caloric test. *Aerospace Med* 1973; 44:444–449.
3. Barnes GR, Benson AJ: Adaptation in the caloric response, in Hood JD (ed): *Vestibular Mechanisms in Health and Disease: VI. Extraordinary Meeting of the Barany Society.* New York, Academic Press, 1978, pp 254–262.
4. Kubo T, Ohira S, Shiraishi I, et al: Comparative study of caloric responses induced by different stimulus intensities. *Acta Otolaryngol (Stockh)[suppl]* 1983; 393:65–71.
5. Stahle J, Sahl R: Electronystagmography in Meniere's disease before, during, and after ultrasonic irradiation. *Acta Otolaryngol (Stockh)[suppl]* 1964; 92:154–166.
6. Tuohimaa P: Vestibular disturbance after acute mild head injury. *Acta Otolaryngol (Stockh)[suppl]* 1978: 359:13–52.
7. Norre ME: Some critical remarks on the interpretation of vestibular test results. *Adv Otorhinolaryngol* 1979; 25:149–155.
8. Proctor LR, Walters GJ, Glackin RN: The stimulus controlled caloric test: A reliability study. *Am J Otolaryngol* 1979; 1:39–45.
9. Mizukoshi K, Watanabe, Y, Watanabe, I, et al: Subjective and objective evaluation of medical treatment for Meniere's disease with special reference to the dose response for adenosine triphosphate. *Adv Otorhinolaryngol* 1983; 30:355–361.
10. Henriksson NG: Speed of the slow component and duration in caloric nystagmus. *Acta Otolaryngol (Stockh)[suppl]* 1956; 125:1–29.

11. Proctor LR, Dix RC, Hughes D, et al: Stimulation of the vestibular receptor by means of step temperature changes during continuous aural irrigation. *Acta Otolaryngol (Stockh)* 1975; 79:425–435.
12. Proctor LR, Dix RC: New approach to the thermal stimulation of vestibular receptor. *Ann Otol Rhinol Laryngol* 1975; 84:425–435.
13. Proctor LR, Dix RC, Metz WA: A method for adjusting the stimulus intensity of the air caloric test: Preliminary report. *Trans Am Acad Ophthalmol Otolaryngol* 1976; 82:210–222.
14. Fleming PM, Proctor LR, Dix RC: Results of new air caloric testing method among normal subjects: I. Biphasic testing. *Ann Otol Rhinol Laryngol* 1978; 87:248–256.
15. Proctor LR, Fleming PM, Little RJA: Results of new air caloric testing method among normal subjects: II. Monophasic testing. *Acta Otolaryngol (Stockh)* 1977; 84:178–186.
16. Proctor LR, Metz WA, Dix RC: Construction of a practical and inexpensive air stimulator for caloric vestibular testing. *Laryngoscope* 1976; 86:126–131.
17. Young JH: *Analysis of Vestibular System Responses to Thermal Gradients Induced in the Temporal Bone.* Thesis, Ann Arbor, University of Michigan, 1972.
18. Proctor LR: Clinical experience with a short-acting caloric test. *Laryngoscope* 1985; 95:75–80.
19. Litton WB, McCabe BF: Neural vs. sensory lesion: Vestibular signs. *Laryngoscope* 1966; 76:1113–1127.
20. Torok N: A new parameter of vestibular sensitivity. *Ann Otol Rhinol Laryngol* 1970; 79:808–817.
21. Ghosh P, Kacker SK: Vestibular recruitment and decruitment. *Acta Otolaryngol (Stockh)* 1979; 88:227–234.
22. Gursky EA: *The Growth Function of the Vestibular Ocular Reflex (VOR) in Central Vestibular Disease.* Thesis, Baltimore, Johns Hopkins University, 1985.
23. Frazer RK, Proctor LR, Glackin RN: Refinement of the caloric vestibular test. *JHU/APL Biomedical Research, Development and Engineering.* MQR/82–3, section 14. Baltimore, The Johns Hopkins University, September 1982.
24. Proctor LR, Frazer RK, Glackin RN, et al: "Recruitment/decruitment" of caloric responses: Effect of anatomical variables. *Adv Otolaryngol* 1983; 30:150–155.
25. Proctor LR, Glackin RN: Factors contributing to variability of caloric test scores. *Acta Otolaryngol (Stockh)* 1985; 100:161–171.
26. Proctor LR, Glackin RN, Shimizu H, et al: Reference values for serial vestibular testing. *Ann Otol Rhinol Laryngol* 1986; 95:83–90.
27. Norre ME: The unilateral vestibular hypofunction. *Acta Otorhinolaryngol Belg* 1978; 32(5):510–516.

8

Rotational Testing of the Horizontal Vestibulo-ocular Reflex

James E. Olsson, M.D.

For many years otolaryngologists have experienced frustration in the diagnosis and management of vestibular disorders. This is in part because patients have a great deal of difficulty in accurately describing their symptoms. Secondly, patients may have significant vestibular pathology and yet have no findings on the physical examination. Thirdly, the vestibular mechanism cannot be directly tested. The otolaryngologist has been forced to rely on stimulation techniques such as caloric irrigation of the ears and eye movement analysis. Both are often imprecise.

Motivated by the desire of investigators to improve diagnostic and management abilities of the otolaryngologist and neurologist, several studies recently used computers to analyze eye movements in an attempt to augment the utility of specific test results. These studies are actually based on a continuum of investigations by a small group of vestibular scientists over the past 80–100 years. The purpose of this chapter is threefold: (1) to define some of the systems engineering terms used in describing the output measures in present vestibular testing; (2) to review briefly some highlights of vestibular research that are relative to current computerized rotational testing; and (3) to summarize some of the current clinical uses of rotational testing.

DEFINITIONS

To understand the literature published on current rotational testing, familiarity with various systems engineering terms commonly used in the description of eye movements is necessary. Terms such as *phase, gain, spectral purity, cross correlation,* and *coherence* are used as output measures because they accurately describe eye movements when analyzed with systems engineering techniques by computers.

Gain.—Gain is the ratio of the amplitude of the output to the amplitude of the input. For example, in smooth pursuit tracking tests, the gain would be the ratio of the amplitude of eye movement excursion to target excursion. In rotation testing, the gain would be the ratio of the total amplitude of the eye movement excursion to the total chair rotation excursion. Gain does not take into account timing of these movements. Symmetry measures compare the gain to the left with gain to the right. Symmetry may be measured in terms of total slow-phase gains or peak slow phase gains.

Phase.—Phase describes the temporal (timing) relationship between the input and output. If there is proper timing of the compensatory eye movement to the chair rotation in a rotation test, the eye movement will be 180° out of phase with head movement, or by convention, will be said to have *zero phase lead.*

Spectral Purity.—Spectral purity relates the frequency content of the input to the output. In a pendular tracking test in which input is a single sinusoidal frequency, the output consists mainly of eye movements at the stimulus frequency but also contains other frequencies generated by system imperfections. These imperfections may consist of measurement system noise, normally occurring vestibular-oculomotor system imperfections, or pathologically induced disturbances. A spectral purity of .95 indicates that 95% of the response is at the input frequency.

Coherence Function.—The coherence function measures the extent to which the output is caused by the input. If the system under study is linear and noise-free, the coherence function will be one (1). A coherence of less than 1 indicates that the system is corrupted by noise or is nonlinear.

Power Spectral Analysis.—Power spectral analysis is a mathematical method by which a complex signal is broken into its component frequencies. This analysis permits the accurate computation of eye movement output measures such as phase, gain, and spectral purity. Due to the extremely complex nature of the calculations, power spectral analysis was not practical until the advent of low-cost minicomputers.

Cross Correlation.—Cross correlation is a mathematical method which relates the general dependence of two sets of data. This method helps define the timing relationships between the input to the vestibular-oculomotor system and the eye movement output.

HISTORY

Although several investigators studied the vestibular system in the 1800s, Dodge[1] in 1903 was the first to categorize systematically eye movements. He divided horizontal eye movements into five types:

Type I—rapid movement of the eye toward an object of interest which is eccentric on the retina; Type II—pursuit movement; Type III—coordinate compensatory eye movement; Type IV—dash reactive compensatory movement; Type V—convergence or divergence. To provide more precise information about vestibular and oculomotor disorders, scientists today continue to study all types of eye movements, either in their original description or in combinations and modifications thereof.

In rotational testing, type IV movements are studied. These reactive compensatory movements occur when a patient is rotated with the eyes closed in the light or with the eyes opened in the dark. A compensatory nystagmus is generated with the fast phase in the direction of the acceleration.

Throughout the years investigators labored to provide better instrumentation and more accurate measurement and description of these compensatory eye movements. In 1951 Wendt[2] reviewed previous investigations and noted that the total slow-phase nystagmus response during a 2-second rotation through 65° with eyes closed was approximately 60% of the input. This was the first attempt at quantifying the gain.

In 1963 Cramer,[3] while working at the School of Aerospace Medicine, published a paper examining the phase and sensitivity (gain) of cat eye movement responses to rotation. He noted that above 0.1 Hz the vestibular-oculomotor system operates like an integrating accelerometer. Eye velocity is thus 180° out of phase with head velocity. Although his experiment required laborious hand computation of complex mathematical functions, this study introduced systems engineering techniques to the field of vestibular research.

Melvill Jones and Milsum[4] furthered this approach in 1965 when they examined the physiologic systems which allow the stabilization of images on the retina from the viewpoint of systems engineering. They summarized several experiments and utilized the known anatomical and physiologic facts to predict theoretically the output functions of the oculomotor system, particularly smooth pursuit and the VOR. They noted that the mathematical model of the semicircular canals worked out by van Egmond et al.[5] predicted a constant gain and 0 phase lead over a frequency range of 0.1–5 Hz. They also summarized the results of smooth pursuit experiments, demonstrating the gain and phase leads obtained from models and from experiments on humans.

Niven et al.[6] published the first study of the phase relationships in humans as a result of rotational stimuli. They used low-frequency sinusoidal stimuli at 0.02, 0.03, 0.05, 0.07, 0.10, 0.15, and 0.2 Hz to demonstrate the low-frequency phase characteristics of the human VOR in six subjects.

Because the method of eye movement analysis in all of these experiments was accomplished by hand, such analysis was impractical for clinical use. Nevertheless, as techniques improved for analysis of eye movements, these studies provided a firm theoretical ground work for later investigators.

Of particular importance was the development of techniques to stimulate precisely the semicircular canals. In the 1970s two major advances in instrumentation were accomplished. First, precision dc torque motors became available and permitted more accurate control of rotational stimuli. For the first time it was possible to quantify accurately the stimulus to the semicircular canals. Second, minicomputers had come into common use at more reasonable prices. This permitted investigators to apply systems engineering methods practically, quickly, and more precisely to analyze vestibular-oculomotor responses. These advances led to a host of studies which quantify the VOR as well as smooth pursuit and saccadic eye movements in both normal subjects and patients with vestibular disorders.

RECENT STUDIES

Studies appearing in the literature over the past 15 years related to the vestibular-oculomotor system can generally be grouped into three broad areas. Most have been concerned with rotatory stimuli of the semicircular canals and the resultant eye movement responses. In some studies the rotational stimuli were modified by simultaneously influencing eye movements with visual stimuli. A smaller group of studies examined the smooth pursuit system, attempting to quantify the integrity of the oculomotor system and determine how vestibular disorders are affected by this system. Fewer studies have evaluated the saccadic eye movements.

This chapter reviews the highlights of studies examining the reactive compensatory eye movement responses to rotational stimuli of the horizontal canals. Rotational tests are of major interest because they appear to have several advantages over previous tests. The input to the semicircular canals can be precisely quantified, whereas that from caloric stimulation or positioning tests cannot. However, many types of stimuli may be used, and the best overall type has not yet been definitely identified. The simplest type is sinusoidal (harmonic), but the sum of sinusoids, pseudorandum stimuli, acceleration ramps, and impulse acceleration have also been investigated. The sum of sinusoids is simply several sinusoids added together and used as a stimulus. The pseudorandum stimulus contains a large number of frequency components, usually more than 100. As the number of frequency components simultaneously used as a stimulus increases, however, the amount of power at any given individual frequency decreases; this appears to be important in clinical testing.

The other major parameter to be determined in the stimulus to the canals is the frequency or range of frequencies used. As noted above, it appeared as though the human vestibular-oculomotor system adequately compensates for rotational stimulation at frequencies between approximately 0.1 Hz and 5 Hz. Above 5 Hz, loss of appropriate compensation appears to originate probably from major nonlinearities in the oculomotor system. Most laboratories have selected the low frequencies for stimulation, but higher frequencies have also been examined.

In the middle of the 1970s Wolfe and Kos[7, 9] reported a series of experiments designed to determine whether eye movement responses to acceleration could be used to detect asymmetries in the vestibular system following unilateral labyrinthectomy. Rhesus monkeys were tested using sinusoidal acceleration at 0.04, 0.08, and 1.2 Hz. The monkeys then underwent labyrinthectomy and were later retested. Nystagmic eye movements were recorded with implantable EOG electrodes. Analog and digital techniques were used to measure slow- and fast-phase velocities, amplitudes, and frequencies.

At 13 months postoperatively there was an asymmetry in the slow-phase velocity and amplitude of the response. In addition, there was a longer delay in the reversal of the nystagmus on reversal of the chair movement (e.g., a change in the phase relationships). In later experience the authors used two lower frequencies (0.01 and 0.02 Hz), because 0.04 Hz appeared to demonstrate best the asymmetries after unilateral labyrinthectomy. Analog techniques were developed[9] to measure phase relationships between the rotational stimuli and the slow-phase eye movement responses. These studies demonstrated a gradual diminution postoperatively in the peak slow-phase velocity asymmetry and in the total velocity asymmetry. In addition, the change of the phase relationships was noted to be constant and reliable, particularly at the lower frequencies (0.01, 0.02, and 0.04 Hz).

In 1977 this laboratory began testing normal subjects and patients with vestibular disorders. Based on animal work, discrete, low-frequency stimulations at 0.01, 0.02, 0.04, 0.08, and 0.16 Hz were selected, with a peak velocity of 50°/sec at each frequency.[9–17] These frequencies were chosen on the assumptions that a broad range of low frequencies would be tested and that the lower frequencies would show asymmetries in humans after unilateral vestibular lesions, as they had in monkeys. The output measures included phase, spectral purity, symmetry and gain. Gain appeared to be the most variable, being highly dependent on the mental status of the patient, on calibration errors, as well as on any medications recently ingested by the patient. Phase, however, appeared to be highly repeatable, being less subject to mental changes as long as subject arousal was maintained above threshold. Symmetry was determined by separately integrating the entire slow-phase output to the left and to the right, dividing the left minus the right difference by the total output, and expressing the ratio as a percentage at each frequency. The symmetry was termed "labyrinthine" or "directional preponderance." The phase, spectral purity, gain, and symmetry were then printed in table form (Tables 8–1 and 8–2). This allowed the spectral purity to be examined by the clinician to ensure that the test was valid. If the spectral purity was below 0.8, concern was raised as to whether the patient had a central lesion preventing proper processing of the stimulus or there was an error in testing.

TABLE 8–1.
Harmonic Acceleration Data Analysis Output—LT Neuroma Preoperative*

SKR	Spectral Purity	HD Odd	HD Even	Noise
Frequency 0.01 Hz				
Stimulus	1.00000	0.00000	0.00000	0.00000
Response	0.96715	0.01510	0.00362	0.01412
Gain 0.46409	Phase 43.875		LP 5.03	
Frequency 0.02 Hz				
Stimulus	1.00000	0.00000	0.00000	0.00000
Response	0.97663	0.00990	0.00088	0.01258
Gain 0.61930	Phase 28.414		LP 7.23	
Frequency 0.04 Hz				
Stimulus	0.99999	0.00000	0.00000	0.00000
Response	0.97223	0.00630	0.00767	0.01381
Gain 0.60454	Phase 18.907		LP 13.33	
Frequency 0.08 Hz				
Stimulus	0.99999	0.00000	0.00000	0.00000
Response	0.97318	0.00308	0.00612	0.01762
Gain 0.69426	Phase 14.134		LP 6.90	
Frequency 0.16 Hz				
Stimulus	0.99999	0.00000	0.00000	0.00000
Response	0.96733	0.00223	0.00207	0.02837
Gain 0.62820	Phase 5.183		LP 2.09	

*Computer printout of preoperative acceleration data from a 38-year-old man with a 2.0-cm left acoustic neuroma. HD, harmonic distortion, LP, labyrinthine preponderance (0 = perfect symmetry, minus = right, plus = left). These results are normal.

Two groups of well-defined patients were selected. The first group was composed of those with acoustic neuromas. These were selected because the site of the lesion was examined surgically; it was a known lesion in a known place. The other group was made up of those with classic Meniere's disease. These were selected to see whether the test would be of use in diagnosing a relatively unknown lesion.

In 1981 Olsson et al.[14] published the results of examinations of 24 patients with acoustic neuromas. When used for diagnosis, the harmonic acceleration test identified 67%, whereas caloric examination identified 79% of the patients with tumors. Together the two tests identified 91% of the patients with tumors. All patients immediately postoperatively had a significant shift in the phase measurement, which remained stable up to 3 years after surgery. Also, an asymmetry (directional preponderance) acutely developed. The labyrinthine preponderance returned toward normal values but did not (as a group)

TABLE 8–2.
Harmonic Acceleration Data Analysis Output—LT Neuroma Postoperative*

SKR	Spectral Purity	HD Odd	HD Even	Noise
Frequency 0.01 Hz				
Stimulus	0.99999	0.00000	0.00000	0.00000
Response	0.76781	0.02976	0.02417	0.17826
Gain 0.21842	Phase 70.889		LP −96.00	
Frequency 0.02 Hz				
Stimulus	0.99999	0.00000	0.00000	0.00001
Response	0.89561	0.00619	0.03821	0.05998
Gain 0.36207	Phase 48.295		LP −93.02	
Frequency 0.04 Hz				
Stimulus	0.99999	0.00000	0.00000	0.00001
Response	0.83544	0.01082	0.03532	0.11842
Gain 0.34621	Phase 34.525		LP −86.91	
Frequency 0.08 Hz				
Stimulus	0.99999	0.00000	0.00000	0.00000
Response	0.88909	0.01165	0.03134	0.06792
Gain 0.55280	Phase 24.325		LP −79.78	
Frequency 0.16 Hz				
Stimulus	0.99999	0.00000	0.00000	0.00001
Response	0.58283	0.02354	0.05408	0.33955
Gain 0.33238	Phase 10.721		LP −68.30	

*Computer printout of 7-day postoperative acceleration data from patient in Table 8–1. There is a large phase decrement (increased phase lead) and marked asymmetry (LP) to the right. The spectral purity is down somewhat, as is the gain.

regain complete symmetry. Jenkins et al.[18, 19] confirmed the phase lead advance at low frequencies as well as the change in directional preponderance. In addition, they noted that at 0.2 Hz the phase tended to return to normal. This was confirmed later by Olsson[19] and Wolfe[17] at 0.16 Hz. Jenkins also demonstrated that the gain increases were slower in compensation than the asymmetry. He thought that utilizing asymmetry to help determine the site of a lesion, particularly in a partially compensated state such as an acoustic neuroma, was not particularly useful, because many do not fall outside of the statistical range of normal. However, Moretz et al.[20] noted that in 100% of 18 patients the vestibular evaluation with harmonic acceleration was abnormal. They pointed out that the test had great sensitivity and thus was of use.

It appears that in lesions such as acoustic neuromas the harmonic acceleration testing is useful in following up patients because of gain and asymmetry measures which tend to return to normal as the patient's dizziness improves. There is more debate as to whether it is a useful screening test for these types of lesions.

The group of investigators working at UCLA have published an impressive series of papers on vestibular-oculomotor testing over the past decade.[21–34] While many of their papers are studies of the oculomotor system or responses to multiple stimuli and are beyond the scope of this chapter, the above-cited studies apply to rotational tests.

The UCLA group used single-frequency rotational testing protocols in most of their early studies. They tested patients at 0.5 Hz with different maximum velocities[21–24] and analyzed the gain of these responses, plotting the slow-component velocity. They noted that the gain of the VOR is highly variable. They also noted that the VOR does not influence the optokinetic nystagmus, even in patients with complete unilateral labyrinthine paralysis over a long time. In one study[24] the gain measures identified 10 of 25 patients with significant unilateral labyrinthine weaknesses. The authors noted that the coefficient of variation of rotation measures was smaller than that of caloric testing. They thought that rotational testing was a more precise measure of peripheral disease than caloric examination. In addition, they thought that rotational testing was better than caloric evaluation of patients with bilateral labyrinthine disease and central disease because visual-vestibular interactions could be accurately assessed. In 1980 the group published a method for measurement of the phase, dc bias, magnitude of the fundamental response, and first two harmonics, as well as the slow-component velocity and gain.[25] In 1981, they began to test patients at multiple frequencies (0.0125, 0.025, 0.05, and 0.1 Hz).[26] By 1982 they had added 0.2 Hz.[27, 28] Again, in these tests they noted that the gain rarely identified an individual patient as different from the normal population. The phase measures were noted to be more consistent discriminators than the gain when compared to the normal population. The authors also noted that in patients followed up over time who had acute lesions, the return of symmetry was apparent.

The UCLA group observed that while the results are consistent and patterns are seen, they are also relatively nonspecific. The phase shifts occur in response to both unilateral and bilateral disease as well as to central and peripheral disease, making rotational testing a poor discriminator of location of disease.

The second large group of patients selected by the School of Aerospace Medicine investigators consisted of patients with classic Meniere's disease. They were selected because investigators thought that conventional ENG tests revealed their greatest shortcomings in testing these patients. In the early studies on patients with Meniere's disease,[12] a significant number had decrements in their phase relationships at the lower stimulus frequencies. At 0.16 Hz they almost invariably had normal phase relationships. In addition, they often had significant asymmetry, particularly at the two lower frequencies. In further studies on this group of patients,[13] the responses to harmonic acceleration were compared with the subjective symptoms. The above findings were confirmed. In addition, those patients who had markedly asymmetric responses were more likely to have classic attacks, particularly if directional preponderance was toward the diseased ear. There have been relatively few other studies on patients with Meniere's disease.

To date my experience confirms the above findings. The only use for rotational testing in patients with Meniere's disease is to see whether they are markedly asymmetric. If so, they tend to be much more asymptomatic than if not. The test is thus a monitoring device but not particularly useful in predicting the patient's course over the long term. Further, the original belief that rotational testing might be helpful in selecting patients for endolymphatic surgery has not held up statistically[37] as larger numbers of patients have been investigated. It is, however, remarkably useful for monitoring patients with Meniere's disease after nerve section. This will be illustrated by case reports.

There has been some concern that patients may habituate to low-frequency rotational testing. Barr et al.[38] demonstrated that patients could voluntarily manipulate gain according to the instructions they were given when rotated in the dark with eyes open. Olsson et al.[14] examined this in patients who had a stable vestibular lesion and noted that they indeed could manipulate the gain but that the phase and asymmetry measure (directional preponderance) was not changed by patients (although at times patients could suppress the nystagmus to a degree precluding measurement).[14] Baloh et al.[30] in 1982 examined this question in detail. They noted that if subjects were rotated for one half hour, they found a phase advance and a decreasing gain. However, when the subjects were rotated for the amount of time it takes to run current protocols, there was no habituation.

Of more concern is the fact that Baloh et al.[34] as well as the group at the School of Aerospace Medicine found that the phase advance is a nonspecific response occurring in virtually all lesions of the vestibular system, thus giving no information regarding the etiology or whether the lesion is peripheral or central. It does, however, provide some information as to the severity of the lesion.

Rubin[39] used the low-frequency harmonic testing in numerous patients with industrial accidents and metabolic disease. He thinks that it is very useful as a screening test in difficult cases of metabolic etiology or work injury.

Staller et al.[40] and Cyr et al.[41] investigated the use of low-frequency rotational testing in the pediatric population. Cyr and his group examined patients from age 3 months to 6 years. They demonstrated no age-related differences in gain, phase, or asymmetry at the 0.08-Hz screening frequency. They studied 21 patients who were postmeningitic. They noted again a decrease in the gain and a phase advance as well as an increased asymmetry in these patients. Staller and his group examined 101 otologically normal infants and children; 96 were successfully tested. A maturational trend was determined in subjects up to 10 months of age when measuring the presence of nystagmus, and there was a maturational change in phase-lag measurements up to approximately 4 years of age. The authors concluded that this test can be used in a high number of infants and young children. They provide normative data in this regard.

The following summarizes the advantages and disadvantages of low-frequency harmonic acceleration testing gleaned from the literature. The advantages are: (1) A precise stimulus may be applied to the semicircular canals with adequate energy at each frequency to provide responses with high spectral purity in the evaluation of patients. (2) Patients accept repeated rotation testing better than they do repeated caloric testing. (3) Rotational testing's major use is in the monitoring of known disease processes. (4) Harmonic testing has a limited but definite use in the diagnosis of vestibular disorders.

The disadvantages appear to be: (1) The current cost of equipment is high. (2) As now routinely done, the testing is relatively time consuming. (3) Rotational testing does not appear to replace caloric examination or other tests from the ENG battery. (4) Many changes that occur with vestibular lesions can cause the same nonspecific responses when examined by acceleration testing.

To attempt to overcome some of the disadvantages, a group of investigators at the University of Pittsburgh used pseudorandum binary sequence (PRBS) rotational stimuli as a possible clinical method.[42–45] This approach used a "white noise" signal which was equivalent to mixing 255 stimulus frequencies spread over a two-decade frequency range from 0.02 Hz to 1.67 Hz. Furman et al.[46] found that the phase and gain measures using these similar stimuli were the same in the alert rhesus monkeys as the responses from discrete sinusoidal stimulation. Their results tended to confirm the results found with the discrete frequency test.[20] Authors concluded that the advantages of this protocol were as follows: (1) It could be run in 7 minutes. (2) Many frequency points along with a statistical estimate of their reliability could be computed. (3) All frequency points were obtained under similar testing conditions, since they were run simultaneously. (4) Low-amplitude acceleration inputs could be used, reducing motion sickness. (5) Subjects could not anticipate or predict stimulus direction. A disadvantage, however, was that the asymmetry measure is an estimate average of the test span, which provides only one numerical evaluation. In contrast, harmonic techniques using discrete frequency stimulation gives several symmetry measures.

High-frequency rotation has been used over a long time in two laboratories. In 1979 and 1980 Schwarz and Tomlinson[47] and Tomlinson et al.[48] reported their experience with high-frequency stimulation. They thought the high-frequency stimulation would eliminate the problem of gain variability which was seen at low frequencies due to the voluntary manipulation by the patient and the susceptibility to visual stimulation. They observed that the gain is close to unity above 0.1 Hz and remains so with rotation up to around 6 Hz.[47] They then thought that testing this in patients might show changes in the gain depending on the pathology. In 1982 Hyden et al.,[49] working in the same laboratory, published a study in which they used passive rotation with both high-frequency PRBS and sinusoidal stimulation of the canals utilizing power spectral analysis to calculate gain phase and coherence functions. This showed the gain increased above unity at frequencies greater than 3 Hz. They also demonstrated that the results could be obtained when the patient had his eyes opened and attempted to fix on the earth-fixed visual background. This indicated that the peripheral vision was unable to suppress the VOR at these frequencies. They were, therefore, able to test the patient in the light with eyes open.

In 1984 a group in Linkoping, Sweden,[50] continued to use a similar technique of high-frequency stimulation. Using a computerized hydraulically driven chair which was oscillated horizontally, they tested the patients in the 0.5–4.5-Hz frequency domain. They demonstrated that patients with vestibular loss had normal gains at low-frequency sinusoidal oscillation below 1 Hz; at higher frequencies there were clearly subnormal values. In those patients with bilateral peripheral loss, gain values were low over the entire frequency region when randomized swings were used. Rotational testing appeared better than caloric testing in their series, because it correlated more successfully with the symptoms. They concluded that the caloric test may be sufficient in most cases to determine VOR function, but when there is a suspected bilateral lesion, it is too insensitive and provides no comparison with the healthy side. The rotation testing appeared to evaluate the VOR in these cases in a more precise way.

In 1986 this Swedish group used the above techniques to evaluate volunteers before, during, and after trichloroethylene exposure. The investigators used the oscillatory chair, and various visual suppression tests were accomplished at differing frequencies along with discrete sinusoids and pseudorandom oscillation. They found a decreased ability to suppress the VOR sinusoidal stimulation during exposure when tested with sinusoidal stimulation. Other groups have used sinusoidal stimulation at lower frequencies to devise a visual-vestibular interaction test as well.[32]

CASE REPORTS

The following cases taken from the author's practice demonstrate some of the uses of low discrete frequency harmonic acceleration in the testing of patients with vestibular lesions. While limited, they illustrate the broad range of use demonstrated by the author and others in the literature.

Case 1

A 54-year-old man with long-standing Meniere's disease and frequent classic attacks underwent a right retrolabyrinthine vestibular nerve section for treatment. The patient did extremely well in the hospital and was discharged 6 days postoperatively. He was instructed to begin vestibular exercises in 1 week and return to the office in 1 month. Ten days postoperatively he had a severe myocardial infarction and was admitted to the intensive care unit in another town. He was treated with bed rest and sedation because he was still complaining of dizziness. When he failed to return for his 1-month appointment, he was called, and it was found that he would be unable to return for another month. When he was seen 2½ months after surgery, he returned to the office in a wheelchair. He was still taking diazepam for dizziness and was unable to walk. He was found to have 3 SD of asymmetry on rotational testing. Because of his psychological makeup, it was difficult to get him off the medication and exercising. At ½ year postoperatively he still had 2 SD of asymmetry and was only walking with a walker or wheelchair around the house. This was in spite of the fact that otherwise he had completely recovered from his myocardial infarction.

Comment

This case demonstrates the extreme urgency of the early compensation process. Immobilization and medications may very well inhibit the patient's final compensation if overused in the early postoperative period. This case demonstrates the objective nature of documentation of poor compensation and seems to indicate that the early treatment of the compensatory process is critical.

Case 2

The patient was a 60-year-old woman with a long history of hearing loss in the left ear. She was found to have a left acoustic neuroma approximately 2 cm in diameter. This was removed in June 1978. Postoperatively, she did fairly well but always had mild unsteadiness in the morning which gradually improved during the day. She never felt her head was entirely clear, and if she moved quickly, she would experience slight unsteadiness. She underwent rotational testing postoperatively and was noted to have 2 SD of asymmetry. Between the third and fourth postoperative years, there was a dramatic change in her asymmetry. On the fourth postoperative year, when she came in for her 4-year postoperative check, she was quite symmetric. In reviewing her history with her, it was found that during the past year she had begun babysitting with her infant granddaughter. She spent a tremendous amount of her day on the floor playing with the granddaughter and taking care of her. She noted that her head now felt clear. She had no dizziness and no motion intolerance.

Comment

This case seems to illustrate that a change in stimulation of the vestibular system may result in greater symmetry even at a late stage after the vestibular injury. It appears to indicate that increasing vestibular stimulation, even long after the injury, can result in better compensation. The difference between this case and case 1 appears to be in the mental attitude of the patient. This is a completely unexplored area, but seems to be important in the compensation process.

Case 3

A 70-year-old woman had long-standing Meniere's disease in the left ear. She had a discrimination on audiometric testing averaging 50% PB max on the left. The patient was first seen in July 1977. She had a slight fluctuation of her hearing in the right ear and was given diuretics. She was followed up and expressed a slight fluctuation on the right, but no vertigo, until June 1986. During the summer of 1986, she began to have markedly fluctuating hearing with a rapid decrease in both pure tone average and discrimination in the right ear. She continued to have very poor discrimination in the left ear and a pure tone average of 65 dB. She was given numerous medications from June to October 1986 without help. In September 1986 she became vertiginous and extremely depressed and desperate. During this period, her rotational testing showed wild swings in symmetry. She had an increase in phase lead. In October 1986 she was given streptomycin and monitored every other day with rotational testing. The gain was followed up carefully. In late October it was noted that her gain began to fall at 18 gm. Streptomycin therapy was stopped, and 7 days later she had a gain of 0.01 at 0.08 Hz and 0.16 Hz. She had slight oscillopsia and a wide-based gait. By January 1987, she had no oscillopsia; her gait was good. Her gain was 0.2 at 0.08 and 0.16 Hz.

Comment

This case demonstrates the use of rotational testing in the monitoring of patients on vestibular-destructive drugs. At times the use of rotational testing to monitor the gain can be very useful in these patients in avoiding long-term oscillopsia with nausea. Interestingly, the patient's hearing in the ear with long-standing Meniere's disease improved dramatically. She went from a PB max of around 50% up to PB max of around 90%. This treatment has made it possible to utilize hearing aids on both ears.

Case 4

A 58-year-old man had right Meniere's disease for several years. He had failed medical therapy and was considered for a nerve section. Prior to sectioning his nerve he was given a visual-vestibular interaction test with rotational testing. It was noted that he could very effectively suppress his gain. He underwent a retrolabyrinthine nerve section in March 1982. Within two months he was functioning effectively with a mild unsteadiness and no classic attacks. He had 2 SD of asymmetry at that point. However, on his 6-month follow-up, he was still unsteady, even though he had been doing his vestibular exercises religiously. In addition, he had taken no vestibular suppressive medications. Evaluation with rotation again documented 2 SD of asymmetry. He was therefore treated by physical therapy daily with intense vestibular exercises. However, this did not seem to change his symptoms or his rotational testing results. Therefore, in January 1983, he underwent a translabyrinthine nerve section. Postoperatively, he had a very slight amount of dizziness. However, within 6 months he again had 2 SD of asymmetry. His symptoms continued to be a slight unsteadiness with some motion intolerance. He was treated with a small amount of vestibular suppressant, diazepam, 1 mg twice daily. However, this made him feel worse, and on rotational testing he had a greater asymmetry. He was treated with glycopyrrolate (Robinul), 1 mg twice daily, which made him feel slightly better, but the rotational testing was still about 2 SD from the norm. This testing result has continued to the present.

Comment

This case illustrates that the symptomatology and the rotational testing in a vestibular injury correlate well. It also demonstrates that in spite of the physician's not understanding the problem with the patient, the results of testing are consistent and indicate an unknown problem in vestibular compensation, even though the patient had good visual suppression of his VOR.

Case 5

A 26-year-old Spanish man fell from an oil rig and had a closed head injury. He had symptoms of unsteadiness and mild motion intolerance when moving quickly. He had a mild positional nystagmus of 5–7°/sec in every position. He had a phase advance of 2 SD at 0.01 and 0.02 Hz and 2 SD of asymmetry throughout the frequency range. He had a 30% reduced vestibular response on the right side. Past history indicated he had suffered a severe vestibular neuronitis five years prior to the accident but had had no difficulty with vertigo by history from two months after this episode until the accident. The insurance company maintained that his current symptomatology was due to his previous labyrinthitis, and the patient maintained that it was due to his accident.

Comment

Rotational testing provided some insight into the origin of his asymmetry and symptoms. Since he became markedly asymmetric later, it was more likely that the pathology, at least in part, was coming from his injury. If it had not, he should have been somewhat symptomatic for the entire time since his vestibular neuronitis. This would have been highly unlikely in a man in his 20s.

SUMMARY

Although many other groups have published individual papers utilizing rotation testing in the vestibular system, this brief review has attempted to examine the work of those groups that have used this technique over a considerable time. Many similarities can be found in the results of these groups.

It appears that there are consistent and measurable changes in response to vestibular disease, enabling the physician to monitor the patient with predictable results. Unfortunately, the changes in gain, asymmetry, and phase appear to be nonspecific. The same decrement may occur in the output measure from a great variety of vestibular lesions. This in general is the difficulty with all vestibular testing. However, rotational testing has one great advantage in monitoring patients. One can provide a precise stimulus to the patient, and it is generally agreed among investigators that a more precise output measure can be obtained utilizing rotational testing than conventional ENG. If the patient has a known disease, therefore, more precise monitoring of that patient's progress is possible with rotational testing.

In certain isolated cases rotational testing can be extremely effective in determining whether a patient has a vestibular lesion. This can be very useful in complicated cases with vague symptoms and in those where on-the-job injury is in question.

REFERENCES

1. Dodge R: Five types of eye movements in the horizontal meridian plane of the field of regard. *Am J Physiol* 1903; 8:307–329.
2. Wendt GR: Vestibular function, in Stevens SS (ed): *Handbook of Experimental Psychology*. New York, John Wiley & Sons, 1951, pp 1191–1223.
3. Cramer RL: The dynamic characteristics of the vestibulo-ocular reflex arc after prolonged stimulation. *Biomed Sci Instrum* 1963; 1:401–406.
4. Melvill Jones M, Milsum JH: Spatial and dynamic aspects of visual fixation. *IEEE Trans BME* 1965; 12:54–62.
5. van Edmond AAJ, Groen JJ, Jongkees LBW: The mechanics of the semicircular canal. *J Physiol* 1949; 110:1–17.
6. Niven JI, Hixson WC, Correia MJ: An experimental approach to the dynamics of the vestibular mechanisms, in *The Role of the Vestibular Organs in the Exploration of Space*. Washington, DC, NASA SP-77, 1965, pp 43–56.
7. Wolfe JW, Kos CM: Nystagmic responses of the rhesus monkey to rotational stimulation following unilateral labyrinthectomy: A preliminary

report. *Trans Am Acad Ophthalmol Otolaryngol* 1976; 82:ORL60–ORL69.

8. Engelken EJ, Wolfe JW: Analog signal processing of eye movements for on-line digital computer analysis. *Physiol Behav* 1977; 18:157–158.
9. Wolfe JW, Kos CM: Nystagmic responses of the rhesus monkey to rotational stimuli following unilateral labyrinthectomy: Final report. *Trans Am Acad Ophthalmol Otolaryngol* 1977; 84:ORL38–ORL45.
10. Wolfe JW, Olsson JE, Engelken EJ, et al: Vestibular responses to bithermal caloric and harmonic acceleration. *Ann Otol Rhinol Laryngol* 1978; 87:861–867.
11. Wolfe JW, Engelken EJ, Kos CM: Low-frequency harmonic acceleration as a test of labyrinthine function: Basic methods and illustrative cases. *Trans Am Acad Ophthalmol Otolarnygol* 1978; 86:ORL130–ORL139.
12. Wolfe JW, Engelken EJ, Olsson JE: Low-frequency harmonic acceleration in the evaluation of surgical treatment of Meniere's disease. *Adv Otorhinolaryngol* 1979; 25:192–196.
13. Olsson JE, Wolfe JW: Comparison of subjective symptomatology and responses to harmonic acceleration in patients with Meniere's disease. *Ann Otol Rhinol Laryngol* 1981; 90(suppl 86):15–17.
14. Olsson JE, Wolfe JW, Engleken EJ: Responses to low-frequency harmonic acceleration in patients with acoustic neuromas. *Laryngoscope* 1981; 91:1270–1277.
15. Wolfe JW, Engelken EJ, Olsson JE: Low-frequency harmonic acceleration in the evaluation of patients with peripheral labyrinthine disorders, in Honrubia V, Brazier M (eds): *Nystagmus and Vertigo: Clinical Approaches to the Patient With Dizziness*. New York, Academic Press, 1982, pp 95–105.
16. Engelken EJ, Stevens KW, Wolfe JW: Application of digital filters in the processing of eye movement data. *Behav Res Methods Instr* 1982; 14(3):314–319.
17. Olsson JE, Wolfe JW: Responses to rotational stimulation of the horizontal canals from patients with acoustic neuromas. *Acta Otolaryngol (Stockh) [Suppl]* 1984; 406:203–208.
18. Jenkins HA, Honrubia V, Baloh RH: Evaluation of multiple-frequency rotatory testing in patients with peripheral labyrinthine weakness. *Am J Otolaryngol* 1982; 3:182–188.
19. Jenkins HA: Long-term adaptive changes of the vestibulo-ocular reflex in patients following acoustic neuroma surgery. *Laryngoscope* 1985; 95:1224–1234.
20. Moretz WH Jr, Orchik DJ, Shea JJ Jr, et al: Low-frequency harmonic acceleration in the evaluation of patients with intracanalicular and cerebellopontine angle tumors. *Otolaryngol Head Neck Surg* 1986; 95:324–332.
21. Honrubia V, Baloh RW, Lau CG, et al: The patterns of eye movements during physiologic vestibular nystagmus in man. *Trans Am Acad Ophthalmol Otolaryngol* 1977; 84:ORL339–ORL347.

22. Lau CG, Honrubia V, Jenkins HA, et al: Linear model for visual-vestibular interaction. *Aviat Space Environ Med* 1978; 49:880–885.
23. Baloh RW, Yee RD, Honrubia V: Internuclear ophthalmoplegia: II. Pursuit, optokinetic nystagmus and vestibulo-ocular reflex. *Arch Neurol* 1978; 35:490–493.
24. Baloh RW, Sills AW, Honrubia V: Impulsive and sinusoidal rotatory testing: A comparison with results of caloric testing. *Laryngoscope* 1979; 89:646–654.
25. Baloh RW, Langhofer L, Honrubia V, et al: On-line analysis of eye movements using a digital computer. *Aviat Space Environ Med* 1980; 51(6):563–567.
26. Baloh RW, Yee RD, Kimm J, et al: Vestibulo-ocular reflex in patients with lesions involving the vestibulo-cerebellum. *Exp Neurol* 1981; 72(1):141–152.
27. Jenkins HA, Honrubia V, Baloh RH: Evaluation of multiple-frequency rotatory testing in patients with peripheral labyrinthine weakness. *Am J Otolaryngol* 1982; 3:182–188.
28. Honrubia V, Jenkins HA, Baloh RW, et al: Evaluation of rotatory vestibular tests in peripheral labyrinthine lesions, in Honrubia V, Brazier MAB (eds): *Nystagmus and Vertigo: Clinical Approaches to the Patient With Dizziness*. New York, Academic Press, 1982, pp 57–77.
29. Honrubia V, Baloh RW, Yee RD, et al: Identification of the location of vestibular lesions on the basis of vestibulo-ocular reflex measurements. *Am J Otolaryngol* 1980; 1(4):291–301.
30. Baloh RW, Henn V, Jager J: Habituation of the human vestibulo-ocular reflex with low-frequency harmonic acceleration. *Am J Otolaryngol* 1982; 3:235–241.
31. Baloh RW, Honrubia V, Yee RD, et al: Changes in the human vestibulo-ocular reflex after loss of peripheral sensitivity. *Ann Neurol* 1984; 16:222–228.
32. Baloh RW, Lyerly K, Yee RD, et al: Voluntary control of the human vestibulo-ocular reflex. *Acta Otolaryngol (Stockh)* 1984; 97:1–6.
33. Honrubia V, Jenkins HA, Baloh RW, et al: Vestibulo-ocular reflexes in peripheral labyrinthine lesions: I. Unilateral dysfunction. *Am J Otolaryngol* 1984; 5:15–26.
34. Baloh RW, Hess K, Honrubia V, et al: Low and high frequency sinusoidal rotational testing in patients with peripheral vestibular lesions. *Acta Otolaryngol (Stockh)* [*Suppl*] 1984; 406:189–193.
35. Hess K, Baloh RW, Honrubia V, et al: Rotational testing in patients with bilateral peripheral vestibular disease. *Laryngoscope* 1985; 95:85–88.
36. Honrubia V, Marco J, Andrews J, et al: Vestibulo-ocular reflexes in peripheral labyrinthine lesions: III. Bilateral dysfunction. *Am J Otolaryngol* 1985; 6:342–352.
37. Olsson JE, Shagets FW, Wolfe JW: Surgical treatment of vertigo. *ENT Monthly* 1980; 59:17–29.

38. Barr CC, Schultheis LW, Robinson DA: Voluntary, nonvisual control of the human vestibulo-ocular reflex. *Acta Otolaryngol (Stockh)* 1976; 81:365–368.
39. Rubin W: Symposium on low frequency harmonic acceleration, the rotary chair: SHA as a modality for monitoring patient progress. *Laryngoscope* 1981; 91:1282–1285.
40. Staller SJ, Goin DW, Hildebrandt M: Pediatric vestibular evaluation with harmonic acceleration. *Otolaryngol Head Neck Surg* 1986; 95:471–476.
41. Cyr DG, Brookhouser PE, Valente M, et al: Vestibular evaluation of infants and preschool children. *Otolaryngol Head Neck Surg* 1985; 93:463–468.
42. Wall C III, Black FO, O'Leary DP: Clinical use of pseudorandom binary sequence white noise in assessment of the human vestibulo-ocular system. *Ann Otol Rhinol Laryngol* 1978; 87:845–852.
43. O'Leary DP, Dunn RF, Honrubia V: Analysis of afferent responses from isolated semicircular canal of the guitar fish using rotational acceleration white-noise inputs. *J Neurophysiol* 1976; 39:631–659.
44. Black FO, Wall C III: Comparison of vestibulo-ocular and vestibulospinal screening tests. *Otolaryngol Head Neck Surg* 1981; 89:811–817.
45. O'Leary DP, Furman JM, Wolfe JW: Use of pseudorandom angular accelerations in the evaluation of vestibuloocular function, in Honrubia V, Brazier M (eds): *Nystagmus and Vertigo: Clinical Approaches to the Patient With Dizziness.* New York, Academic Press, 1982, pp 107–113.
46. Furman JM, O'Leary DP, Wolfe JW: Application of linear system analysis to the horizontal vestibulo-ocular reflex of the alert rhesus monkey using pseudorandom binary sequence and single frequency sinusoidal stimulation. *Biol Cybern* 1979; 33:159–165.
47. Schwarz DWF, Tomlinson RD: Diagnostic precision in a new rotatory vestibular test. *J Otolaryngol* 1979; 8:544–548.
48. Tomlinson RD, Saunders GE, Schwarz DWF: Analysis of human vestibulo-ocular reflex during active head movements. *Acta Otolaryngol* 1980; 90:184–190.
49. Hyden D, Istl YE, Schwarz DWF: Human visuo-vestibular interaction as a basis for quantitative clinical diagnostics. *Acta Otolaryngol* 1982; 94:53–60.
50. Larsby B, Hyden D, Odkvist LM, et al: Caloric and rotatory tests in patients with uni- and bilateral vestibular loss. *Acta Otolaryngol (Stockh) [Suppl]* 1984; 412:111–112.
51. Larsby B, Tham R, Eriksson B, et al: Effects of trichloroethylene on the human vestibulo-oculomotor system. *Acta Otolaryngol (Stockh)* 1986; 101:193–199.

9

*Rotational Testing: An Overview**

Robert W. Baloh, M.D.

Vicente Honrubia, M.D., D.M.Sc.

Robert D. Yee, M.D.

Kathleen M. Jacobson, B.A.

Rotational testing has become a routine part of the electronystagmographic (ENG) examination at many centers across the country. Test methodology varies from center to center, but the main components of the test battery are similar. In this chapter we describe how rotational testing is performed in our laboratory and briefly summarize the interpretation of results for each component of the test battery.

METHODS

We use direct current (dc) electro-oculography (EOG) for routine clinical recordings. Electrodes are placed at the inner and outer canthi to record horizontal movements and above the eyebrow and below the lower eyelid to record vertical movements and to monitor eye blinks.

*Dr. Baloh is supported by NIH grants NS 09823 and EY 04556. Dr. Honrubia is supported by NIH grant NS 09823. Dr. Yee is supported by NIH grant EY 03737 and the Dolly Green Scholar Award from Research to Prevent Blindness, Inc., New York, New York.

A 6-pole low-pass filter with cutoff frequency of 42 Hz (−3 dB) removes high-frequency noise before the signal enters the analog-to-digital converter. Complete details of the recording system have been reported elsewhere.[1]

The patient is seated in a chair mounted on a motorized rotating table inside a light-tight, electrically shielded room. A cloth drum with 1-in. wide stripes (15° apart) mounted on a black cloth completely surrounds the patient so that the entire visual field is stimulated. An array of 3 LEDs spaced at the center and 15° to the right and left is attached to the chair directly in front of the patient. This allows for rapid calibration in any chair position in the light and in the dark. Frequent calibrations are interspersed throughout the testing procedure to correct for any fluctuations in corneoretinal potential. The rotatory chair, optokinetic drum, and calibration lights are all controlled by the same microprocessor that analyzes the nystagmus response.

For optokinetic nystagmus (OKN) the drum is rotated alone, and the patient is instructed to stare at the stripes directly in front of him but not to follow them as they move around. We routinely use both step and sinusoidal optokinetic stimuli. For the former the optokinetic drum rapidly achieves a constant velocity (routinely 30° and 60°/sec clockwise and counterclockwise), and after 1 minute of stimulation the lights are turned off and optokinetic after nystagmus (OKAN) is recorded. The VOR is tested by rotating the chair sinusoidally in the dark while the subject performs continuous mental arithmetic. Finally, for visual vestibular interaction the subject is rotated in the light with the optokinetic drum stationary (visual vestibulo-ocular reflex or VVOR) and in the dark with the center LED lit (VOR with fixation-suppression, or VOR-Fix). Fixation-suppression of the VOR can also be evaluated by coupling the optokinetic drum and chair, thereby rotating both drum and chair sinusoidally in the light. The computer algorithm generates stimulus frequencies for each test ranging from 0.0125 to 1.6 Hz with peak velocities ranging from 15° to 120°/sec. For rotational testing at high frequencies (≥ .8 Hz) the peak velocity that can be achieved without distortion of the sinusoidal waveform is dependent on the weight of the subject. For screening purposes we routinely use 0.05 Hz and a peak velocity of 60°/sec.

Complete details of the on-line digital computer analysis techniques have been reported elsewhere.[1] In brief, the eye position signal (digitized at a rate of 200 samples/sec) is differentiated to yield an instantaneous velocity record. Fast components (saccades) are identified on the basis of their characteristic velocity profile and the direction of the stimulus movement. After the fast components are removed, the gaps in the remaining slow eye velocity record are filled by connecting points on each side of the missing segment with a linear regression line. A fast Fourier transform is then performed, giving a dc offset term, the magnitude and phase of the fundamental, and the percent harmonic distortion [magnitude of the first 5 harmonics divided by (magnitude of fundamental plus magnitude of first 5 harmonics)] × 100 (Fig 9–1, left side). To assess symmetry of response plots of slow-component eye velocity vs. stimulus velocity are created by overlaying the same cycles used for frequency analysis (see Fig 9–1, right side). The gain in each direction is then calculated using the mean slow-phase eye velocity in a 2°/sec window at the peak stimulus velocity. Typical responses of a normal subject to the four standard rotational tests are shown in Figure 9–2 (left side). In each case the peak stimulus velocity is 60°/sec. All responses are symmetric. The mean gain ± 1 SD for similar testing in 20 normal subjects is as follows: OKN − 0.83 ± 0.13; VOR − 0.50 ± 0.15; VVOR − 0.99 ± 0.05; and VOR-Fix − 0.03 ± 0.02. The OKN and VVOR responses are in phase with the stimulus but the VOR exhibits a small phase lead at this frequency (normal mean ± 1 SD = 10 ± 4°).

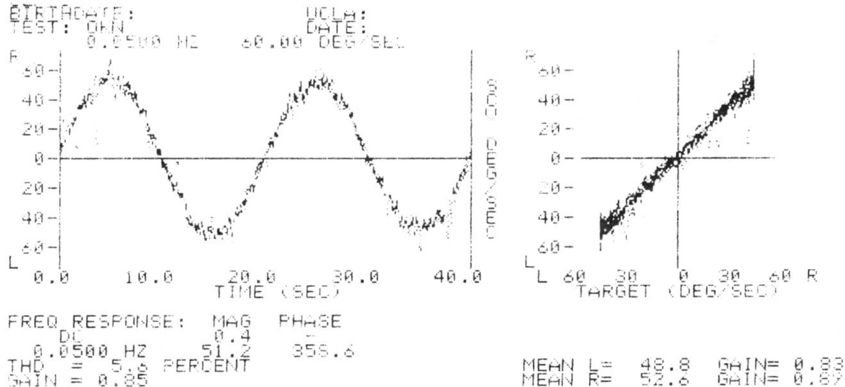

FIG 9–1.

Sample data analysis for sinusoidal optokinetic test. **Left,** plot of slow component velocity (SCV) vs. time. **Right,** overlay plot of SCV vs. drum velocity (same 2 cycles); frequency 0.05 HZ, peak velocity 60°/sec; *Mag,* magnitude, DC, offset value in °/sec, *THD,* percent total harmonic distortion; phase >360° = phase lead, <360°, phase lag; *Gain* **(left side),** magnitude of fundamental/peak chair velocity, *Gain* **(right side),** average peak SCV in each direction/peak drum velocity.

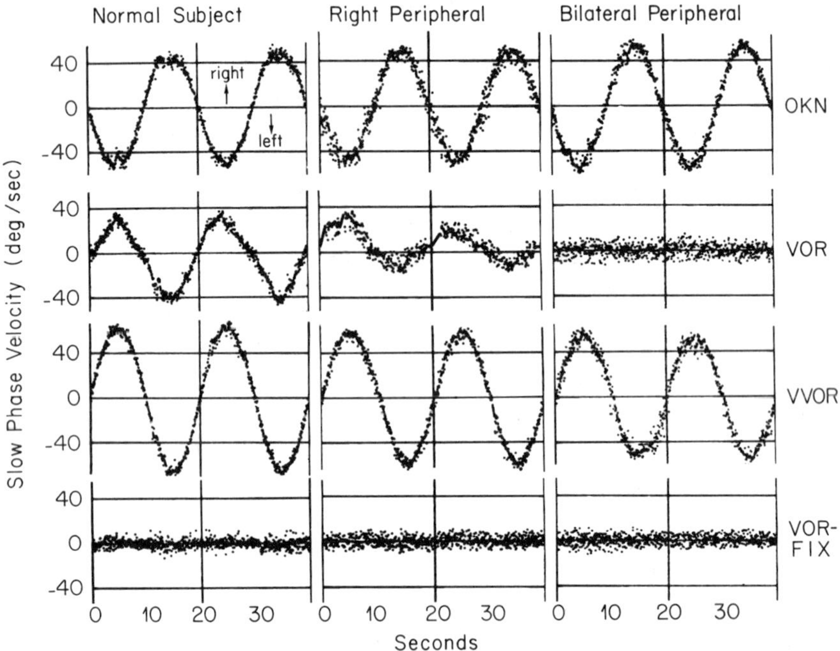

FIG 9–2.
Plots of slow-phase velocity vs. time from the 4 standard sinusoidal rotational tests (0.05 Hz, peak velocity 60°/sec) in normal subject **(left),** patient who underwent right labyrinthectomy **(center),** and patient with bilateral vestibulopathy secondary to ototoxic drugs (right). (From Baloh RW, Sakala S, Yee RD, et al: Quantitative vestibular testing. *Otolaryngol Head Neck Surg* 1984; 92:145–150. Used by permission.)

RESULTS

Optokinetic Nystagmus (OKN)

With one exception, lesions of the peripheral vestibular system (labyrinth and 8th nerve) do not impair optokinetic responses (see Fig 9–2, center and right).[2] Patients with acute unilateral peripheral vestibular lesions show an asymmetry of OKN consistent with a summation of their spontaneous nystagmus and induced OKN. This asymmetry occurs only during the acute phase and disappears within a few days as the spontaneous nystagmus disappears. Patients with bilateral peripheral vestibular loss (e.g., due to ototoxic drug exposure) have normal OKN but diminished or absent OKAN.

Lesions throughout the CNS can lead to abnormal optokinetic nystagmus.[2] Slow- and fast-component abnormalities occur. Any lesion that results in abnormal voluntary saccades will also impair the fast components of OKN. With abnormal fast-component initiation, the eyes deviate in the direction of the slow phase, often becoming pinned in an extreme orbital position. Neurologic disorders producing this phenomenon include congenital oculomotor apraxia, ataxia telangiectasia, Huntington's disease, progressive supranuclear palsy, and olivopontocerebellar atrophy. Each of these conditions is associated with diffuse neuronal loss, although involvement of the basal ganglia may be a common thread.

Lesions involving the visual pursuit pathways lead to abnormalities of the slow phase of optokinetic nystagmus. The main pursuit pathway runs from the occipitoparietal region to the ipsilateral pontine reticular formation with a major relay in the cerebellar flocculus.[2] There may also be a subcortical pathway involving the accessory optic system, although in primates the contribution of this subcortical pathway seems to be minimal. Lesions of the parieto-occipital region and of the pontine reticular formation impair optokinetic slow phases when the stripes move toward the side of the lesion (Fig 9–3, right).[13] Lesions involving the flocculus or other structures in the caudal midline cerebellum invariably lead to a severe bilateral impairment of optokinetic slow phases (see Fig 9–3, center).[4] Patients with lesions of the vestibular nuclei (e.g., the lateral medullary syndrome) have a tonic deviation of the eyes toward the side of the lesion and greater OKN slow-phase velocity in that direction (probably due to a summation of the tonic bias and the OKN slow-phase velocity) (see Fig 9–3, left).[15]

Vestibulo-ocular Reflex

Patients with unilateral lesions of the labyrinth or 8th cranial nerve have two characteristic abnormalities on sinusoidal rotational testing (see Fig 9–2, center).[6] They show (1) an asymmetric gain with decreased slow-phase velocity away from the side of the lesion (i.e., with rotation toward the side of the lesion) and (2) an increased phase advance of eye velocity relative to stimulus velocity at low frequencies of rotation (0.05 Hz and lower). The asymmetry is most pronounced with an acute lesion and often disappears as compensation occurs, whereas the increased phase lead at low frequencies remains indefinitely.[7]

With bilateral peripheral vestibular lesions rotational responses are symmetrically diminished (see Fig 9–2, right). Typically, the response gain is much lower for low frequencies than for high frequen-

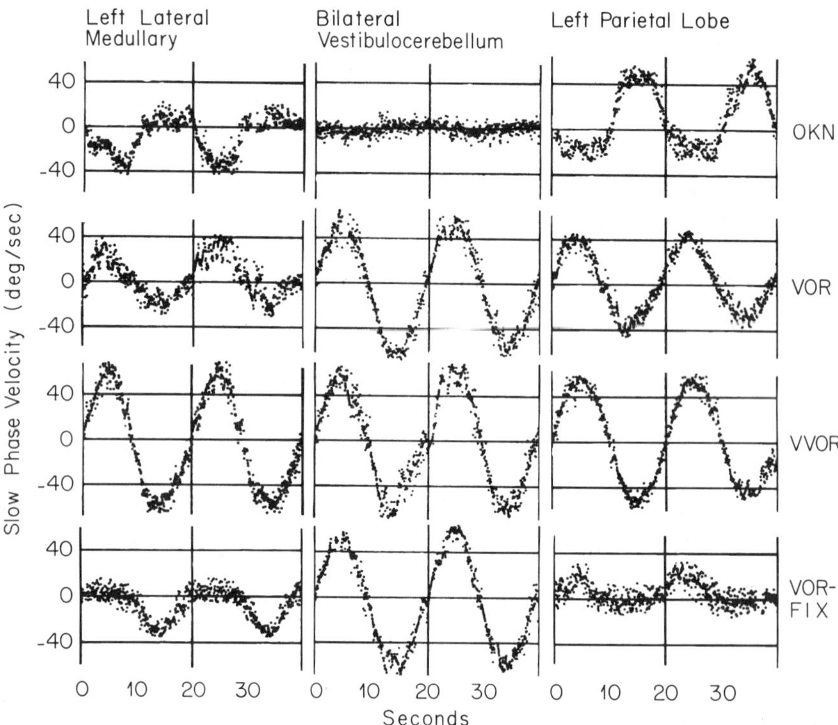

FIG 9–3.

Plots of slow-phase velocity vs. time from the 4 standard sinusoidal rotational tests (0.05 Hz, peak velocity 60°/sec) in patient with infarction of the left lateral medullary region **(left),** patient with caudal midline cerebellar atrophy **(center),** and patient with glioma in deep parietal lobe on left side **(right).** (From Baloh RW, Sakala S, Yee RD, et al: Quantitative vestibular testing. *Otolaryngol Head Neck Surg* 1984; 92:145–150. Used by permission.)

cies of rotation. A patient may have no response to rotational testing at low frequencies or to standard bithermal caloric testing and yet have normal rotational responses above 1 Hz.[6] In those subjects in whom VOR responses are present at low frequencies there is a marked increase in phase lead of eye velocity relative to head velocity.

Visual-Vestibular Interaction

When a normal subject is rotated in the light with the surrounding optokinetic drum stationary, the gain (peak eye velocity/peak stimulus velocity) is near 1 for a wide range of frequencies and peak velocities.[8]

In this case there is a synergistic interaction of the VOR and optokinetic systems. At low frequencies (< 0.05 Hz) the optokinetic system dominates and the gain of the VVOR can be near 1, even if there is a complete loss of vestibular function bilaterally. However, for higher frequencies ($\geqslant$ than 1 Hz) the VOR becomes more important, and the gain of the optokinetic system rapidly falls off. Therefore, at low frequencies the VVOR test is primarily a test of the optokinetic system, whereas at high frequencies it is primarily a test of the VOR. As shown in Figures 9–2 and 9–3, the VVOR responses at intermediate frequencies can be near normal despite major abnormalities in the OKN or VOR responses as long as the combination of the two is adequate to compensate for the chair movement.

Normal subjects are able to suppress the VOR with fixation as long as the frequency and peak velocity of rotation do not exceed some critical value. Patients with abnormal OKN will invariably have abnormal fixation-suppression of the VOR (see Fig 9–3). If they exhibit impaired OKN slow phases to the right, they will be unable to inhibit VOR slow phases to the left (see Fig 9–3, right).[9] Patients with lesions of the flocculus and caudal midline cerebellum typically have profound impairment of optokinetic nystagmus and almost complete inability to suppress the VOR with fixation (see Fig 9–3, center).[4] In these patients the VOR and VOR-Fix responses are almost identical.

CONCLUSIONS

Even with modern rotational devices using sophisticated analysis techniques, the caloric test is still indispensable for identifying unilateral peripheral vestibular lesions. The degree of asymmetry of rotatory-induced nystagmus seen with partial unilateral lesions is often not outside the normal range, and even in patients with complete unilateral peripheral lesions symmetry of response returns with compensation. An increased phase shift of the VOR at low frequencies of sinusoidal stimulation is a more persistent finding, but this only indicates a vestibular dysfunction, not the side of the lesion or whether it is central or peripheral. Further, it is a nonspecific finding that can even be seen in normal subjects if they are habituated by prolonged periods of rotation.

Rotational testing is particularly helpful for identifying bilateral peripheral vestibular loss (e.g., ototoxic drug exposure), since both labyrinths are stimulated simultaneously and the degree of remaining function is accurately quantified. Because the variance associated with normal rotatory responses is less than that associated with caloric responses, diminished function is identified earlier. Further, artifactually diminished caloric responses occasionally occur in patients with angular narrow external canals or with highly pneumatized temporal bones. Since a rotatory stimulus is unrelated to these factors, rotatory-induced nystagmus is normal in such patients. Patients with absent caloric responses may have decreased but measurable rotatory-induced nystagmus, particularly at higher stimulus velocities. The ability to identify remaining vestibular function, even if minimal, is an important advantage of rotatory testing, particularly when the physician is contemplating ablative surgery or monitoring the effects of ototoxic drugs.

Optokinetic and visual vestibular interaction testing is particularly useful for evaluating patients with suspected CNS lesions. When combined with quantitative tests of visual ocular control (saccades and smooth pursuit), this test can often localize the site and extent of the lesion. Characteristic patterns of response are associated with lesions at different levels of the CNS.

REFERENCES

1. Baloh RW, Langhofer L, Honrubia V, et al: On-line analysis of eye movements using a digital computer. *Aviat Space Environ Med* 1980; 51:563–567.
2. Baloh RW, Yee RD, Honrubia V: Clinical abnormalities of optokinetic nystagmus, in Lennerstrand G, Zee DS, Keller EL (eds): *Functional Basis of Ocular Motility Disorders*. New York, Pergamon Press, 1982, pp 311–320.
3. Baloh RW, Yee RD, Honrubia V: Optokinetic nystagmus and parietal lobe l9sions. *Ann Neurol* 1979; 7:269–276.
4. Baloh RW, Yee RD, Kimm J, et al: The vestibulo-ocular reflex in patients with lesions involving the vestibulocerebellum. *Exp Neurol* 1981; 72:141–152.
5. Baloh RW, Yee RD, Honrubia V: Eye movements in patients with Wallenberg's syndrome. *Ann NY Acad Sci* 1981; 374:600–613.
6. Baloh RW, Honrubia V, Yee RD, et al: Changes in the human vestibulo-ocular reflex after loss of peripheral sensitivity. *Ann Neurol* 1984; 16:222–228.
7. Wolfe JW, Engelken EJ, Olsson JE: Low-frequency harmonic acceleration in the evaluation of patients with peripheral labyrinthine disorders, in Honrubia V, Brazier M (eds): *Nystagmus and Vertigo: Clinical Approaches to the Patient With Dizziness*. New York, Academic Press Inc, 1982, pp 95–106.

8. Baloh RW, Sakala S, Yee RD, et al: Quantitative vestibular testing. *Otolaryngol Head Neck Surg* 1984; 92:145–150.
9. Dichgans J, von Reutern GM, Rommelt J: Impaired suppression of vestibular nystagmus by fixation in cerebellar and noncerebellar patients. *Arch Psychiatr Nervenkr* 1978; 226:183–199.

PART THREE

Smooth Eye Movements: Normal, Abnormal

10

*Smooth Pursuit Disorders: Physiological and Anatomical Considerations**

James A. Sharpe, M.D., F.R.C.P.(C.)
Mark J. Morrow, M.D.

Smooth ocular pursuit serves to maintain the image of small, slowly moving target at the fovea. This eye movement system is critical in achieving optimal visual acuity by matching smooth eye movement velocity with target velocity. Visual acuity starts to decrease when the velocity of retinal image slip exceeds about 2°/sec.[1] When pursuit eye velocity is lower than target velocity, a series of catch-up saccades compensates for the limited smooth eye movement response. Since this *saccadic pursuit* is a sensitive sign of brain disease when it occurs at low target speeds, the pursuit system provides a valuable parameter of brain dysfunction for neurologists, otolaryngologists, and ophthalmologists. In this chapter, we present clinical considerations of the physiological and anatomical substrates of smooth pursuit and discuss its disorders.

*Supported by the Medical Research Council of Canada Grants ME5509 and MT5404 (Dr. Sharpe), and by National Institutes of Health Research Service Award EY-06040 and a Chisholm Memorial Fellowship, University of Toronto (Dr. Morrow).

PHYSIOLOGICAL CONSIDERATIONS

When normal subjects track constant velocity targets, smooth eye movements become admixed with increasing numbers of saccades at target velocities over 30°–40°/sec.[2, 3] Even at lower speeds, eye and target velocities are not perfectly matched.[4, 5] Maximum values of pursuit eye acceleration and velocity are far below the capacity of the ocular motor system during saccades. Humans can attain smooth eye movement accelerations of up to about 1,200°/sec^2 and velocities of up to 150°/sec during pursuit of predictable sinusoidal targets[6] and velocities of up to 90°/sec with constant velocity targets.[7] The disparity between the motor output of the saccadic and pursuit systems suggests limits on the sensory analysis of target motion information or on the premotor processing of pursuit commands.

The difference between target and eye velocity, retinal slip velocity, is the principal stimulus for smooth pursuit. This velocity error determines the changes in eye velocity (eye accelerations) that match foveal and target image velocity. Acceleration error and position error serve as complementary stimuli; initial pursuit responses are faster for accelerating targets,[8, 9] and smooth pursuit can be elicited by targets that jump to-and-fro without a smooth velocity component, acting as position errors,[10] or by a visual afterimage positioned off the fovea.[11] Smooth pursuit is a selective motor system that is typically activated by a small target moving across a stationary background. Once pursuit is initiated, the background is no longer stationary relative to the eyes. This relative background movement produces an optokinetic stimulus opposite to the direction of target movement. This optokinetic "drag" causes only slight reduction in smooth pursuit velocity when pursuit against structured and featureless backgrounds are compared.[5, 12, 13] Background visual texture also reduces the initial acceleration of pursuit toward a moving target dot,[14] but this does not result from optokinetic stimulation by the background, since the eyes are fixed during the interval in which target motion determines the acceleration response[8]; this effect of visual background demonstrates an operation of motion detection in the pursuit system.

Smooth pursuit is not entirely dependent on retinal images. Although very few individuals can voluntarily pursue an imaginary target smoothly in darkness,[15] normal subjects can pursue a retinal afterimage placed on or near the fovea.[11, 16] An internal percept of target motion contributes to effective smooth pursuit. Normal subjects improve pursuit with increasing predictability of target motion,[17, 18] and they can pursue an intermittently disappearing target if its trajectory is predictable.[19] Lisberger and associates[20] termed the process that sustains eye velocity in the absence of retinal velocity error, velocity memory. Smooth eye movements can also be elicited by proprioceptive cues, such as attempting fixation of one's own moving hand in the dark,[21] or by central percepts of target information, such as are derived from watching randomly moving dot video patterns,[22] or the occluded center of a rolling wheel that is marked by several small lamps along its rim.[23] Sequential illumination of a stationary stimulus pattern can also elicit smooth eye movement; this is called sigma-pursuit.[24]

Models of Smooth Pursuit

Most control system analyses of smooth pursuit present negative feedback models in which smooth eye movement decreases retinal slip, thereby reducing the eye velocity command. Simple negative feedback models are inadequate, however, since they predict large ocular oscillations as eye velocity falls when retinal slip is reduced to zero.[25] In fact, pursuit velocity is sustained in the absence of retinal velocity error. This *velocity memory*[20] can be explained by an extra-retinal (internal) representation of target motion, derived from the efferent command for smooth pursuit movement, called efference copy or corollary discharge.[26] This type of model[20, 26] employs a positive feedback loop that sums the efference copy of smooth eye velocity with retinal slip information to yield an internal estimate of target velocity.

The internal positive feedback loop cancels the outer negative visual feedback loop.[20, 25] A system without the benefit of negative feedback must be monitored by parametric adjustments of its errors on a trial-by-trial basis. The plasticity of the VOR (see chapter 1 for a discussion of parametric adjustment of the VOR) exemplifies such long-term correction of errors in an ocular motor system. Optican and associates[27] demonstrated that the pursuit system also undergoes plastic changes in response to weakness of an extraocular muscle. For example, when a patient with a left 6th nerve paralysis is forced to track with his left eye by patching his right eye, the output of the system increases over several days so that leftward pursuit by the left eye increases to nearly match target velocity. Then, if the patch is switched to the left eye, leftward pursuit with the right eye is increased in velocity. Its velocity exceeds target velocity, demonstrating parametric change in the pursuit system. Recently, Robinson and colleagues[25] refined models of pursuit by adding an internal negative feedback loop that subtracts current eye velocity from desired eye velocity to yield an eye velocity error signal that drives the eyes to the limits of their acceleration saturation. Their model[25] is consistent with motor plasticity[27] and incorporates both acceleration[6] and velocity[7] saturation properties of smooth pursuit.

Measurement of Pursuit

The testing of smooth pursuit requires attention to stimulus conditions. To assess foveal smooth pursuit, target illumination should be in the photopic (> 5 cd/m^2) or mesopic ($> 10^{-3}$ cd/m^2) range, since the fovea is blind to dim targets.[28] However, after dark adaptation, human subjects can effectively track dim targets which stimulate only scotopic vision by maintaining the target image on the peripheral retina.[29] To ensure that one is testing only pursuit and not the optokinetic system, the target must be small (1–20 minutes of arc) so that it can be confined to the fovea. Target motion must be of sufficient amplitude to allow some maintenance of steady state pursuit; $\pm 10°$ from the midposition at frequencies from 0.25 to 1.0 Hz is suitable. The head should be firmly immobilized or recorded by means of a helmet and potentiometer or a magnetic search coil.[30, 31] In natural settings, smooth pursuit is a combination of smooth head and eye tracking. Combined eye and head pursuit can be measured when subjects are encouraged to track with the head, provided that the head and eyes are both accurately recorded,[32, 33] but measurement of ocular tracking alone is the standard test of the pursuit system. Electro-oculography (EOG) with skin electrodes,[34, 35] infrared limbus reflection devices mounted on spectacle frames,[3, 12] or magnetic search coil techniques using an annular scleral contact lens[31, 32] are all readily employed in clinical laboratories. With EOG or search coil methods, patients can wear spectacles that correct any refractive error to ensure optimal acuity of the moving target. Since inattention impairs pursuit,[36] subjects must be alert, and vigilance should be encouraged.

Most investigators have analyzed steady-state characteristics of pursuit in response to constant velocity or sinusoidal targets. The most appropriate measure of the system is its gain, the ratio of its output (eye velocity) to its input (target velocity). The ideal gain of pursuit is 1.0. Gain can be measured using computer algorithms to determine average smooth eye movement velocity, or the mode velocity (the velocity at which the eyes spend the largest proportion of time) in each direction for several target cycles.[34] Since pursuit is variable throughout repeated cycles of target motion, measurement of many cycles is desirable. For manual analysis from polygraph recordings, we prefer to determine the mean of 15 or more half-cycles of pursuit in each direction, using maximal smooth eye movement velocity for each half-cycle to calculate gain.[3] One can also measure the slopes of smooth eye movements, determine the duration of the slopes, and establish a weighted average for gain.[12]

Computer analysis requires algorithms that recognize and remove saccades[34, 37] or interactive programs that allow the investigator to place cursors at the beginning and end of each uninterrupted smooth eye movement displayed on a graphics terminal and thereby delete saccades from the analysis.[32, 38] A cumulative smooth eye movement trace can be generated by filling the gaps left after saccades are deleted.[37, 39] Eye and target motion can be phase matched, and computer algorithms can then match smooth eye movements with corresponding target segments to compute average gain[38] or maximal gain[32] for each half-cycle. With this method, gain can be determined at selected target velocities for several time bins within a target sinusoid.[38]

Since eye acceleration limits the pursuit response,[6] it is appropriate to quantify the upper limits of smooth pursuit velocity or acceleration in response to sine wave targets that differ in frequency and amplitude; target acceleration can thus be varied while holding peak velocity constant.[6, 38, 40] Velocity saturation can also be measured when subjects track large amplitude constant velocity targets.[7] Attempts to assess smooth pursuit by the number of so-called velocity arrests[36, 41] or the number[42] or amplitudes[35] of saccades in a tracking record, or the cross-correlation coefficients between eye and target position[43] measure saccades or a combination of saccades and pursuit, but do not quantify smooth eye motion.[44] Measurement of phase lag between eye and target positions[45, 46] has not proved useful in clinical laboratories.

Measurement of initial smooth eye acceleration responses to slowly moving targets can be utilized to study the sensory limb of the pursuit system and its open loop properties before eye motion alters its performance.[8] Rashbass[47] introduced step-ramp stimuli, where a target rapidly "steps" away from the fovea, then "ramps" at a constant velocity toward the fovea, to evoke smooth eye acceleration prior to any corrective saccades. Because the latency of smooth pursuit is shorter than for saccades, the smooth eye movement usually occurs first. Step-ramp responses demonstrate that the pursuit system preferentially responds to velocity, not position errors, since the eye accelerates away from the target position[9, 47] (Fig 10–1,A). However, for

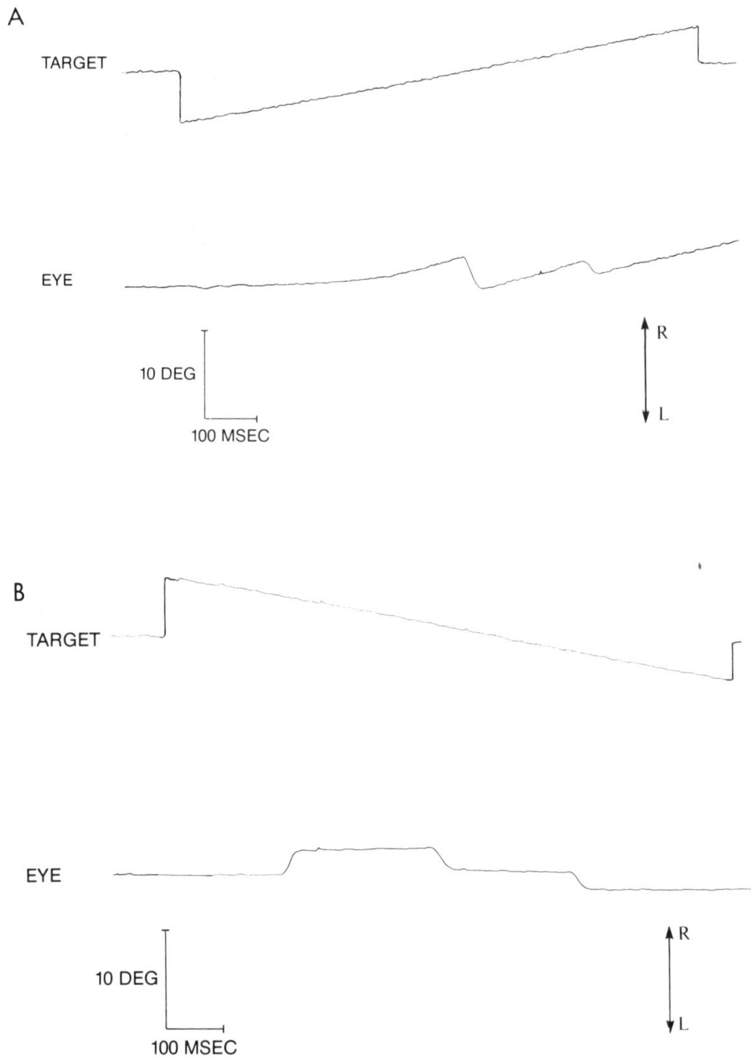

FIG 10–1.
Pursuit initiation in response to step-ramp stimuli. Magnetic search coil recordings of eye movements to target steps away from fixation (6° to the left and right, respectively), followed by constant velocity ramps of 10°/sec toward fixation in patient with left parietotemporal lesion. (**A,** normal response: eyes beginning to accelerate to the right approximately 200 msec after target ramp begins. A corrective saccade follows the initial acceleration to foveate the target. **B,** abnormal response: minimal smooth eye acceleration to the left. Multiple saccades are used to refixate the target.

small target steps, a small initial acceleration may be elicited in the direction of the position error.[10, 48] Robinson and colleagues[25] suggested that the initial response to target position error might result from central interpretation of a small target jump as a velocity error. Initial eye acceleration is delayed for 100–125 msec after a target moves; because of this latency, the first 100–125 msec of the acceleration reflects the response of the pursuit system to the target motion that occurred while the eyes were still.[8, 20] That is, the initial acceleration response to target motion is a measure of the system response before it begins to correct retinal slip. Responses to retinal images located away from the fovea can be measured using step-ramp stimuli. Targets that move rapidly toward the fovea elicit faster initial acceleration responses than those moving away, and targets close to the fovea evoke faster accelerations than eccentric targets.[8, 9]

Saccadic pursuit of slowly moving targets indicates paresis of smooth pursuit, which corresponds to subnormal smooth eye movement gain. Pursuit paresis is a sensitive indicator of brain dysfunction. Saccadic pursuit in all directions does not specify involvement of any particular neural structures, since much of the brain seems to participate in generating pursuit. Focal brain lesions typically cause asymmetric pursuit. Analyses of steady-state pursuit reveal two fundamental patterns of dysfunction. Gain may be preferentially lowered at high target accelerations,[38, 40] indicating that the deficit is subnormal acceleration saturation. In other cases, pursuit gain is uniformly low at all target velocities, implying involvement of an element controlling the steady-state gain of the system.[38, 49] Both low steady-state gain and subnormal acceleration saturation occur in some conditions.[38, 40, 50, 51] Analysis of pursuit initiation[8, 9, 20, 52, 53] offers a means of measuring the system before eye velocity is fed back to alter subsequent eye motion. It thereby reveals the open loop operation of brain pathways that generate pursuit, and it assesses motion detection qualities of the brain.[52, 53] This motion detection is an operation of the afferent limb of the pursuit system.

ANATOMICAL CONSIDERATIONS

Afferent Pursuit Pathways

The afferent limb of the smooth pursuit system comprises the pathway from retina to lateral geniculate nucleus, to striate cortex, and then to extrastriate visual areas. At least 13 discrete cortical areas with retinotopic "maps" of the visual fields have been identified in the monkey; these are organized into two parallel pathways, one concerned with analyzing motion, the other with processing form and color.[54–56] The striate visual cortex relays signals to ipsilateral parietal and temporal lobe cortex.[56] Visual information that mediates ocular tracking is also transmitted to the opposite cerebral hemisphere via the corpus callosum.[57] A proposed scheme for the flow of information from afferent to efferent pursuit pathways is presented in Figure 10–2.

In the monkey, the motion detection pathway includes the middle temporal visual area (MT) of the superior temporal sulcus, which receives inputs from striate cortex. From MT, signals are relayed to adjacent areas of the superior temporal sulcus and parietal cortex. These adjacent pathways include the middle superior temporal visual area (MST) and inferior parietal lobule (IPL or area 7a).[56] Both MST and IPL project to the frontal eye fields.[56, 58] MT, MST, and IPL contain neurons that respond selectively to image motion on the retina and are direction sensitive.[54, 59, 60] Although these regions are fairly well defined in the monkey, their homologues in the human cerebral cortex are uncertain.

Lesions of simian striate cortex or MT cause pursuit deficits that

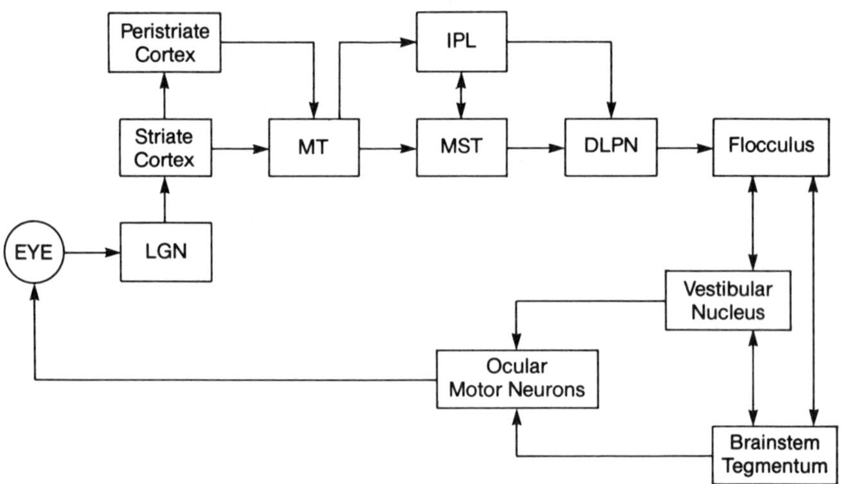

FIG 10–2.

Putative pursuit pathway. Scheme of cortical hierarchy of visual motion processing and motor pathways for smooth pursuit, based on experimental data in monkeys. Homologous areas in man are uncertain. *LGN,* lateral geniculate nucleus; *MT,* middle temporal area of superior temporal sulcus; *MST,* middle superior temporal area; *IPL,* inferior parietal lobule; *DLPN,* dorsolateral pontine nucleus.

are related to target position on the retina; pursuit eye movements achieve normal speed and accuracy unless the target falls on the region of the visual field represented by the damaged area.[53, 61] In contrast, lesions of area MST cause defective ipsilateral pursuit independent of target location on the retina.[62] While striate cortex and MT have a sensory role in pursuit, MST and IPL seem to participate at a stage that is neither purely sensory nor purely motor. Unilateral lesions of the frontal eye fields cause ipsilateral pursuit defects, whereas bilateral lesions cause severe, symmetric disturbances.[63, 64] Combined lesions of the frontal eye fields and IPL cause greater impairment than either alone,[65] implying redundancy of their function.

Efferent Pursuit Pathways

The cerebral cortex projects to the cerebellum and brain stem through specific corticopontocerebellar pathways. Neurons of IPL and MST project to the ipsilateral dorsolateral pontine nucleus (DLPN).[56, 66] Neurons in DLPN encode signals related to target direction, velocity, and position.[67, 68] The DLPN projects to the cerebellar flocculus and vermis.[69] Stimulation of the cerebellar flocculus, vermis, and certain hemispheric areas elicits smooth eye movements.[70] This implicates a pathway from the cerebellum to brain stem circuits that generates these eye movements (see Fig 10–2). The flocculus and vermis receive inputs that encode eye and target velocity and provide outputs that govern smooth pursuit.[71, 72]

Axons from the flocculus inhibit neurons in the medial vestibular nucleus.[73] These vestibular neurons discharge in relation to smooth pursuit and VOR movements. Chemical lesions of the simian medial vestibular nucleus and nucleus propositus hypoglossi abolish the position component of horizontal pursuit responses[74] to optokinetic stimulation. The conversion of eye velocity commands to eye position commands is performed by the mathematical process of integration. In the absence of a position command, the eyes drift back toward the orbital midposition at a rate determined by the elastic restoring forces of orbital soft tissue and ocular muscles. Lesions of the prepositus hypoglossi and medial vestibular nuclei also eliminate eye position holding after horizontal saccades and VOR stimulation,[74] indicating that these structures compose the final common integrator of horizontal eye velocity commands. Both the eye velocity command and the integrated eye position command are transmitted to ocular motor neurons.

Another area located ventral to the abducens nucleus contains neurons which increase their firing rate during ipsilateral smooth pursuit.[75] Cells of the dentate nucleus and the y-group of the vestibular nuclear complex increase their rates of discharge during upward smooth pursuit and stimulation of neurons at these sites produces smooth upward eye movements.[76] The interstitial nucleus of Cajal[77] also contains neurons that modulate their firing during vertical smooth pursuit. The medial longitudinal fasciculus and probably the brachium conjunctivum relay vertical pursuit commands rostrally from the vestibular nuclei and y-group to vertically acting motor neurons in the third and fourth nerve nuclei.[78–80] Apart from these pathways, precise routes by which motor commands are relayed to ocular motor neurons are uncertain. Several redundant parallel pathways probably compose the efferent limb of the pursuit system. Physiologic roles of other structures, such as the basal ganglia,[45, 49] that participate in pursuit are unknown.

CLINICAL CONSIDERATIONS

Cerebral Hemispheric Lesions

Extensive unilateral cerebral hemispheric lesions profoundly impair ipsilateral pursuit,[81, 82] but contralateral pursuit gain can actually be higher than the ideal value of unity.[50, 81] This gain asymmetry is associated with slow contralateral drift of the eyes; corrective fast phases produce ipsilateral beating nystagmus that we call pursuit paretic nystagmus. The drift is not fast enough to explain the augmentation of contralateral pursuit gain.[50] In addition to ipsilateral pursuit defects, extensive unilateral cortical ablations in monkeys produce subnormal velocity saturation of contralateral pursuit, although eye velocities up to the saturation point exceed target velocities.[83] Vertical pursuit in either direction is also significantly impaired. Although the contralateral and vertical pursuit impairment resolves, it suggests that each hemisphere participates in horizontal high-velocity pursuit in both directions and in vertical pursuit. In humans who have undergone surgical hemidecortication for epilepsy, ipsilateral gain is impaired at all target velocities,[81] suggesting involvement of steady-state gain. Retention of some ipsilateral pursuit after hemidecortication implicates redundant pursuit pathways, either in subcortical structures or in the contralateral hemisphere. The following case illustrates the effects of a large cerebral hemispheric lesion on pursuit.

A 35-year-old man presented with right visual field loss that he noticed at age 18. Examination showed a complete right homonymous hemianopia, spontaneous left beating nystagmus in primary position, and mild right limb clumsiness. Severe leftward pursuit impairment was re corded by the magnetic search coil technique (Fig 10–3). Analysis of pursuit initiation showed marked asymmetry (see Fig 10–1). Radiologic studies revealed a cystic structure within the left parietal and temporal lobes (Fig 10–4).

Isolated parietal lobe lesions cause predominantly ipsilateral pursuit deficits[50, 84–86]; although acute unilateral parietal lobe damage can cause bilateral pursuit defects, oculographic study shows that gain is lower toward the side of the lesion.[85] While extensive parietal lesions may lower ipsilateral pursuit gain at all target velocities,[50] more limited lesions reduce it only at high target accelerations.[40] Parietal lobe lesions also decrease initial eye acceleration toward the side of damage.[50] These pursuit asymmetries are independent of hemianopic vi-

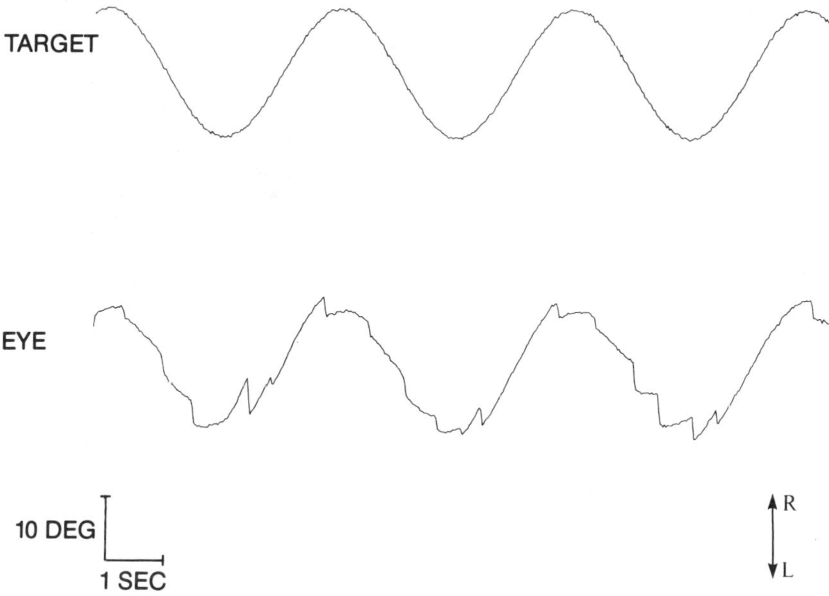

FIG 10–3.
Steady-state sinusoidal pursuit response of patient with left parietotemporal lesion using magnetic search coil technique. Stimulus is a sine wave target with 20° peak-to-peak amplitude at 0.25 Hz. Smooth eye velocities to the right exceed target velocity, requiring "back-up" saccades. To the left, "catch-up" saccades are necessary due to eye velocity being slower than target velocity.

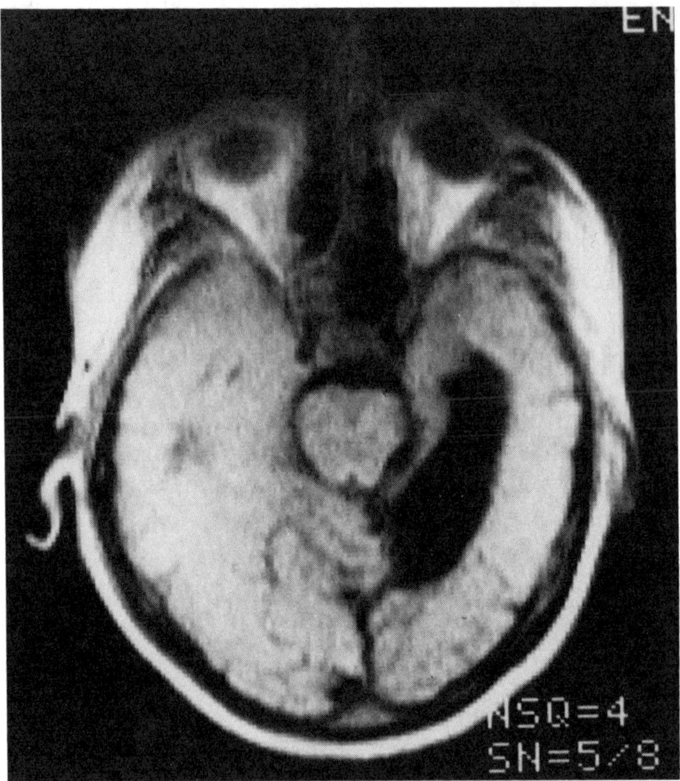

FIG 10–4.
Magnetic resonance image showing large cystic structure involving deep temporal and parietal lobes of left hemisphere of the patient whose oculographic records are shown in Figures 10–1 and 10–3.

sual field defects, which are often associated, since patients with hemianopia can have symmetric smooth pursuit[87] and patients without hemianopia can have asymmetric pursuit.[50, 85] In monkeys, smooth pursuit is present after bilateral striate cortex ablation, suggesting that accessory visual pathways and extrastriate cortex are sufficient to generate it.[88] Since reports of pursuit deficits from parietal lobe lesions in humans have not correlated quantitative oculography with pathologic localization, homologues of the human and simian cortical topography concerned with pursuit remain uncertain. One report[89] suggests that a small area including superior parietal lobule and angular gyrus is crucial for pursuit in man.

Frontal lobe lesions may cause horizontal pursuit paresis that appears to be symmetric on clinical examination, but quantitative eye movement recordings demonstrate lower pursuit gain toward the side of damage.[90, 91] Lesions in the posterior thalamus cause ipsilateral pursuit gain reduction.[92, 93] This may be caused by involvement of descending corticopontine fibers[66] or by damage to the pulvinar, which transmits and receives fibers from MT.[56]

Omnidirectional pursuit paresis occurs in diffuse neurodegenerative diseases (Table 10–1), but patterns of dysfunction differ. For example, in Parkinson's disease[49] and progressive supranuclear palsy,[94] pursuit gain is reduced at all target velocities, implicating the basal ganglia in the control of the steady-state gain element of pursuit. Huntington's disease also impairs pursuit.[95] In Alzheimer's disease, pursuit gain is reduced uniformly for a variety of target velocities, but, in addition, when target velocity is held constant and target acceleration is increased, pursuit gain decreases markedly.[96] The cortical degeneration of Alzheimer's disease involves both the gain element of pursuit

TABLE 10–1.
Smooth Pursuit Paresis

Unidirectional (ipsilateral)
Parietal lobe lesions
Posterior thalamic lesions
Midbrain and pontine tegmental lesions
Cerebellar lesions, particularly floccular
Omnidirectional
Diffuse cerebral, cerebellar or brain stem disease
Alzheimer's disease
Parkinson's disease
Huntington's disease
Progressive supranuclear palsy
Psychiatric disorders (schizophrenia, affective disorders)
Cerebellar degenerations
Sedative-hypnotic or anticonvulsant drugs
Alcohol
Barbiturates
Benzodiazepines
Carbamazepine
Chloral hydrate
Lithium
Methadone
Phenytoin
Senescence
Inattention, fatigue

and the saturating nonlinear element that limits smooth eye acceleration.

Numerous qualitative studies in the psychiatric literature suggest that defective pursuit accompanies schizophrenia.[36, 41, 97] Reduced gain is also reported in unaffected relatives of schizophrenics.[98] Recent quantitative studies[98, 99] of smooth pursuit gain indicate that paresis of smooth pursuit, not related to drug effects, does occur in schizophrenics, but that it is nonspecific, as it also occurs in affective disorders.

Brain Stem Lesions

Information concerning midbrain pathways that transmit pursuit commands from the cerebral cortex to the pontine tegmentum is meager. Matsuo et al.[100] reported loss of pursuit after unilateral destruction of the medial pretectum. This deficit did not occur with kainic acid lesions of this area. Since kainic acid kills local neurons but spares axons of remote neurons, this suggests that axons mediating smooth pursuit traverse the medial pretectum. In patients with unilateral lesions of the midbrain reticular formation, Zackon and Sharpe[101] identified impaired pursuit in both horizontal directions, but ipsilateral pursuit gain was lower. Unilateral lesions of the pontine tegmentum abolish ipsilateral pursuit[102] but both bidirectional pursuit paresis from unilateral caudal pontine damage[103] and contralateral pursuit paresis from unilateral rostral pontine damage[104] have been reported in patients. These observations suggest the possibility of a double decussation of pursuit pathways as they descend from the midbrain to the caudal pontine tegmentum.[102] However, ipsilateral projections from the cerebral hemisphere to the cerebellum and brain stem are consistent with most observations from human and animal studies.

Chemical lesions of the paramedian pontine reticular formation with kainic acid abolish saccades but preserve smooth pursuit and the VOR in monkeys.[105] Selective infarction of the midline and paramedian pontine reticular formation, confirmed by neuropathologic study in one patient, caused paralysis of saccades and nystagmus fast phases in all directions, while sparing smooth pursuit and the VOR.[106] These findings demonstrate that the paramedian pontine reticular formation contains neurons which generate saccades but not smooth eye movements. No focal brain stem lesion has been documented to cause an isolated deficit of smooth pursuit without affecting other smooth eye movements or saccades.

Paralysis or reduced gain of upward smooth pursuit is caused by dorsal midbrain lesions.[102, 107] Both upward and downward pursuit palsies result from ventral midbrain damage confined to the paramedian tegmentum.[108] Lesions of the medial longitudinal fasciculus cause both internuclear ophthalmoplegia and paresis of vertical smooth eye movements[109, 110]; this attests to the importance of the medial longitudinal fasciculus as an ascending tract carrying vertical pursuit commands.[78, 79] Neuropathologic correlations with quantitative eye movement recordings will be required to establish roles of other brain stem structures in the regulation of smooth pursuit.

Cerebellar Lesions

Diffuse cerebellar degenerations cause omnidirectional pursuit paresis.[51, 111, 112] Horizontal and vertical pursuit is impaired only at high target velocities in mild disease, while it is equally deranged for all velocities in more advanced degeneration.[51] Horizontal pursuit is symmetrically impaired, but vertical pursuit is worse downward.[51] Hemicerebellectomy in monkeys severely degrades ipsilateral pursuit.[113] Bilateral ablation of the flocculus and paraflocculus[114] causes less pursuit paresis than does total cerebellectomy,[115] implying that other cerebellar regions participate in generating pursuit. Cerebellopontine angle tumors can impair pursuit ipsilaterally or bilaterally[116, 117]; ipsilateral pursuit impairment is likely the result of compression of the ipsilateral flocculus, while bilateral impairment has been attributed to brain stem and bilateral floccular compression.[117]

Unilateral infarction of the rostral cerebellum, in the distribution of the superior cerebellar artery, causes asymmetry of the amplitude of saccades. Contralateral saccades are hypermetric and ipsilateral saccades are hypometric[118]; this saccadic asymmetry causes spurious pursuit asymmetry. Although pursuit gain is lowered equally in both horizontal directions, larger amplitude contralateral catch-up saccades and undershooting ipsilateral catch-up saccades make the tracking record asymmetric (Fig 10–5). One could sum the amplitudes of all saccades in each direction and subtract the sum from the amplitude of total eye excursion to estimate the efficacy of smooth pursuit. However, measurement of the ratio of smooth eye movement velocity to target velocity is less demanding. Determination of actual smooth eye movement gain, rather than estimates of the frequency or amplitudes of catch-up saccades, readily detects genuine smooth pursuit asymmetry.

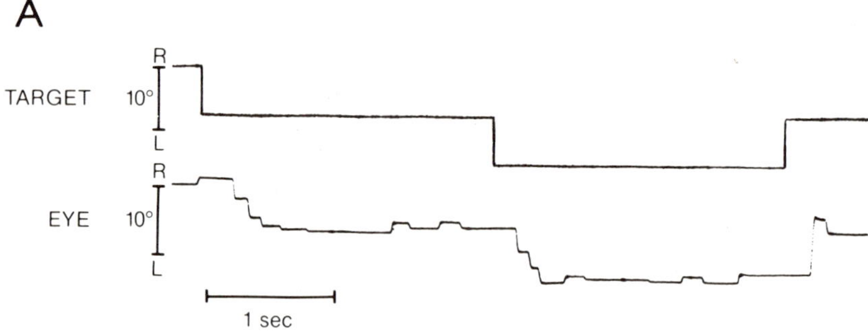

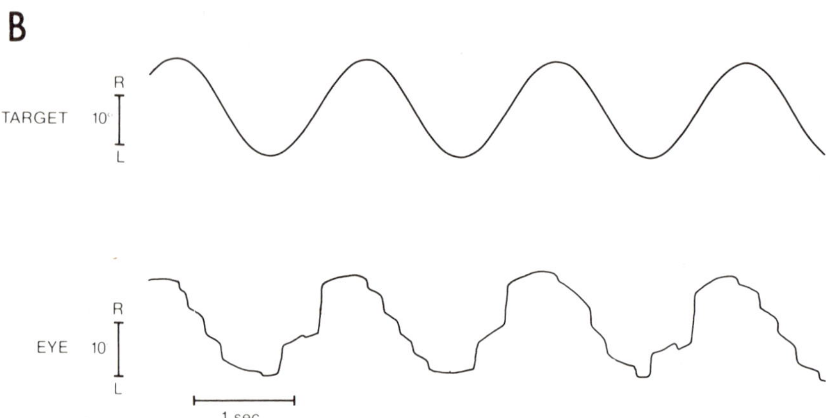

FIG 10–5.
Oculographic recording in rostral cerebellar infarction from occlusion of left superior cerebellar artery. **A,** saccades contralateral to the cerebellar infarct (rightward) overshoot the target, and saccades ipsilateral to the infarct are hypometric. **B,** horizontal pursuit shows compensatory catch-up saccades in both directions. Although actual smooth pursuit velocities were symmetric to the right and left, the hypermetric rightward saccades and the hypometric leftward saccades caused a spurious appearance of smooth pursuit asymmetry. (Adapted from Ranalli PJ, Sharpe JA: Contrapulsion of saccades and ipsilateral ataxia: A unilateral disorder of the rostral cerebellum. *Ann Neurol* 1986; 20:311–316. Used by permission.)

Pursuit Paresis Caused By Drugs

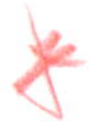

Asymmetry of pursuit signifies a focal brain lesion, while omnidirectional pursuit paresis is a common manifestation of diffuse brain disease. However, drugs are the most frequent cause of omnidirectional pursuit impairment in otherwise neurologically intact patients.

Most medications that are known to degrade smooth pursuit are sedatives or anticonvulsants (see Table 10–1). Rigorous quantitative oculographic study demonstrates that alcohol[119] impairs smooth pursuit. Less quantitative studies suggest that methadone,[120] chloral hydrate,[121] benzodiazepines,[43, 122] barbiturates,[122, 123] and lithium[124] reduce smooth pursuit gain. Qualitative evidence is available to support clinical observation that phenytoin[125] and carbamazepine[126] also degrade pursuit. Medications which impair pursuit gain tend to do so at all target velocities.[43, 119, 120]

Aging and Smooth Pursuit

Smooth pursuit is an age-dependent motor system. Compared with young adults, smooth pursuit gain is significantly reduced in subjects over age 65.[3, 127, 128] The latency of initiation of pursuit is increased in the elderly.[3] The efficacy of pursuing sinusoidal and triangular waveform targets was compared in a study of middle-aged (mean age, 50) and elderly subjects (mean age, 77) in our laboratory.[38] All smooth eye movements were matched with corresponding target velocities to compute gain throughout the target excursions; saccades were removed. Pursuit of both triangular and sinusoidal targets had lower gain in the elderly. Triangular pursuit gain was lower than sinusoidal pursuit gain (Fig 10–6). The difference was attributed to very high acceleration demands of triangular waveforms at their turnaround points; sinusoidal target motion imposes smoothly changing and smaller acceleration demands. We advocate the use of sine wave targets in clinical laboratory tests of the pursuit system, since the effects of acceleration on smooth eye movements can be assessed by changing the frequency or amplitude of target motion. This is appropriate, because the normal pursuit system responds to changes in target velocity with changes in eye velocity.[6]

When sine wave targets having the same peak velocities are presented at varying amplitudes and frequencies (Fig 10–7), the pattern of eye motion appears different (compare Fig 10–7A, B, and C, where targets have peak velocities of 31°/sec), although smooth eye movement gain is virtually the same. Laboratory workers cannot simply inspect oculographic tracings to reliably determine that smooth pursuit is impaired. Comparison of pursuit at fixed target frequencies shows a uniform reduction in gain, independent of target velocity, in the elderly (Fig 10–8). Although velocity saturation occurs in young subjects when they track large-amplitude ramp targets over 90°/sec,[7] no velocity saturation is reached at target velocities up to 63°/sec in

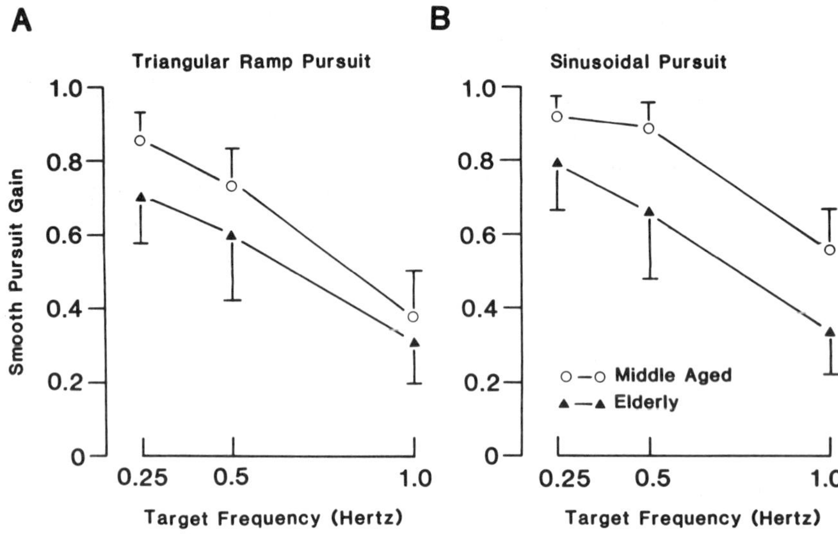

FIG 10–6.
Plots of smooth pursuit gain vs. target frequency for triangular pursuit **(A)** and sinusoidal pursuit **(B)** in 10 middle-aged *(open circles)* and 11 elderly *(filled triangles)* subjects. Target amplitudes are ± 10°. *Error bars* indicate 1 SD. (From Zackon DH, Sharpe JA: Smooth pursuit in senescence: Effects of target velocity and acceleration. *Acta Otolaryngol (Stockh)* 1987; 104:290–297. Used by permission.)

middle-aged or elderly subjects.[38] However, when target acceleration is increased to 795°/sec^2 under conditions of identical peak target velocity, smooth eye movement velocity does fall in the elderly (Fig 10–9)[38] to values well below those in young subjects.[6] Senescent tracking is degraded by involvement of the steady-state gain element of the pursuit system at low target acceleration demands and by acceleration saturation at high demands.

Cerebral cortical atrophy,[129] cerebellar Purkinje cell loss[130] and atrophy of extraocular muscles[131] are senescent changes that could affect the steady-state gain. In addition, loss of neurons in the nigrostriatal pathway[132] is a feature of aging that might alter the gain element in a manner analogous to that proposed for pursuit impairment in Parkinson's disease.[49] Loss of cerebral cortical neurons is probably the structural correlate of lowered acceleration responses[38] in aging, as in parietal lobe lesions and Alzheimer's disease. These experiments indicate that the diagnosis of impaired pursuit must be qualified by the age of the patient before it can be attributed to drugs or brain disease.

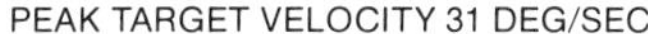

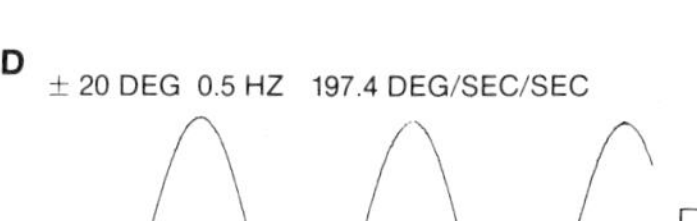

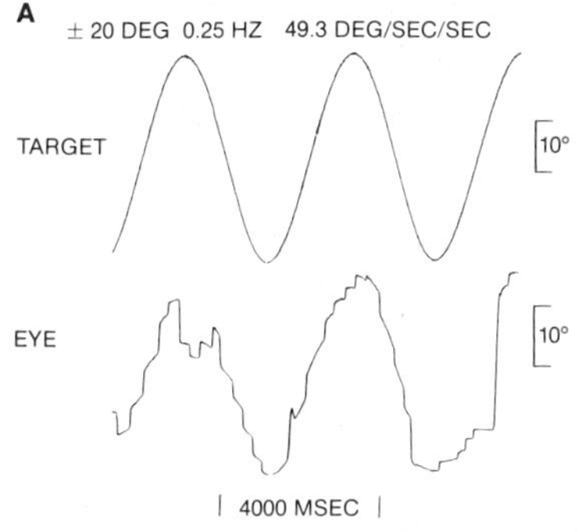

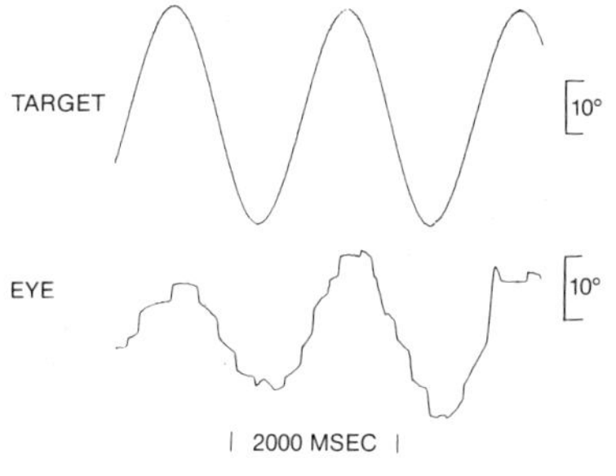

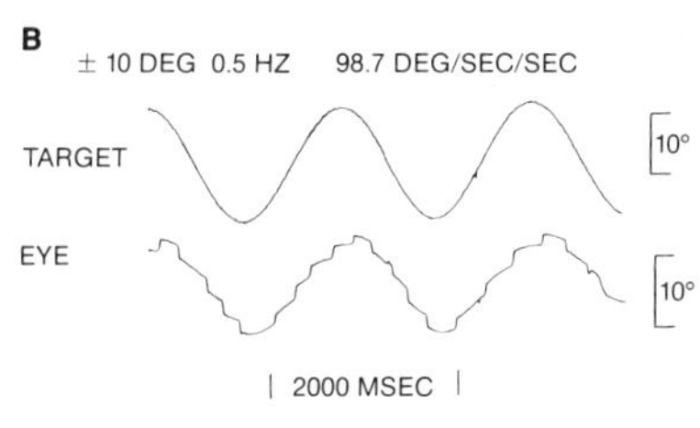

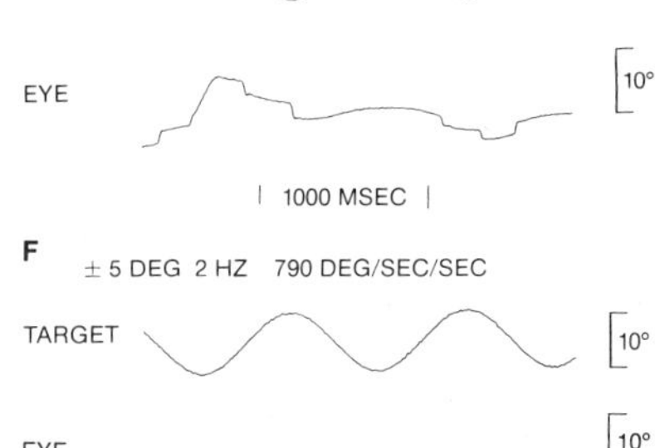

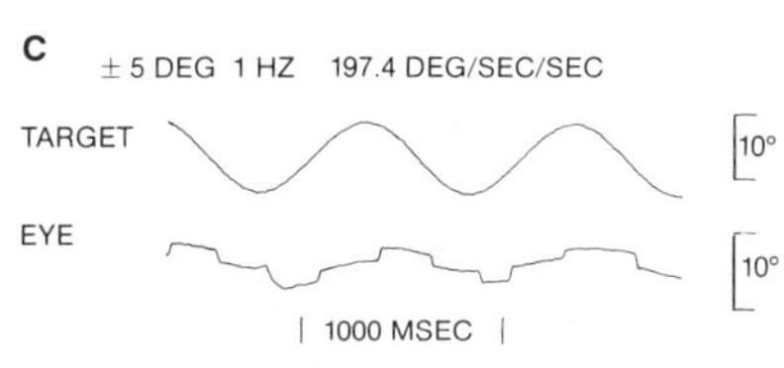

FIG 10–7.
Tracking records of an elderly male subject for targets having uniform peak velocities of 31 °/sec **(left column, A–C)** and 63°/sec **(right column, D–F)** at different frequencies and amplitudes with increasing target accelerations. Although tracking records appeared different, actual smooth eye movement velocity gain did not fall appreciably until target accelerations reached 395° and 790°/sec^2 (**E** and **F**). (Adapted from Zackon DH, Sharpe JA: Smooth pursuit in senescence: Effects of target velocity and acceleration. *Acta Otolaryngol (Stockh)* 1987; 104:290–297.

SUMMARY

Sustained foveation of slowly moving targets is the cardinal function of smooth pursuit. The pursuit system responds primarily to retinal velocity errors, and its response is limited by acceleration and

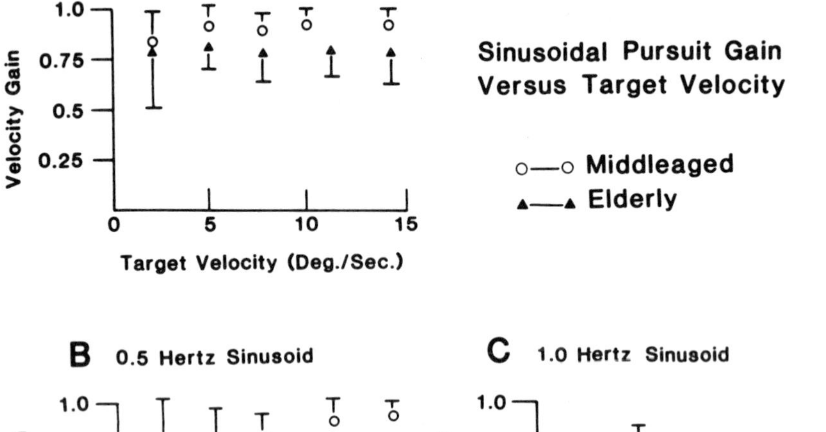

FIG 10–8.
Smooth pursuit gain is plotted against target velocity for sinusoidal targets at fixed frequencies (**A,** 0.25 Hz; **B,** 0.5 Hz; **C,** 1.0 Hz). Target amplitudes are ± 10°. Elderly subjects show uniform reduction in the steady-state gain at different target velocities at each frequency. Values are means for 10 middle-aged and 11 elderly subjects. *Error bars* signify 1 SD. (From Zackon DH, Sharpe JA: Smooth pursuit in senescence: Effects of target velocity and acceleration. *Acta Otolaryngol (Stockh)* 1987; 104:290–297. Used by permission.)

velocity saturation. Smooth pursuit is quantified by its gain, the ratio of smooth eye movement velocity to target velocity. Analysis of the initiation of pursuit can assess the open loop operation and motion detection properties of the system. Afferent pursuit pathways that participate in target motion analysis include the inferior parietal and superior temporal lobes. These cortical regions relay pursuit commands to the dorsolateral pons and cerebellar flocculus. Velocity commands are transmitted to the brain stem, where they are integrated to eye position commands in the medial vestibular and prepositus hypoglossi nuclei. Position and velocity commands are then delivered to ocular motor neurons.

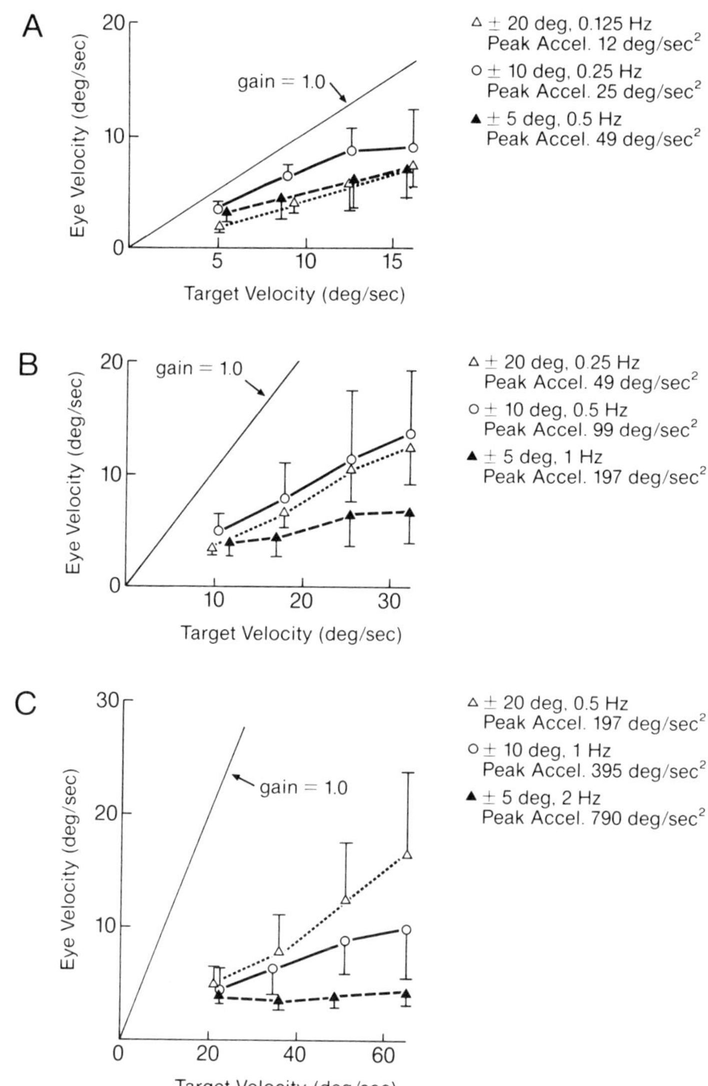

FIG 10–9.
Under conditions of identical *peak* target velocities (**A,** 16°/sec; **B,** 31°/sec; and **C,** 63°/sec), smooth eye movement velocities do not saturate as target velocity increases within a sinusoid. Smooth pursuit velocities are significantly reduced when target acceleration increases to 790°/sec^2. *Error bars* indicate 1 SD. Values are means for 4 elderly subjects (average age, 81 years). (From Zackon DH, Sharpe JA: Smooth pursuit in senescence: Effects of target velocity and acceleration. *Acta Otolaryngol (Stockh)* 1987; 104:290–297. Used by permission.)

Cerebral hemispheric lesions, principally those involving the parietal lobe, lower ipsilateral pursuit gain and acceleration saturation. Cerebral hemispheric degenerations impair smooth pursuit in all directions. Unilateral lesions of the midbrain and pontine tegmentum lower ipsilateral pursuit gain. Internuclear ophthalmoplegia is associated with paresis of vertical pursuit. Dorsal midbrain lesions may impair upward pursuit, while ventral midbrain lesions cause paresis of upward and downward pursuit. Cerebellar lesions, particularly those involving the vestibulocerebellum, degrade ipsilateral pursuit. Advancing age and many sedative and anticonvulsant drugs impair pursuit in all directions. Smooth pursuit paresis is a most sensitive indicator of brain dysfunction. It is detected clinically by the presence of saccadic tracking of slowly moving targets and quantified readily by oculography.

REFERENCES

1. Murphy BJ: Pattern thresholds for moving and stationary gratings during smooth eye movements. *Vision Res* 1978; 18:521–530.
2. Robinson DA: The mechanics of human smooth pursuit eye movement. *J Physiol (Lond)* 1965; 180:569–591.
3. Sharpe JA, Sylvester TO: Effect of aging on horizontal smooth pursuit. *Invest Ophthalmol Vis Sci* 1978; 17:465–468.
4. Kowler E, Murphy BJ, Steinman RM: Velocity matching during smooth pursuit of different targets on different backgrounds. *Vision Res* 1978; 18:603–605.
5. Collewijn H, Tamminga EP: Human smooth and saccadic eye movements during voluntary pursuit of different target motions on different backgrounds. *J Physiol (Lond)* 1984; 351:217–250
6. Lisberger SG, Evinger C, Johanson GW, et al: Relationship between eye acceleration and retinal image velocity during foveal smooth pursuit in man and monkey. *J Neurophysiol* 1981; 46:229–249.
7. Meyer CH, Lasker AG, Robinson DA: The upper limit of human smooth pursuit velocity. *Vision Res* 1985; 25:561–563.
8. Lisberger SG, Westbrook LE: Properties of visual inputs that initiate horizontal smooth pursuit in monkeys. *J Neurosci* 1985; 5:1662–1673.
9. Tychsen L, Lisberger SG: Visual motion processing for the initiation of smooth-pursuit eye movements in humans. *J Neurophysiol* 1986; 56:953–968.
10. Pola J, Wyatt HJ: Target position and velocity: The stimuli for smooth pursuit eye movements. *Vision Res* 1980; 20:523–534.
11. Kommerell G, Taumer R: Investigations of the eye tracking system through stabilized retinal images. *Bibl Ophthalmol* 1972; 82:288–297.

12. Kaufman SR, Abel LA: The effects of distraction on smooth pursuit of normal subjects. *Acta Otolaryngol (Stockh)* 1986; 102:57–64.
13. Yee RD, Daniels SA, Jones OW, et al: Effects of an optokinetic background on pursuit eye movements. *Invest Ophthalmol Vis Sci* 1983; 24:1115–1122.
14. Keller EL, Khan NS: Smooth-pursuit initiation in the presence of a textured background in the monkey. *Vision Res* 1986; 26:943–955.
15. Heywood S: Voluntary control of smooth eye movements and their velocities. *Nature* 1972; 238:408–410.
16. Heywood S, Churcher J: Eye movements and the afterimage—I. Tracking the afterimage. *Vision Res* 1971; 11:1163–1168.
17. Michael JA, Melvill Jones G: Dependence of visual tracking capability upon stimulus predictability. *Vision Res* 1966; 6:707–716.
18. Bahill TA, McDonald JD: Smooth pursuit eye movements in response to predictable target motions. *Vision Res* 1983; 23:1573–1583.
19. Becker W, Fuchs AF: Prediction in the oculomotor system: Smooth pursuit during transient disappearance of a visual target. *Exp Brain Res* 1985; 57:562–575.
20. Lisberger SG, Morris EJ, Tychsen L: Visual motion processing and sensory-motor integration for smooth pursuit eye movements. *Ann Rev Neurosci* 10:97–129, 1987
21. Gauthier GM, Hofferer J-M: Eye tracking of self-moved targets in the absence of vision. *Exp Brain Res* 1976; 26:121–139.
22. Ward R, Morgan MJ: Perceptual effect of pursuit eye movements in the absence of a target. *Nature* 1978; 274:158–159.
23. Steinbach MJ: Pursuing the perceptual rather than the retinal stimulus. *Vision Res* 1976; 16:1371–1376.
24. Behrens F, Collewijn H, Grusser O-J: Velocity step responses of the human gaze pursuit system: Experiments with sigma-movement. *Vision Res* 1985; 25:893–905.
25. Robinson DA, Gordon JL, Gordon SE: A model of the smooth pursuit eye movement system. *Biol Cybern* 1986; 55:43–57.
26. Yasui S, Young LR: Perceived visual motion as effective stimulus to pursuit eye movement system. *Science* 1975; 190:906–908.
27. Optican LM, Zee DS, Chu FC: Adaptive responses to ocular muscle weakness in human pursuit and saccadic eye movements. *J Neurophysiol* 1985; 54:110–122.
28. Le Grand Y: Spectral luminosity, in Jameson LM, Hurvich M (eds): *Handbook of Sensory Physiology*. Berlin, Springer, 1972, vol 7, pp 413–433.
29. Winterson BJ, Steinman RM: The effect of luminance on human smooth pursuit of perifoveal and foveal targets. *Vision Res* 1978; 18:1165–1172.
30. Robinson DA: A method of measuring eye movement using a scleral search coil in a magnetic field. *IEEE Trans Biomed Elec* 1963; BME-10:137–144.

31. Collewijn H, Van Der Mark R, Jansen TC: Precise recording of human eye movements. *Vision Res* 1975; 15:447–450.
32. Leigh RJ, Sharpe JA, Ranalli PJ, et al: Comparison of smooth pursuit and combined eye-head tracking in human subjects with deficient labyrinthine function. *Exp Brain Res* 1987; 66:458–464.
33. Collewijn H, Conijn P, Tamminga EP: Eye-head coordination in man during the pursuit of moving targets, in Lennerstrand G, Zee DS, Keller EL (eds): *Functional Basis of Ocular Motility Disorders*. Oxford, Pergamon Press, 1982, pp 369–378.
34. Baloh RW, Konrad HR, Sills AW, et al: Quantitative measurement of smooth pursuit eye movements. *Ann Otol Rhinol Laryngol* 1976; 85:111–119.
35. Schalen L: Quantification of tracking eye movements in normal subjects. *Acta Otolaryngol (Stockh)* 1980; 90:404–413.
36. Shagass C, Roemer RA, Amadeo M: Eye-tracking performance and engagement of attention. *Arch. Gen. Psychiatry* 1976; 33:121–125.
37. Tomlinson RD, Blakeman A: A finite impulse response filter for the computer analysis of eye movement recordings, in preparation.
38. Zackon DH, Sharpe JA: Smooth pursuit in senescence: Effects of target velocity and acceleration. *Acta Otolaryngol (Stockh)* 1987; 104:290–297.
39. Meiry JL: The vestibular system and human dynamic space orientation. *Washington DC NASA CR* 628, 1966.
40. Leigh RJ, Tusa RJ: Disturbance of smooth pursuit caused by infarction of occipitoparietal cortex. *Ann Neurol* 1985; 17:185–187.
41. Holzmann PS, Proctor LR, Hughes DW: Eye-tracking patterns in schizophrenia. *Science* 1973; 181:179–181.
42. Hutton JT, Nagel JA, Loewenson RB: Eye-tracking dysfunction in Alzheimer's type dementia. *Neurology* 1984; 34:99–102.
43. Rothenberg SJ, Selkoe D: Specific oculomotor deficit after diazepam: II. Smooth pursuit eye movements. *Psychopharmacology* 1981; 74:237–240.
44. Ziegler AS, Abel LA, Dell'Osso LF: To say "bad" isn't good enough—non-specificity of the LN (S/N) ratio for smooth pursuit analysis. *Invest Ophthalmol Vis Sci* 1986; 27(suppl):58.
45. Melvill Jones G, DeJong JD: Visual tracking of sinusoidal target movement in Parkinson's disease, in *D.R.B. Aviation Medical Research Unit (Department of Physiology)*. Montreal, McGill University, 1974–1976, vol 5, pp 271–288.
46. Thickbroom GW, Black JJ: Eye motion kinetics in moving target pursuit: A system for detection of oculomotor abnormalities in neurological disorders. *Int J Biomed Comput* 1980; 11:427–439.
47. Rashbass C: The relationship between saccadic and smooth pursuit tracking eye movements. *J Physiol (Lond)* 1961; 159:326–338.
48. Carl JR, Gellman RS: Adaptive responses in human smooth pursuit, in

Keller EL, Zee DS (eds): *Adaptive Processes in Visual and Oculomotor Systems.* Oxford, Pergamon Press, 1986, pp 335–339.

49. White OB, Saint-Cyr JA, Tomlinson RD, et al: Ocular motor deficits in Parkinson's disease: II. Control of the saccadic and smooth pursuit systems. *Brain* 1983; 106:571–587.
50. Leigh RJ, Thurston SE: Recovery of ocular motor function in humans with cerebral lesions, in Keller EL, Zee DS (eds): *Adaptive Processes in Visual and Oculomotor Systems.* Oxford, Pergamon Press, 1986, pp 231–238.
51. Zee DS, Yee RD, Cogan DG, et al: Ocular motor abnormalities in hereditary cerebellar ataxia. *Brain* 1976; 99:207–234.
52. Tychsen L, Lisberger SA: Maldevelopment of visual motion processing in humans who had strabismus with onset in infancy. *J Neurosci* 1986; 6:2485–2508.
53. Newsome WT, Wurtz RH, Dursteler MR, et al: Deficits in visual motion processing following ibotenic acid lesions of the medial temporal visual area of the Macaque monkey. *J Neurosci* 1985; 5:825–840.
54. Maunsell JH, Van Essen DC: Functional properties of neurons in middle temporal visual area of the macaque monkey: I. Selectivity for stimulus direction, speed, and orientation. *J Neurophysiol* 1983; 49:1127–1147.
55. Van Essen DC, Maunsell JH: Hierarchical organization and functional streams in the visual cortex. *Trends Neurosci* 1983; 6:370–375.
56. Maunsell JH, Van Essen DC: The connections of the middle temporal visual area (MT) and their relationship to a cortical hierarchy in the macaque monkey. *J Neurosci* 1983; 3:2563–2586.
57. Pasik P, Pasik T: Optokinetic nystagmus: An unlearned responses altered by section of the chiasma and corpus callosum in monkeys. *Nature* 1964; 203:609–611.
58. Pandya DN, Kuypers HG: Cortico-cortical connections in the rhesus monkey. *Brain Res* 1969; 13:13–36.
59. Komatsu H, Wurtz RH: Distribution of pursuit cells in the medial superior temporal area (MST) of the monkey. *Soc Neurosci Abstr* 1986; 12:1182.
60. Sakata H, Shibutani H, Kawano K: Functional properties of visual tracking neurons in posterior parietal association cortex of the monkey. *J Neurophysiol* 1983; 49:1364–1380.
61. Segraves MA, Goldberg ME, Deng S-Y, et al: No notion of motion: Monkeys with unilateral striate lesions have long term deficits in the utilization of stimulus velocity information by the oculomotor system, in Keller EL, Zee DS (eds): *Adaptive Processes in Visual and Oculomotor Systems.* Oxford, Pergamon Press, 1986, pp 217–221.
62. Dursteler MR, Wurtz RH, Yamakazi DS: Pursuit and OKN deficits following ibotenic acid lesions in the medial superior temporal area (MST) of monkey. *Soc Neurosci Abstr* 1986; 16:1182.

63. Keating EG, Gooley SG, Kenny DV: Impaired tracking and loss of predictive eye movements after removal of the frontal eye fields. *Soc Neurosci Abstr* 1985; 11:472.
64. Lynch JC, Allison JC: A quantitative study of visual pursuit deficits following lesions of the frontal eye fields in rhesus monkeys. *Soc Neurosci Abstr* 1985; 15:473.
65. Lynch JC, Allison JC, Hines RS, et al: Oculomotor impairment following combined lesions of parieto-occipital cortex and frontal eye fields in rhesus monkeys. *Soc Neurosci Abstr* 1986; 12:1086.
66. Glickstein M, Cohen JL, Dixon B, et al: Corticopontine visual projections in macaque monkeys. *J Comp Neurol* 1980; 190:209–229.
67. Suzuki DA, Keller EL: Visual signals in the dorsolateral pontine nucleus of the alert monkey: Their relationship to smooth pursuit eye movements. *Exp Brain Res* 1984; 53:473–478.
68. Suzuki DA, Keller EL, Yee RD: Smooth-pursuit eye movement related visual and visuo-motor responses in dorsolateral pontine nucleus of alert monkey. *Soc Neurosci Abstr* 1985; 11:473.
69. Brodal P: Further observations on the cerebellar projections from the pontine nuclei and the nucleus reticularis tegmenti pontis in the rhesus monkey. *J Comp Neurol* 1982; 204:44–55.
70. Ron S, Robinson DA: Eye movements evoked by cerebellar stimulation in the alert monkey. *J Neurophysiol* 1973; 36:1004–1022.
71. Lisberger SG, Fuchs AF: Role of primate flocculus during rapid behavioral modification of vestibulo-ocular reflex: I. Purkinje cell activity during visually guided horizontal smooth-pursuit eye movements and passive head rotation. *J Neurophysiol* 1978; 41:733–763.
72. Suzuki DA, Noda H, Kase M: Visual and pursuit eye movement related activity in the posterior vermis of the cerebellum. *J Neurophysiol* 1981; 46:1120–1139.
73. Lisberger SG, Pavelko TA: Functional properties of brainstem cells inhibited from the cerebellar flocculus in monkey. *Soc Neurosci Abstr* 1984; 10:988.
74. Cannon SC, Robinson DA: The final common integrator is in the prepositus and vestibular nuclei, in Keller EL, Zee DS (eds): *Adaptive Processes in Visual and Oculomotor Systems*. Oxford, Pergamon Press, 1986, pp 307–311.
75. Eckmiller R, Mackeben M: Pre-motor single unit activity in the monkey brainstem correlated with eye velocity during pursuit. *Brain Res* 1980; 184:210–214.
76. Chubb MC, Fuchs AF: Contribution of y group of vestibular nuclei and dentate nucleus of cerebellum to generation of vertical smooth eye movements. *J Neurophysiol* 1982; 48:75–99.
77. King WM, Fuchs AF, Magnin M: Vertical eye movement-related responses of neurons in midbrain near interstitial nucleus of Cajal. *J Neurophysiol* 1981; 46:549–562.

78. Pola J, Robinson DA: Oculomotor signals in the medial longitudinal fasciculus of the monkey. *J Neurophysiol* 1978; 41:245–259.
79. Tomlinson RD, Robinson DA: Signals in the vestibular nucleus mediating vertical eye movements in the monkey. *J Neurophysiol* 1984; 51:1121–1136.
80. Carpenter MB, Cowie RJ: Connections and oculomotor projections of the superior vestibular nucleus and cell group 'y'. *Brain Res* 1985; 336:265–287.
81. Sharpe JA, Lo AW, Rabinovitch HE: Control of the saccadic and smooth pursuit systems after cerebral hemidecortication. *Brain* 1979; 102:387–403.
82. Troost BT, Daroff RB, Weber RB, et al: Hemispheric control of eye movements: II. Quantitative analysis of smooth pursuit in a hemispherectomy patient. *Arch Neurol* 1972; 27:449–452.
83. Tusa RJ, Zee DS, Herdmann SJ: Recovery of oculomotor function in monkeys with large unilateral cortical lesions, in Keller EL, Zee DS (eds): *Adaptive Processes in Visual and Oculomotor Systems.* Oxford, Pergamon Press, 1986, pp 209–216.
84. Larmande P, Prier S, Masson M, et al: Perturbation de la poursuite oculaire et lesions parieto-occipitales unilaterales. *Rev Neurol (Paris)* 1980; 136:345–353.
85. Sharpe JA: Cerebral ocular motor deficits, in Lennerstrand G, Zee DS, Keller EL (eds): *Functional Basis of Ocular Motility Disorders.* Oxford, Pergamon Press, 1982, pp 479–488.
86. Baloh RW, Yee RD, Honrubia V: Optokinetic nystagmus and parietal lobe lesions. *Ann Neurol* 1980; 7:269–276.
87. Sharpe JA, Deck JHN: Destruction of the internal sagittal stratum and normal smooth pursuit. *Ann Neurol* 1978; 4:473–476.
88. Zee DS, Tusa RJ, Herdman SJ, et al: The acute and chronic effects of bilateral occipital lobectomy upon eye movements in monkey, in Keller EL, Zee DS (eds): *Adaptive Processes in Visual and Oculomotor Systems.* Oxford, Pergamon Press, 1986, pp 267–274.
89. Pierrot-Deseilligny C, Gray F, Brunet P: Infarcts of both inferior parietal lobules with impairment of visually guided eye movements, peripheral visual inattention and optic ataxia. *Brain* 1986; 109:81–97.
90. Pyykko I, Dahlen A-I, Schalen L, et al: Eye movements in patients with speech dyspraxia. *Acta Otolaryngol (Stockh)* 1984; 98:481–489.
91. Sharpe JA, Bondar RL, Fletcher WA: Contralateral gaze deviation after frontal lobe haemorrhage. *J Neurol Neurosurg Psychiatry* 1985; 48:86–88.
92. Brigell M, Babikian V, Goodwin JA: Hypometric saccades and low-gain pursuit resulting from a thalamic hemorrhage. *Ann Neurol* 1984; 15:374–378.
93. Hirose G, Kosoegawa H, Saeki M, et al: The syndrome of posterior thalamic hemorrhage. *Neurology* 1985; 35:998–1002.

94. Troost BT, Daroff RB: The ocular motor defects in progressive supranuclear palsy. *Ann Neurol* 1977; 2:397–403.
95. Leigh RJ, Newman SA, Folstein SE, et al: Abnormal ocular motor control in Huntington's disease. *Neurology* 1983; 33:1268–1275.
96. Fletcher WA, Sharpe JA: Smooth pursuit dysfunction in Alzheimer's disease. *Neurology* 1988; 38:272–277.
97. Lipton RB, Levy DL, Holzman PS, et al: Eye movement dysfunction in psychiatric patients: A review. *Schizophr Bull* 1983; 9:13–32.
98. Abel LA, Hertle RW, Meltzer HY: Smooth pursuit in psychiatric disease: Are there specific defects in patients and their relatives? *Soc Neurosci Abstr* 1986; 12:1091.
99. Yee RD, Baloh RW, Marder SR, et al: Eye movements in schizophrenia. *Invest Ophthalmol Vis Sci* 1986; 27(suppl):58.
100. Matsuo V, Buttner-Ennever J, Cohen B, et al: Effect of pretectal lesions on components of the horizontal optokinetic response. *Soc Neurosci Abstr* 1983; 9:749.
101. Zackon DH, Sharpe JA: Midbrain paresis of horizontal gaze. *Ann Neurol* 1984; 16:495–504.
102. Daroff RB, Hoyt HF: Supranuclear disorders of ocular control systems in man: Clinical, anatomical and physiological correlations, in Bach-y-Rita P, Collins CC, Hyde JE (eds): *The Control of Eye Movements*. New York, Academic Press, 1971, pp 175–235.
103. Pierrot-Deseilligny C, Chain F, Serdaru M, et al: The "one and a half syndrome": Electro-oculographic analyses of five cases with deductions about the physiological mechanisms of lateral gaze. *Brain* 1981; 104:665–699.
104. Pierrot-Deseilligny C, Chain F, Gray F, et al: Les paralysies de la lateralite d'origine protuberantielle. *Rev Neurol (Paris)* 1979; 135:741–762.
105. Henn V, Lang W, Hepp K, et al: Experimental gaze palsies in monkeys and their relation to human pathology. *Brain* 1984; 107:619–636.
106. Hanson MR, Hamid MA, Tomsak RL, et al: Selective saccadic palsy caused by pontine lesions: Clinical, physiological, and pathological correlations. *Ann Neurol* 1986; 20:209–217.
107. Baloh RW, Furman JM, Yee RD: Dorsal midbrain syndrome: Clinical and oculographic findings. *Neurology* 1985; 35:54–60.
108. Ranalli PJ, Sharpe JA, Fletcher WA: Palsy of upward and downward saccadic, pursuit and vestibular movements with a unilateral midbrain lesion: Pathophysiological correlations. *Neurology* 1988; 38:114–121.
109. Baloh RW, Yee RD, Honrubia, V: Internuclear ophthalmoplegia: II. Pursuit, optokinetic nystagmus and the vestibulo-ocular reflex. *Arch Neurol* 1984; 35:490–493.
110. Ranalli PJ, Sharpe JA: Vertical vestibulo-ocular reflex dysfunction in internuclear ophthalmoplegia. *Neurology* 1987; 37(suppl 1):307.
111. Baloh RW, Konrad HR, Honrubia V: Vestibulo-ocular function in patients with cerebellar atrophy. *Neurology* 1975; 25:160–168.

112. Baloh RW, Yee RD, Honrubia V: Late cortical cerebellar atrophy: Clinical and oculographic features. *Brain* 1986; 109:159–180.
113. Westheimer G, Blair SM: Functional organization of primate oculomotor system revealed by cerebellectomy. *Exp Brain Res* 1974; 21:463–472.
114. Zee DS, Yamasaki A, Butler PH, et al: Effects of ablations of flocculus and paraflocculus on eye movements in primate. *J Neurophysiol* 1981; 46:878–899.
115. Optican LM, Robinson DA: Cerebellar-dependent adaptive control of primate saccadic system. *J Neurophysiol* 1980; 44:1058–1076.
116. Baloh RW, Konrad HR, Dirks D, et al: Cerebellar-pontine angle tumors: Results of quantitative vestibulo-ocular testing. *Arch Neurol* 1976; 33:507–512.
117. Nedzelski JM: Cerebellopontine angle tumors: Bilateral flocculus compression as cause of associated oculomotor abnormalities. *Laryngoscope* 1983; 93:1251–1260.
118. Ranalli PJ, Sharpe JA: Contrapulsion of saccades and ipsilateral ataxia: A unilateral disorder of the rostral cerebellum. *Ann Neurol* 1986; 20:311–316.
119. Baloh RW, Sharma S, Moskowitz H, et al: Effect of alcohol and marijuana on eye movements. *Aviat Space Environ Med* 1979; 50:18–23.
120. Rothenberg S, Schottenfeld S, Selkoe D, et al: Specific oculomotor deficit ater acute methadone. *Psychopharmacology* 1980; 67:229–234.
121. Levy DL, Lipton RB, Holzman PS: Smooth pursuit eye movements: Effects of alcohol and chloral hydrate. *J Psychiatr Res* 1981; 16:1–11
122. Norris H: The action of sedatives on brain stem oculomotor systems in man. *Neuropharmacology* 1971; 10:181–191.
123. Holzman PS, Levy DL, Uhlenhuth EH, et al: Smooth pursuit eye movements and diazepam, CPZ, and secobarbital. *Psychopharmacology (Berlin)* 1975; 44:111–115.
124. Levy DL, Dorus E, Shaughnessy R, et al: Pharmacologic evidence for specificity of pursuit dysfunction to schizophrenia: Lithium carbonate associated with abnormal pursuit. *Arch Gen Psychiatry* 1985; 42:335–341.
125. Bittencourt RM, Gresty MA, Richens A: Quantitative Assessment of smooth-pursuit eye movements in healthy and epileptic subjects. *J Neurol Neurosurg Psychiatry* 1980; 43:1119–1124.
126. Umeda Y, Sakata E: Equilibrium disorder in carbamazepine toxicity. *Ann Otolaryngol* 1977; 86:318–322.
127. Spooner JN, Sakala SM, Baloh RW: Effect of aging on eye tracking. *Arch Neurol* 1980; 37:575–576.
128. Hutton JT, Nagel JA, Loewenson RB: Variables affecting eye tracking performance. *Electroencephalogr Clin Neurophysiol* 1982; 56:414–419.
129. Creasy H, Rapoport SI: The aging human brain. *Ann Neurol* 1985; 17:2–10.

130. Hall TC, Miller AKH, Corsellis JAN: Variations in the human Purkinje cell population according to age and sex. *Neuropathol Appl Neurobiol* 1975; 1:267–292.
131. Miller JE: Aging changes in extraocular muscle, in Lennerstrand G, Bach-y-Rita P (eds): *Basic Mechanisms of Ocular Motility and their Clinical Implications*. Oxford, Pergamon Press, 1975, pp 47–61.
132. McGeer PL, McGeer EG, Suzuki JS: Aging and extrapyramidal function. *Arch Neurol* 1977; 34:33–35.

11

*The Vertical Vestibulo-ocular Reflex**

Paul J. Ranalli, M.D., F.R.C.P.(C.)
James A. Sharpe, M.D., F.R.C.P.(C.)

The VOR subserves vision by generating conjugate smooth eye movements that are equal in velocity and opposite in direction to head movements. As a result, the eyes remain stationary with respect to the world, and images of the surrounding world remain stable on the retina. Visual acuity is dependent on the accuracy of the VOR. As the eyes and head move in opposite directions, the ratio of eye velocity to head velocity, or the VOR gain, must approximate unity. The horizontal VOR has been the subject of intensive investigation and its function is well defined.[1–4] Vertical head motion during such activities as walking or running has a frequency content ranging from 1 to 4 Hz.[5–7] Study of the vertical VOR in human subjects has been limited by the imprecision of EOG or infrared recording techniques. The magnetic search coil method[8, 9] provides accurate recording of vertical eye motion without eyelid artifacts. In this chapter, we consider anatomical and physiologic principles of the human vertical VOR, present data concerning its dynamic operations, and discuss clinical correlates of its disorders.

*Supported by Medical Research Council of Canada grants ME5509 and MT5404 (Dr. Sharpe) and a Medical Research Council of Canada Fellowship in Neuro-ophthalmology (Dr. Ranalli).

ANATOMICAL CONSIDERATIONS

Vertical head acceleration stimulates the anterior and posterior semicircular canals, while changes in head pitch stimulate otolithic receptors. Head motion excites primary vestibular fibers of the 8th nerve, the first-order neurons which project to the vestibular nuclei. Two major pathways, the medial longitudinal fasciculus (MLF) and brachium conjunctivum (BC), transmit signals from second-order VOR neurons in the vestibular nuclei to the third-order neurons of the four pairs of ocular motor nuclei concerned with vertical eye movements: the trochlear nuclei, innervating the superior oblique muscles, and the oculomotor subnuclei serving superior rectus, inferior rectus, and inferior oblique muscles. Detailed knowledge of the synaptology of the direct vertical VOR is available from studies of mechanical or electrical stimulation of individual semicircular canals and ampullary nerves in the cat[10, 11] and rabbit,[12, 13] while the monkey has been incompletely studied. The classic division of the VOR into a "direct" disynaptic three-neuron arc and an "indirect" polysynaptic reticular and cerebellar pathway[11, 14] from the labyrinths to the ocular muscles has been modified by the finding in monkeys[15, 16] that eye velocity signals of the direct pathway and eye position signals of the indirect pathway share the MLF.

Direct Vertical VOR

Three general principles pertain to central vertical VOR connections: (1) Each semicircular canal innervates extraocular muscles in its own plane, resulting in contraction of one extraocular muscle in each eye, called the prime mover, and relaxation of its antagonist. (2) Excitatory projections are contralateral, while inhibitory projections are ipsilateral. (3) Anterior canal and saccule excitatory signals are partly conveyed through the BC, while all other information ascends in the brain stem tegmentum. Pathways mediating the direct vertical VOR are summarized in Table 11–1.

Anterior Canal.—Anterior canal excitation is conveyed via second-order neurons of the superior vestibular nucleus through the BC, the MLF, and a ventral tegmental pathway, to the contralateral inferior oblique and superior rectus motor neurons[12, 17–21] (Figs 11–1 and 11–2). That is, stimulation of one anterior canal excites the ipsilateral superior rectus and contralateral inferior oblique muscles; their motor

TABLE 11–1.
Direct Connections of the Vertical Vestibulo-Ocular Reflex*

Receptor	Effect	Relay Nucleus	Pathway	Motor Nucleus	Ocular Muscle
Anterior canal	Excitation	SVN	BC, c-MLF, or VTD	c-III	i-SR c-IO
	Inhibition	SVN	i-MLF	i-IV i-III	c-SO i-IR
Posterior canal	Excitation	MVN	c-MLF	c-IV c-III	i-SO c-IR
	Inhibition	SVN	i-MLF	i-III	i-IO c-SR
Utricle	Excitation	? LVN ? IVN	MLF	c-VI c-IV c-III	c-LR i-SO c-IR c-IO i-SR
				i-III	i-MR
Saccule	Excitation	y-group, LVN	BC	? b-III ? b-IV	?

*Direct vestibulo-ocular projections as determined by electrophysiologic studies in rabbit, cat, and monkey. SVN, superior vestibular nucleus; MVN, medial vestibular nucleus; LVN, lateral vestibular nucleus; AC, anterior canal; PC, posterior canal; BC, brachium conjuctivum; MLF, medial longitudinal fasciculus; i, ipsilateral; c, contralateral; b, bilateral; III, oculomotor nucleus; IV, trochlear nucleus; VI, abducens nucleus; VTD, ventral tegmental decussation; SR, superior rectus; IR, inferior rectus; SO, superior oblique; IO, inferior oblique; MR, medial rectus; LR, lateral rectus.

neurons are contralateral to the canal.[12] Reciprocal inhibition of anterior canal signals is relayed by superior vestibular nucleus neurons that ascend in the ipsilateral reticular formation and MLF to the ipsilateral trochlear nucleus and inferior rectus subnucleus.[22, 23] Bilateral stimulation of the ampullary nerves of the anterior canals drives the eyes straight up.[10] The anterior canals activate the upward VOR during downward head motion.

Posterior Canal.—Posterior canal excitatory signals are relayed by neurons in the rostral part of the medial vestibular nucleus through the contralateral MLF to the trochlear nucleus and inferior rectus subnucleus[12, 24–26] (see Fig 11–2). The trochlear nucleus innervates the opposite eye and the inferior rectus subnucleus innervates the ipsilateral eye. Thus, one posterior canal activates the superior oblique muscle of the ipsilateral eye and the inferior rectus muscle of the contralateral eye. Signals mediating reciprocal inhibition to antagonist muscles are relayed by the superior and rostral part of the medial ves-

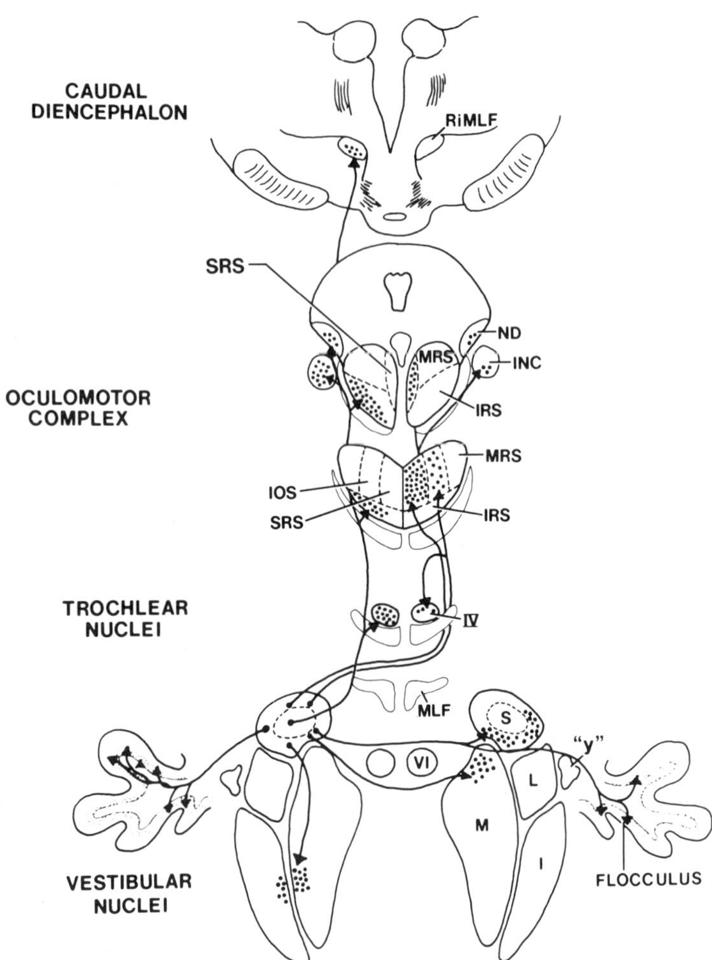

FIG 11–1.
Superior vestibular nucleus *(S)* efferents. S neurons project to ipsilateral medial *(M)* and inferior *(I)* vestibular nuclei and to contralateral rostral M and peripheral S. *SRS,* superior rectus subnucleus; *MRS,* medial rectus subnucleus; *IRS,* inferior rectus subnucleus; *IOS,* inferior oblique subnucleus; *ND,* nucleus Darkschewitsch; *INC,* interstitial nucleus of Cajal. (From Carpenter MB, Cowie RJ: Connections and oculomotor projections of the superior vestibular nucleus and cell group 'y.' *Brain Res* 1985; 336:265–287. Used by permission.)

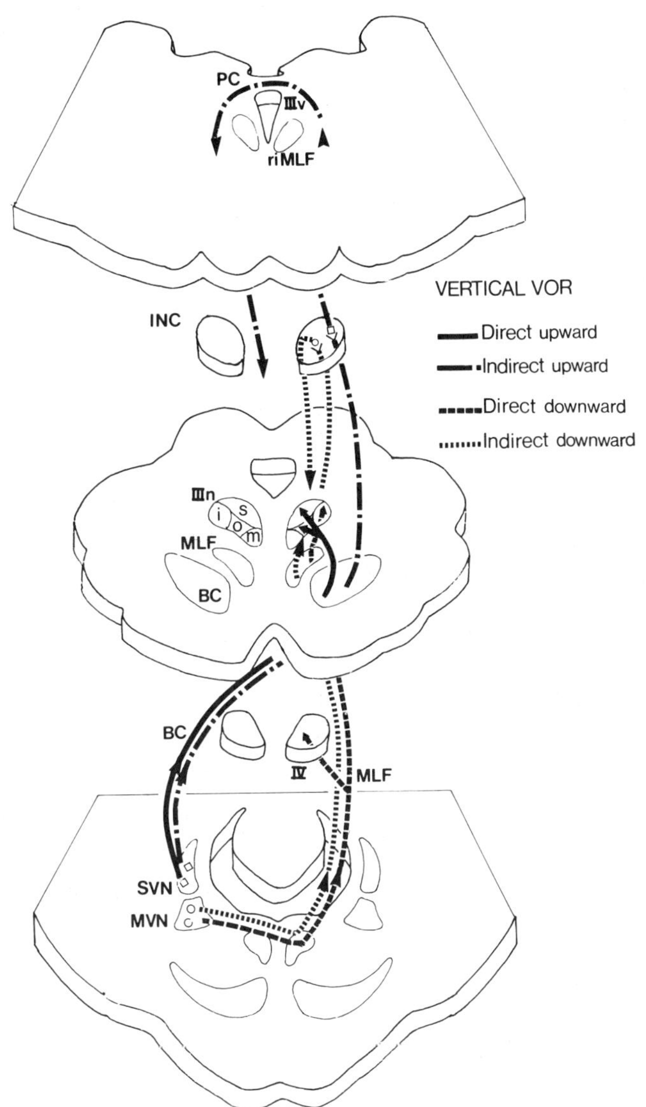

FIG 11–2.

Anatomical schema for the central projections mediating the vertical VOR in man. VOR signals reach the midbrain through the brachium conjunctivum *(BC),* medial longitudinal fasiculus *(MLF),* and a ventral tegmental decussation (not shown). *PC,* posterior commissure; *riMLF,* rostral interstitial nucleus of the medial longitudinal fasciculus; *INC,* interstitial nucleus of Cajal; *IIIn,* oculomotor nucleus; *o,* inferior oblique subnucleus; *i,* inferior rectus subnucleus; *s,* superior rectus subnucleus; *m,* medial rectus subnucleus; *IV,* trochlear nucleus; *SVN,* superior vestibular nucleus; *MVN,* medial vestibular nucleus. (From Ranalli PJ, Sharpe JA, Fletcher WA: Palsy of upward and downward saccadic pursuit and vestibular movements with a unilateral midbrain lesion: Pathophysiological correlations. *Neurology* 1988; 38:114–122. Used by permission.)

tibular nucleus via the ipsilateral reticular formation and MLF,[23] and via crossing fibers in the oculomotor nucleus,[26] to the superior rectus and inferior oblique subnuclei. Bilateral stimulation of the ampullary nerves of the posterior canals drives the eyes straight down.[10] The posterior canals activate the downward VOR during upward head motion.

Superior Vestibular Nucleus.—Connections of this nucleus subserve anterior canal excitatory signals, and, when either the anterior or posterior canals are disfacilitated, inhibitory signals. Eye movements induced by unilateral stimulation of this nucleus and spontaneous nystagmus following its destruction are in a plane parallel to the ipsilateral anterior canal.[27, 28] In addition to primary vestibular afferents, the superior vestibular nucleus receives signals from other vestibular nuclei, the vestibulocerebellum, and the interstitial nucleus of Cajal (INC)[21] (see Fig 11–1).

Medial Vestibular Nucleus.—Projections of this nucleus are consistant with the excitatory and inhibitory pathways mediating the VOR in the plane of the posterior semicircular canal[23, 29] (see Fig 11–2). Lesion studies have been less specific in determining the function of this nucleus.[28] Afferents to the medial vestibular nucleus arise from the perihypoglossal nuclear complex, other vestibular nuclei, the vestibulocerebellum, the oculomotor nuclei, and the INC.[29, 30]

Inferior Vestibular Nucleus.—This nucleus receives afferents from all contralateral vestibular nuclei (except the lateral nucleus) and bilateral projections from the oculomotor and perihypoglossal nuclei.[29] Its efferent fibers project to the contralateral trochlear and oculomotor nuclei, and it has reciprocal connections with the ipsilateral nodulus, uvula, and anterior vermis of the cerebellum. Its ocular motor function is unknown.

Lateral Vestibular Nucleus.—Its neurons project primarily to the spinal cord via the vestibulospinal tract. Ascending uncrossed projections which terminate in the ipsilateral medial rectus subnucleus[29] may mediate signals from excitation of the utricle or horizontal semicircular canal.

Medial Longitudinal Fasciculus.—Burst-tonic fibers that originate in the abducens nucleus are interneurons mediating adducting saccades. However, lesion studies[29, 32] show that many second-order vestibular neurons contribute to the MLF, and that their axons contact the motor neurons of vertical muscles (see Fig 11–1 and 11–2). The considerable fiber degeneration seen in the MLF after lesions of the vestibular nucleus must largely represent second-order vestibular neurons.

Otolithic-Ocular Reflexes.—These reflexes contribute gravity information to the vertical VOR when the head is upright. Much is unknown about the synaptic arrangement of the otolithic reflexes. Stimulation of one utricular nerve results in vertical ocular divergence and contralateral ocular torsion; the ipsilateral eye deviates up, the contralateral eye down, and the upper corneal meridians of both eyes rotate to the opposite side.[31] Stimulation of the saccular nerve activates both the lateral vestibular nucleus and the y-group of the vestibular nucleus,[33] but its effect on eye movements is not clear. The anatomy of an inhibitory otolithic-ocular reflex is unknown but is probably polysynaptic.[34]

Y-Group of the Vestibular Nucleus.—The y-group consists of a pair of dorsolateral accessory vestibular nuclei[18, 21, 35–37] implicated in the generation of vertical eye movements (see Fig 11–1). Ventral y receives primary vestibular afferents from the saccule[38] and a heavy innervation from the flocculus.[39] Neurons of the dorsal y, also known as the "infracerebellar nucleus," project through the ventral tegmental pathway[37] to the oculomotor[40–43] and trochlear[44] nuclei bilaterally and greater contralaterally. Stimulation of dorsal y produces monosynaptic excitation of ipsilateral superior rectus and contralateral inferior oblique muscles, consistent with participation of dorsal y in the anterior canal excitatory pathway.[45] Since saccular afferents innervate ventral y, and the dorsal y projects to vertical ocular motor nuclei, a projection from ventral y to dorsal y has been postulated,[36] but not yet demonstrated, to complete the sacculo-ocular reflex circuit.

Dentate Nucleus.—This deep cerebellar nucleus projects to the oculomotor nucleus, particularly its vertical subnuclei.[46, 47] In monkeys, electrical stimulation of the dentate nucleus elicits upward eye movements.[48, 49] Neurons with activity related to upward eye velocity and upward head velocity have been recorded in y-group, the dentate nucleus, and adjacent white matter, suggesting that this region forms a functional unit that participates in upward gaze.[39, 50]

The Indirect Vertical VOR and the Neural Integrator

Primary vestibular afferents supply the vestibular nucleus only with a head velocity signal. Since the final output of the VOR is an eye position command, the vestibular eye velocity command must be integrated, in the mathematical sense, to yield the eye position command; both eye velocity and position commands must then be delivered to the motor neuron in a fixed ratio.[13] The nucleus prepositus hypoglossi and the interstitial nucleus of Cajal (INC) have the appropriate anatomical connections to contribute to the integration of vertical eye velocity commands into eye position commands. The concept of an anatomical indirect VOR, described by Lorente de Nó in 1933,[14] is paralleled by the concept of a physiological indirect VOR. The direct VOR pathway transmits the head (eye) velocity signals, while the indirect VOR participates in the integration of the eye velocity signals to eye position signals, which are then transmitted to ocular motor neurons. In modern terms, structures that perform the neural integration and relay the position commands can be considered the anatomical substrate of the indirect VOR.

The INC are paired accessory ocular motor nuclei in the midbrain periaqueductal gray matter that seem to be a crucial link in the indirect vertical VOR pathway. Each INC receives disynaptic inhibitory and excitatory potentials from the vestibular nerve, via the ipsilateral and contralateral MLF, respectively.[51] The ipsilateral inhibitory pathway is derived from the superior vestibular nucleus,[21] while both the superior and medial vestibular nuclei contribute to the contralateral excitatory pathway[29] (see Figs 11–1 and 11–2). Neurons of the INC project monosynaptically to contralateral vertical ocular motor neurons,[42] but the route of these vertical smooth eye movement pathways in the midbrain is unknown. Efferent INC fibers also send information to the superior and medial vestibular nuclei, the nucleus prepositus hypoglossi, and the inferior olivary nucleus.[51]

Lesions of the posterior commissure in monkey[52] and man[53] completely abolish all upward eye movements above the midline, including vestibular movements induced by oculocephalic stimulation. This indicates that signals mediating the upward VOR are relayed dorsally through the posterior commissure prior to innervation of the oculomotor nuclei. The final pathway of the downward VOR is unknown, but likely descends directly from the INC to the oculomotor and trochlear nuclei (see Fig 11–2).

The paired rostral interstitial nuclei of the medial longitudinal fasciculus (riMLF) lie just rostral to the INC. They contain medium-lead burst neurons for vertical saccades[54] and nystagmus quick phases and receive bilateral (predominantly ipsilateral) superior vestibular nucleus afferents to their medial caudal portion, directly adjacent to the INC[21, 55] (see Fig 11–1). Since fibers of passage from the riMLF traverse the INC, the contribution of riMLF to the indirect vertical VOR pathway is difficult to isolate from lesion and stimulation studies. Each riMLF mediates vertical nystagmus quick phases[56, 57] by ipsilateral projections to vertically acting motor neurons in the oculomotor and trochlear nuclei.

Neurons in riMLF are maximally activated in specific canal planes. For example, downward head pitch in the plane of one anterior canal drives the eyes upward by vestibular slow phases mediated by the contralateral superior rectus and inferior oblique motor neurons. The ipsilateral riMLF is activated to generate the appropriate downward fast phases via projections to ipsilateral inferior rectus and superior oblique motor neurons. Similarly, upward head pitch in the plane of one posterior canal, which drives the eyes downward by vestibular slow phases mediated by the contralateral inferior rectus and superior oblique motor neurons, also activates the ipsilateral riMLF to generate the appropriate upward fast phases via projections to the ipsilateral superior rectus and inferior oblique motor neurons. In either case, the riMLF ipsilateral to the stimulated canal creates the correct fast phase signals.[57]

The nucleus prepositus hypoglossi is one of the perihypoglossal nuclei in the medulla; it projects exclusively excitatory connections to ocular motor neurons mediating signals to all vertical eye muscles.[58] The nucleus prepositus hypoglossi and medial vestibular nucleus compose the site of the neural integrator[59] for all horizontal eye movements; these structures mathematically integrate eye velocity signals into the tonic eye position signal necessary to maintain the eye in an eccentric position against the elastic restoring forces of orbital muscles. This final common integrator also contributes to the integration of vertical saccades[59]; its role in the vertical VOR has not been tested, and the site of integration of vertical smooth eye movement velocity commands to position commands is unknown. Several nuclear groups contain units with activity related to vertical eye position: y-group,[39, 50] the flocculus,[60] nucleus prepositus hypoglossi,[58] and the INC.[61]

Vestibulo-cerebello-vestibular pathways will likely be shown to play an important role in the indirect vertical VOR. The flocculus has reciprocal connections with the vestibular nuclei that participate in vertical smooth eye movements,[21, 39] and it receives primary vestibular afferents, as well as visual projections via climbing fibers from the inferior olivary nucleus[62] and mossy fibers from pontine nuclei[63] in cat and rabbit. The fastigial nuclei receive vestibular inputs concerned with the otoliths.

Finally, the indirect vertical VOR may utilize other circuits, for example, internuclear commissural pathways between the vestibular nuclei, which mediate crossed inhibition between canal pairs[64–66] and excitatory polysynaptic circuits within the vestibular nucleus.[67]

PHYSIOLOGICAL CONSIDERATIONS

Vertical head velocity signals are recorded in the MLF, confirming its role as the middle leg (interneuron) of the three-neuron reflex arc.[15, 16] The MLF is more than a simple vestibular relay. In addition to carrying a head velocity (vestibulo-ocular) signal, it transmits the integrated tonic eye position, as well as vertical pursuit eye velocity signals, and its fibers pause during saccades or nystagmus quick phases in any direction.[16] Because of these properties, these MLF neurons are called tonic-vestibular-pause cells. The pause in activity during saccades observed in tonic-vestibular-pause cells and other vestibular neurons may be due to inputs from inhibitory burst neurons at the pontomedullary reticular formation that are known to project to the vestibular nucleus in the cat.[68]

Single-unit studies of vestibular nucleus reveal a variety of cells which modulate with vertical eye movements.[67, 69–71] Vertical tonic-vestibular-pause cells in the vestibular nucleus have firing rates similar to the tonic-vestibular-pause cells of the MLF.[16, 71] Many of these cells can be activated antidromically by stimulation of the MLF,[71] identifying the tonic-vestibular-pause unit as the interneuron of the vertical VOR.

Cancellation of the Vertical VOR

The tonic-vestibular-pause signal cannot provide the only smooth eye movement input to ocular motor neurons. During pursuit with the head free, the VOR must be cancelled, and the eyes remain stationary in the orbit; ocular neurons do not change their discharge rate during VOR cancellation.[3] Nonetheless, tonic-vestibular-pause neurons in the vestibular nuclei that project in the MLF do carry a head velocity signal despite cancellation of the reflex.[69, 71] Therefore, ocular motor neurons must receive another input to cancel the head velocity signal from the vestibular nuclei. During cancellation of the horizontal VOR, the unwanted vestibular drive has been thought to be cancelled by a pursuit signal, since horizontal pursuit and cancellation are dynamically similar,[72–75] and because patients with defective smooth pursuit typically have defective cancellation.[76] However, VOR gain can be modulated in ways that do not seem to involve the pursuit system, such as changing VOR gain by altering mental set during head shaking in the dark,[1] or cancelling the VOR while tracking unpredictably moving targets.[77]

A signal that cancels the vertical VOR might be represented by the upward head velocity signal recorded in y-group and the dentate nucleus during passive vertical rotation in monkeys.[39, 50] Neurons in this region also carry an upward pursuit signal, and are silent during the vertical VOR tested in darkness. This head velocity signal, with some modification, might be used to cancel the oppositely directed vertical eye velocity signal carried by the MLF. Cancellation of the MLF eye velocity signal might occur in rostral midbrain nuclei, such as the INC, or at the ocular motor nuclei. Bilateral lesions of the MLF in monkeys abolish the vertical VOR and the ability to sustain eccentric vertical fixation, leading to vertical gaze-evoked nystagmus.[78] Slight recovery of the vertical VOR occurs after one month, suggesting sparing of an alternate extrafascicular pathway, such as the BC.

The INC likely participates in the vertical VOR. It contains burst and tonic vertical neurons which carry eye velocity and position signals.[61] INC neurons may provide an integrated signal of eye position to vertical ocular motor neurons, to which they project. The INC may be part of a "distributed" integrator network for the vertical VOR. Consistent with this view, bilateral INC lesions in cats result in increased VOR phase lead during sinusoidal rotation in pitch.[79]

Ocular Tilt Reaction

Stimulation of the midbrain tegmentum of monkeys near the INC produces the ocular tilt reaction, a triad of head tilting, skew deviation, and ocular torsion.[80] The tilt is toward the side of INC stimulation; that is, the head inclines ipsilaterally, the ipsilateral eye is depressed, the contralateral eye elevates, and the 12 o'clock corneal meridians rotate conjugately in the direction of the lower skewed eye. The ocular tilt reaction is similar to that produced by stimulation of the contralateral utricular nerve.[31] In one patient, an ocular tilt reaction occurred transiently toward the side of a utricle destroyed during stapedectomy.[81]

A transient ocular tilt reaction has been observed in a patient with a midbrain abscess[82] and in another patient with multiple sclerosis in whom the lesion was not localized.[83] Compression of one side of the midbrain and posterior commissure by tumor resulted in contralateral head tilt and upward gaze palsy.[84] We have observed an ocular tilt reaction which was directed away from the side of a unilateral infarct of the INC and riMLF in a patient who had spontaneous vertical and torsional nystagmus that resembled one half cycle of seesaw nystagmus.[85] These cases suggest that lesions of the midbrain disrupt the otolith-ocular reflex.

Velocity Storage in the Vertical VOR

When the canal-derived vertical VOR is isolated from the otolithic vestibular input by rotating a cat lying on its side about a vertical axis, a unilateral INC lesion abolishes storage of nystagmus slow-phase velocity after perrotary stimulation of the downward VOR and reduces it for the upward VOR. Perrotary nystagmus during prolonged rotation and post-rotary slow phases after the head stops are attributed to a velocity storage integrator that is responsible for extending the duration (time constant) and the low-frequency response of the VOR[86]; it is distinct from the neural integrator (discussed above) that yields eye position signals from head velocity signals. Thus, the INC seems to be an element of both the velocity storage integrator and the velocity-to-position integrator of vertical smooth eye motion.

Symmetry of the Vertical VOR: Effect of Otolithic Reflexes

The horizontal VOR is symmetric to the left and right, but studies of the vertical VOR of cats[87–90] and monkeys[91] show an asymmetric response to head acceleration. When cats are placed on their sides and rotated about a vertical axis, to eliminate gravitational changes and otolith-ocular reflexes, the upward VOR has greater gain, a longer time constant, and less phase lead than downward VOR. The VOR time constant is the period after a sustained rotation is stopped, at which two thirds of the stored slow-phase velocity of nystagmus has discharged. Oscillation in pitch with the head erect allows the otoliths to contribute to the downward VOR and reduces asymmetries in gain and phase lead between upward and downward VOR in the cat[89] and monkey.[92] Another study of the vertical VOR in monkeys rotated on their sides showed symmetry of upward and downward VOR gain and phase lead over a wide frequency range (0.01–1.0 Hz).[93]

Adaptation and Plasticity of the VOR

The remarkable accuracy of the VOR is achieved through an adaptive mechanism that senses errors in the performance of the VOR and gradually adjusts its gain.[94] The performance of the VOR is judged by the absolute standard of minimal image motion across the retina during head turns. Confronted with persistent visual errors, the VOR is able to make short-term and long-term adaptive adjustments to its gain.[95–97] This regulatory function is said to be adaptive because it responds to errors with a change that reduces those errors. In addition, these changes are plastic; that is, the new value of gain persists until a different mismatch of visual and vestibular inputs causes the VOR to change again. The anatomical site of this modification is as yet undetermined. A controversy exists over whether the site of motor learning of the VOR is entirely confined to the flocculus,[98] or whether the flocculus merely provides the error signal to a learning site somewhere in the brain stem.[99] Most experimental work on adaptation and plasticity of the VOR has concerned the horizontal VOR; however, recent microstimulation mapping of the monkey flocculus has identified "microzones" related to vertical and torsional eye movements which are distinct from the microzone associated with adaptive changes in horizontal vestibular eye movements.[98, 100] Enduring dysfunction of the VOR and spontaneous nystagmus in patients gives evidence of lesions involving the brain stem or cerebellar sites of this adaptive mechanism.

Initiation of the Vertical VOR

The initiation of the vertical VOR has a complex time course. Following a latency of 15 msec, the first 15 msec of vertical VOR in cats is symmetric and resistant to visual adaptation.[90] During the subsequent 15 msec (30 msec after head motion starts), downward smooth eye movement velocity exceeds upward, and VOR gain can be augmented or diminished by visual adaptation. Eye velocity rapidly increases to a peak equal in magnitude and opposite in direction to head velocity, then decays within 1 second to a plateau velocity of approximately 0.6 gain; upward plateau velocity exceeds downward by 15%.[90] The initial 15-msec segment of vertical VOR may represent the rapidly mediated, nonadaptable direct VOR pathway, while the adaptable indirect pathway, which likely traverses a polysynaptic circuit, has an initiation latency of 30 msec. Snyder and King[90] provide evidence that the indirect pathway is subject to plastic adaptation in the face of persistant errors of retinal image motion.

Human Studies

Information concerning the vertical VOR in man is meager. Rotation in pitch has been performed with subjects sitting upright,[100] lying on their sides,[72] sitting with their heads inclined sideways,[101] or inclined forward and rotated to orient the sagittal head plane in pitch, while the body is rotated in yaw.[102] These studies have two major limitations: passive sinusoidal stimulation is confined to frequencies lower than those generated by most natural voluntary head movements,[5–7] and EOG, an imprecise method of recording vertical eye movement, was used. In general, the vertical VOR demonstrates gains similar to those of horizontal VOR but greater phase leads[101] and shorter time constants.[72, 101, 102] When upward and downward VOR were compared, the data were conflicting: upward VOR gain was reported to be higher[72] or lower[102]; upward and downward time constants were similar. In a study of the human vertical VOR during active head movement, gain of 0.91 and phase lag of 7° at 1 Hz was recorded by infrared oculography[103]; upward and downward VOR were not distinguished. We have studied the dynamics of the vertical VOR in normal subjects.[104]

We investigated 14 normal subjects ranging in age from 21 to 35 years, with a mean age of 28.5 years (SD ± 3.5). Subjects sat upright in a fixed chair and actively pitched their heads sinusoidally at 0.25–2 Hz, paced by a programmed timer signal. Head and eye motion were measured by the magnetic search coil technique,[8] with head motion recorded by a coil mounted on a head band and eye motion by a scleral contact annulus.[9] The VOR was measured in darkness; subjects were instructed to imagine a stationary target. Eye movements recorded with the head erect represent the sum of otolith organ responses to changes in gravity and semicircular canal reflexes to head acceleration. The attempt to imagine a stationary target during active head movements adds voluntary enhancement,[1] and active head motion introduces planned eye movements to the VOR; however, this method reduces the variability in the VOR observed during passive whole body rotation while subjects perform mental arithmetic. Visual enhancement of the VOR was measured while subjects viewed an actual stationary target.

Vertical VOR gain in darkness ranged from 0.85 to 0.96 (Fig 11–3); with a fixation target, gain increased to a range of 0.96–1.12, with most gains above 1.0 (Fig 11–4). At the target distance tested, gains above 1.0 for the visually enhanced VOR can be explained by translational eye movements generated by dynamic otolith-ocular re-

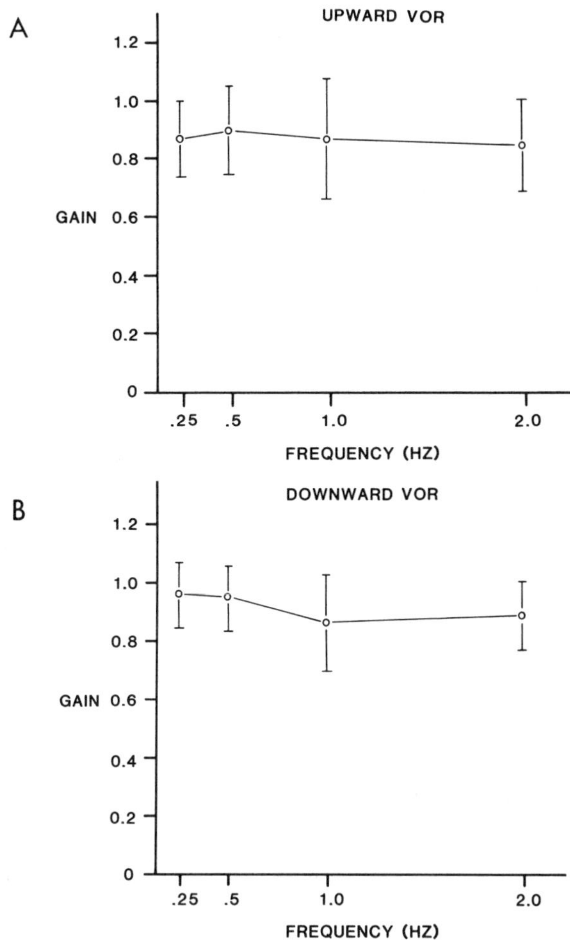

FIG 11–3.
Vertical VOR in normal subjects. **(A)** upward and **(B)** downward vertical VOR gain vs. frequency of head movement. Values are mean gain ± 1 SD.

flexes.[105] Mean downward VOR gains were greater than mean upward gains in darkness, but the difference was not statistically significant. Upward and downward gains were symmetric with a fixation target. No frequency dependence was observed within the bandwidth tested. The eyes were 180° out of phase with the head, defined as 0° phase lag, at frequencies from 0.25 to 2 Hz (Fig 11–5). These gain and phase values are similar to those observed for the vertical VOR in monkeys tested by passive rotation in the head on side position.[93]

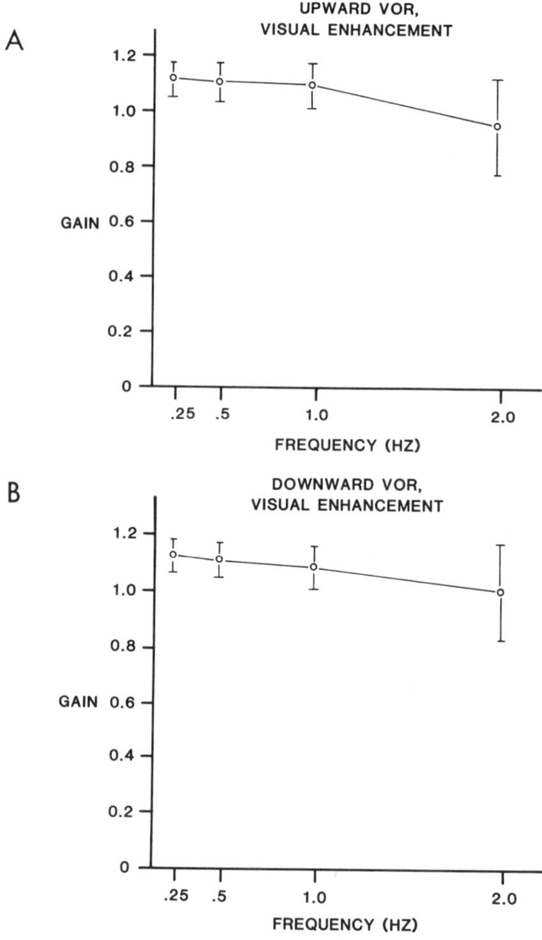

FIG 11–4.
Visual enhancement of the vertical VOR in normal subjects. **(A)** upward and **(B)** downward visual enhancement of the vertical VOR. Values are mean gain ± 1 SD.

During pursuit with the freely moving head at frequencies below 0.5 Hz, subjects cancelled 76%–78% of their vertical VOR gains measured in darkness (Fig 11–6). At higher frequencies of head-free pursuit, ability to cancel the VOR decreases, as peak target accelerations approach the saturation limits of the pursuit system.[75] Attempts at head free pursuit of a target moving at 2 Hz (peak target acceleration of 1,579°/sec^2) generated little cancellation of the vertical VOR. Upward and downward VOR cancellation was symmetric.

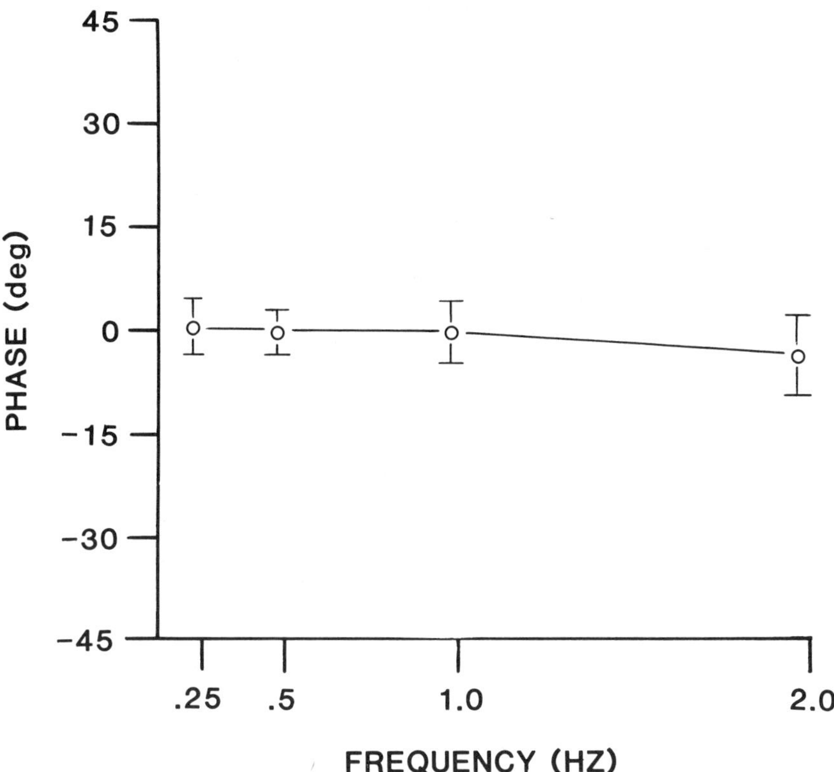

FIG 11–5.
Vertical VOR phase is close to 0° at all frequencies. Values are mean phase for both upward and downward smooth eye movements in darkness. *Error bars* indicate 1 SD.

CLINICAL CORRELATES

Dysfunction of the vertical VOR occurs in patients with focal and degenerative disease and metabolic encephalopathies affecting the brain stem and cerebellum. The effects of disease can be grouped anatomically as follows.

Midbrain

Over 30 cases of vertical gaze paresis associated with autopsy-proved mesencephalic lesions have been documented.[106, 107] Of these, only two employed EOG to determine the relative contribution of saccades, pursuit, and VOR to the vertical gaze paresis. Both were cases

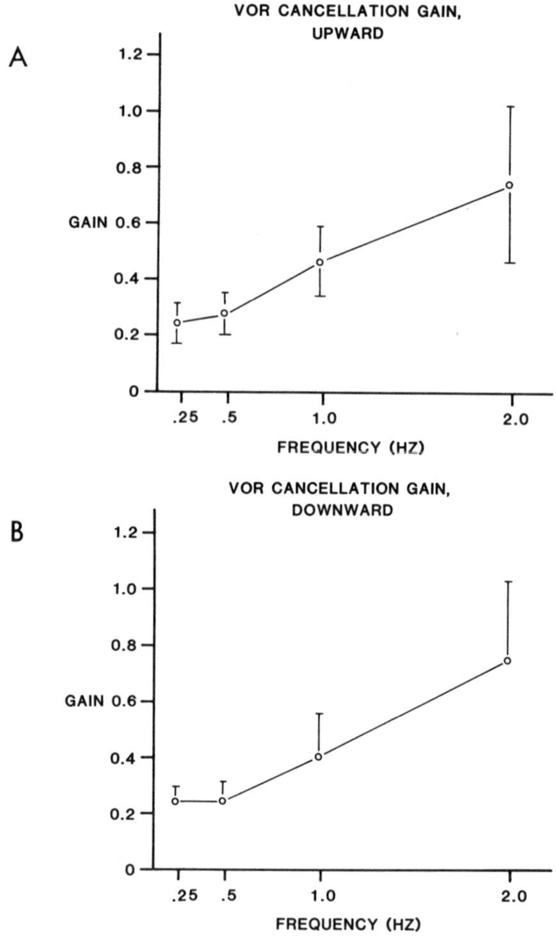

FIG 11–6.
VOR gain during vertical eye-head tracking in normal subjects. **(A)** upward and **(B)** downward vertical VOR gain during cancellation vs. frequency of head movement. Values are gain ± 1 SD.

of bilateral midbrain infarction with partial or complete paresis of vertical saccades and pursuit; vertical VOR amplitude appeared full, but gain and phase were not measured.[106, 107] An EOG study[108] of midbrain lesions that caused varying degrees of vertical saccadic palsy revealed relative preservation of the vertical VOR, but smooth eye movements were not quantified.

We measured reduced gain, limited amplitude, and abnormal

phase lead of the vertical VOR by the magnetic search coil technique in a patient with a discrete unilateral infarction involving the INC and riMLF, confirmed by neuropathologic examination.[85] This observation implies that signals mediating the vertical VOR traverse, and are partially integrated by the INC.[85] The lesion spared the ocular motor nuclei, indicating that *supranuclear* lesions of the rostral midbrain can impair the vertical VOR; this varies from traditional teaching that supranuclear lesion spare the vertical VOR.[109, 110] The misconception largely results from the usual method of testing the vertical VOR at the bedside: the "oculocephalic" maneuver, in which the patient's head is passively flexed and extended while fixating on a target in a well-lit room. The eye movements that result represent not only the vertical VOR, but also visual enhancement of this reflex by smooth pursuit and optokinetic reflex mechanisms. Moreover, although the examiner may judge the amplitude of oculocephalic eye movements to be normal, the gain and phase of the vertical VOR are not measured at the bedside. Complete assessment of vertical VOR dysfunction requires oculographic recording and quantification of vertical VOR movements performed in darkness.

Medial Longitudinal Fasciculus

Bilateral lesions of the MLF cause bilateral internuclear ophthalmoplegia (INO), consisting of binocular paresis of adduction and gaze-evoked abducting nystagmus. Bilateral INO is associated with impairment of the vertical VOR and smooth pursuit, and vertical gaze-evoked nystagmus. Reduced vertical VOR gain with low-frequency head movement was recorded by EOG in four patients[111] and by search coil oculography at 1 Hz in another patient.[112] Absence of the vertical VOR and intact vertical pursuit was claimed in a case of locked-in syndrome and bilateral INO due to tegmental pontine hemorrhage[113]; however, visual fixation was not controlled during VOR testing.

We recorded reduced gain and abnormal phase lag of the vertical VOR at frequencies up to 2 Hz in a group of patients with unilateral or bilateral INO.[114] VOR gain increased when the patients viewed a stationary target, but remained below the ideal gain of unity, indicating defective visual enhancement of the reflex. Despite a subnormal vertical VOR, patients with INO were unable to adequately cancel this reflex when they pursued a vertical target with combined head and eye motion.[114] Impairment of the vertical VOR in patients with INO is consistent with that observed in experimental lesions of the MLF,[78] and indicates that vertical VOR, vertical eye position, and VOR cancelation signals in man are carried, at least in part, by the MLF.

Cerebellum and Lower Brain Stem

Spontaneous vertical nystagmus is a characteristic sign of lesions of the vestibulocerebellum or lower brain stem. An imbalance of vertical smooth pursuit or vestibular tone likely underlies the development of upbeat or downbeat nystagmus; however, few quantitative measurements of vertical smooth eye movements have been performed.[115, 116]

Downbeat nystagmus occurs with dysgenesis of the vestibulocerebellum and medulla in the Arnold-Chiari malformation,[115, 117] hereditary and acquired cerebellar degeneration,[115, 118, 119] multiple sclerosis,[117, 119] hydrocephalus,[120] familial periodic ataxia,[121] electrolyte disturbance,[122] and toxic levels of lithium[123] or anticonvulsants.[124, 125] No cause is found in up to 40% of cases,[118] many of which may have restricted cerebellar degenerations. The pathogenesis of downbeat nystagmus is unknown, but probably involves the selective effect of lesions on downward VOR[117] or pursuit[115] pathways. Excitatory central projections from the posterior,[29] but not anterior,[21] semicircular canals cross in the floor of the fourth ventricle. Therefore, a lesion in the dorsal midline of the medulla would be expected to cause a loss of downward vestibular tone, resulting in an upward slow-phase drift and downbeat nystagmus. This hypothesis has been confirmed by the occurrence of downbeat nystagmus after experimental midsagittal section of the medulla in monkeys.[126] Bilateral lesions of the flocculus[127] or nodulus[128] also cause downbeat nystagmus, possibly reflecting loss of inhibitory influence of Purkinje cells on anterior canal[127] or otolithic-ocular[129] relays, respectively.

The intensity of downbeat nystagmus often varies with the position of the head in pitch. This position-dependent asymmetry was recorded in a patient with downbeat nystagmus and a hyperactive upward VOR during pitch rotation in the upright position.[116] Symmetry of the vertical VOR and disappearance of spontaneous downbeat nystagmus occurred in the supine position. The authors proposed[116] that asymmetric vertical semicircular canal reflexes were subject to modulation by otolith-ocular reflexes. This supported a role for otolithic influence on the imbalanced vertical vestibular tone that causes downbeat nystagmus.[117] Downbeat nystagmus might also result from a disturbance of the neural integrator of vertical smooth eye movements, but this has not been confirmed by measurement of reduced gain and reduced time constant of the downward integrator. A pathologically elevated gain of the neural integrator for upward smooth eye movements was proposed as the cause of downbeat nystagmus with exponentially increasing slow phases in a patient with paraneoplastic cerebellar degeneration.[130]

Upbeat nystagmus in the primary position has been associated with lesions in the medullary and pontine tegmentum,[131, 132] the inferior olive and perihypoglossal nuclei,[133] diffusely in the lower brain stem,[134] and as a manifestation of Wernicke's disease[135] or meningitis.[136] Tobacco smoking can induce spontaneous upbeat nystagmus in normal subjects in darkness.[137] Involvement of the brachium conjunctivum and anterior vermis of the cerebellum has also been postulated to cause upbeat nystagmus,[138, 139] by disrupting upward VOR and pursuit projections. Imbalance of the VOR causes the eyes to glide down. Lesions causing upbeat nystagmus have been the most discretely localized in the tegmentum of the pontomedullary junction[131, 132]; they are more ventral than the dorsal tegmental lesions associated with downbeat nystagmus.[126] Upbeat nystagmus in these cases may result from interruption of upward vestibular signals carried by the ventral tegmental pathway,[21] while sparing downward vestibular signals crossing within the more dorsal decussation of the MLF.[126] The downward slow phase drift of upbeat nystagmus is usually linear, but an increasing exponential waveform was recorded in a patient with a cerebellar cyst, in whom upbeat nystagmus increased on downgaze.[140]

Sustained upgaze or downgaze can accompany coma following hypoxic encephalopathy due to cardiac arrest,[141] subarachnoid hemmorhage,[142] or sedative drug intoxication.[143] This may signify tonic imbalance of vertical vestibular tone that is sustained when saccades and quick phases are paralyzed in coma.

SUMMARY

The vertical VOR serves to maintain stable vision by generating compensatory eye movements for the high-frequency active and passive head movements that accompany daily activities such as walking and running. The direct vertical VOR consists of a three-neuron arc. Head velocity signals from the anterior and posterior semicircular canals and otoliths are delivered to second-order neurons located in the superior and rostral medial vestibular nuclei, then relayed via the medial longitudinal fasciculus, brachium conjunctivum, and ventral tegmental pathway to the oculomotor and trochlear nuclei. The reflex requires integration of eye velocity commands to position commands, velocity storage, and extension of its low-frequency response by indirect polysynaptic circuits, which are shared by the interstitial nucleus of Cajal, nucleus prepositus hypoglossi, and vestibular nuclei.

The upward and downward VOR is symmetric and demonstrates near-unity gain and perfect phase compensation for head movements ranging between 0.25 and 2 Hz in normal human subjects. The reflex can be canceled during vertical head-free pursuit below 0.5 Hz; cancelation deteriorates at higher frequencies. Lesions of the brain stem and cerebellum impair the vertical VOR. Internuclear ophthalmoplegia is accompanied by reduced vertical VOR gain, abnormal phase lag, and impaired cancellation. Discrete supranuclear lesions of the rostral midbrain, involving the interstitial nucleus of Cajal, cause reduced gain and abnormal phase lead, providing evidence that the rostral midbrain contains indirect pathways subserving integration of the vertical VOR.

REFERENCES

1. Barr CC, Schultheis LW, Robinson DA: Voluntary, non-visual control of the human vestibulo-ocular reflex. *Acta Otolaryngol (Stockh)* 1976; 81:365–375.
2. Tomlinson RD, Saunders GE, Schwarz DWF: Analysis of human vestibulo-ocular reflex during active head movements. *Acta Otolaryngol (Stockh)* 1980; 90:184–190.
3. Skavenski AA, Robinson DA: Role of abducens neurons in vestibuloocular reflex. *J Neurophysiol* 1973; 36:724–738.
4. Pellionisz A: Tensorial aspects of the multidimensional approach to the vestibulo-oculomotor reflex and gaze, in Berthoz A, Melvill Jones G (eds): *Adaptive mechanisms in gaze control. Facts and theories.* New York, Elsevier, 1985, pp 281–296.
5. Grossman GE, Abel LA, Thurston SE, et al: Frequency and velocity ranges of natural head rotations. *Soc Neurosci Abstr* 1986; 12:251.
6. Gresty MA: Coordination of head and eye movements to fixate continuous and intermittent targets. *Vision Res* 1974; 14:395–403.
7. Gresty MA, Hess K, Leech J: Disorders of the vestibulo-ocular reflex producing oscillopsia and mechanisms compensating for loss of labyrinthine function. *Brain* 1977; 100:693–716.
8. Robinson DA: A method of measuring eye movement using a scleral search coil in a magnetic field. *IEEE Trans Biomed Elect* 1963; BME-10:137–145.
9. Collewijn H, van der Mark F, Jansen TC: Precise recording of human eye movements. *Vision Res* 1975; 15:447–450.

10. Cohen B, Suzuki J, Bender MB: Eye movements from semicircular canal nerve stimulation in the cat. *Ann Otol Rhinol Laryngol* 1964; 73:153–170.
11. Szentagothai J: The elementary vestibulo-ocular reflex arc. *J Neurophysiol* 1950; 13:395–407.
12. Ito M, Nisimaru N, Yamamoto M: Pathways for the vestibulo-ocular reflex excitation arising from semicircular canals of rabbits. *Exp Brain Res* 1976; 24:257–271.
13. Robinson DA: Control of eye movements, in Brooks VB (ed): *Handbook of Physiology: Vol II, Part 2. The Nervous System*. Baltimore, American Physiological Society, Williams & Wilkins, 1981, pp 1275–1320.
14. Lorente de Nó R: Vestibulo-ocular reflex arc. *Arch Neurol Psychiatr* 1933; 30:245–291.
15. King WM, Lisberger SG, Fuchs AF: Response of fibers in medial longitudinal fasciculus (MLF) of alert monkeys during horizontal and vertical conjugate eye movements evoked by vestibular or visual stimuli. *J Neurophysiol* 1976; 39:1135–1149.
16. Pola J, Robinson DA: Oculomotor signals in medial longitudinal fasciculus of the monkey. *J Neurophysiol* 1978; 41:245–259.
17. Abend WK: Functional organization of the superior vestibular nucleus of the squirrel monkey. *Brain Res* 1977; 132:65–84.
18. Highstein SM, Reisine H: Synaptic and functional organization of vestibulo-ocular reflex pathways. *Prog Brain Res* 1979; 50:431–442.
19. Yamamoto M, Shimoyama I, Highstein SM: Vestibular nucleus neurons relaying excitation from the anterior canal to the oculomotor nucleus. *Brain Res* 1978; 148:31–42.
20. Hirai N, Uchino Y: Superior vestibular nucleus neurons related to the excitatory vestibulo-ocular reflex of anterior canal origin and their ascending course in the cat. *Neurosci Res* 1984; 1:73–79.
21. Carpenter MB, Cowie RJ: Connections and oculomotor projections of the superior vestibular nucleus and cell group 'y.' *Brain Res* 1985; 336:265–287.
22. Uchino Y, Suzuki S: Axon collaterals to the extraocular motoneuron pools of inhibitory vestibulo-ocular neurons activated from the anterior, posterior and horizontal semicircular canals in the cat. *Neurosci Lett* 1983; 37:129–135.
23. Graf W, Ezure K: Morphology of vertical canal related second order vestibular neurons in the cat. *Exp Brain Res* 1986; 63:35–48.
24. Uchino Y, Hirai N, Watanabe S: Vestibulo-ocular reflex from the posterior canal nerve to extraocular motoneurons in the cat. *Exp Brain Res* 1978; 32:377–388.
25. Uchino Y, Hirai N, Suzuki S, et al: Properties of secondary vestibular neurons fired by stimulation of ampullary nerve of the vertical, anterior or posterior semicircular canals in the cat. *Brain Res* 1981; 223:273–286.
26. Graf W, McCrae RA, Baker R: Morphology of posterior canal related

secondary vestibular neurons in rabbit and cat. *Exp Brain Res* 1983; 52:125–138.

27. Tokumasu K, Goto K, Cohen B: Eye movements from vestibular nuclei stimulation in monkeys. *Ann Otolaryngol* 1969; 78:1105–1119.
28. Uemura T, Cohen B: Effects of vestibular nuclei lesions on vestibulo-ocular reflexes and posture in monkeys. *Acta Otolaryngol (Stockh)* [*Suppl*] 1973; 315:1–71.
29. Carleton SC, Carpenter MB: Afferent and efferent connections of the medial, inferior and lateral vestibular nuclei in the cat and monkey. *Brain Res* 1983; 278:29–51.
30. Pompeiano O, Walberg F: Descending connections to the vestibular nuclei: An experimental study in the cat. *J Comp Neurol* 1957; 108:465–503.
31. Suzuki JI, Tokumasu K, Goto K: Eye movements from single utricular nerve stimulation in the cat. *Acta Otolaryngol (Stockh)* 1969; 68:350–362.
32. Tarlov E: Anatomy of the two vestibulo-ocular projection systems, in Brodal A, Pompeiano O (eds): *Progress in Brain Research: Basic Aspects of Central Vestibular Mechanisms.* Amsterdam, Elsevier, 1972, vol 37, pp 471–491.
33. Hwang JC, Poon WF: An electrophysiological study of the sacculo-ocular pathways in cats. *Jpn J Physiol* 1981; 25:241–251.
34. Blanks RHI, Anderson JH, Precht W: Response characteristics of semicircular canal and otolith systems in cat: II. Response of trochlear motoneurons. *Exp Brain Res* 1978; 32:509–528.
35. Brodal A, Pompeiano O: The vestibular nuclei in the cat. *J Anat* 1957; 91:438–455.
36. Frederickson CJ, Trune DR: Cytoarchitecture and saccular innervation of nucleus y in the mouse. *J Comp Neurol* 1986; 252:302–322.
37. Sato Y, Kawasaki T: Target neurons of floccular caudal zone inhibition in Y-group nucleus of vestibular nuclear complex. *J Neurophysiol* 1987; 57:460–480.
38. Gacek RR: The course and termination of first order neurons supplying vestibular endorgans in the cat. *Acta Otolaryngol (Stockh)* 1969; 254:1–66.
39. Chubb MC, Fuchs AF: The role of the dentate nucleus and y-group in the generation of vertical smooth eye movements. *Ann NY Acad Sci* 1981; 374:446–454.
40. Gacek RR: Location of brainstem neurons projecting to the oculomotor nucleus in the cat. *Exp Neurol* 1977; 57:725–749.
41. Graybiel AM, Hartwieg EA: Some afferent connections of the oculomotor complex in the cat: An experimental study with tracer techniques. *Brain Res* 1971; 81:543–551.
42. Steiger H-J, Buttner-Ennever JA: Oculomotor nucleus afferents in the monkey demonstrated with horseradish peroxidase. *Brain Res* 1979; 160:1–15.

43. Stanton GB: Afferents to oculomotor nucleus from area 'y' in Macaca mulata: An anterograde degeneration study. *J Comp Neurol* 1980; 192:377–385.
44. Gacek RR: Location of trochlear vestibulo-ocular neurons in the cat. *Exp Neurol* 1978; 59:479–491.
45. Ghelarducci B, Highstein SM, Ito M: Origin of the preoculomotor projections through the brachium conjunctivum and their functional roles in the vestibulo-ocular reflex, in Baker R, Berthoz A (eds): *Control of Gaze by Brain Stem Neurons*. Amsterdam, Elsevier, 1977, pp 167–175.
46. Carpenter MB, Strominger NL: Cerebello-oculomotor fibres in the rhesus monkey. *J Comp Neurol* 1964; 123:211–230.
47. Highstein SM: The organization of the vestibulo-oculomotor and trochlear reflex pathways in the rabbit. *Exp Brain Res* 1973; 17:285–300.
48. Cohen B, Goto K, Shanzer S, et al: Eye movements induced by electrical stimulation of the cerebellum in the alert cat. *Exp Neurol* 1965; 13:145–162.
49. Ron S, Robinson DA: Eye movements evoked by cerebellar stimulation in the alert monkey. *J Neurophysiol* 1973; 36:1004–1022.
50. Chubb MC, Fuchs AF: Contribution of y-group of vestibular nuclei and dentate nucleus of cerebellum to generation of vertical smooth eye movements. *J Neurophysiol* 1982; 48:75–99.
51. King WM, Precht W, Dieringer N: Synaptic organization of frontal eye field and vestibular afferents to the interstitial nucleus of Cajal in the cat. *J Neurophysiol* 1980; 43:912–928.
52. Pasik T, Pasik P, Bender MB: The pretectal syndrome in monkeys: I. Disturbances of gaze and body posture. *Brain* 1969; 92:521–534.
53. Keane JR, Davis RL: Pretectal syndrome with metatstatic malignant melanoma to the posterior commissure. *Am J Ophthalmol* 1970; 82:910–914.
54. Buttner-Ennever JA, Buttner U, Cohen B, et al: Vertical gaze paralysis and the rostral interstitial nucleus of the medial longitudinal fasciculus. *Brain* 1982; 105:125–149.
55. Buttner-Ennever JA, Lang W: Vestibular projections to the monkey thalamus and rostral mesencephalon: An autoradiographic study, in Gualtierotti T (ed): *Vestibular Function and Morphology*. New York, Springer-Verlag, 1981, pp 130–143.
56. Hepp K, Vilis T, Henn V: Vertical and torsional rapid eye movement generation in the riMLF. *Soc Neurosci Abstr* 1986; 12:1187.
57. Vilis T, Hepp K, Schwarz U, et al: Unilateral riMLF lesions impair saccade generation along specific vertical planes. *Soc Neurosci Abstr* 1986; 12:1187.
58. Baker R: Anatomical and physiological organization of brainstem neurons, in Baker R, Berthoz A (ed): *Control of Gaze By Brain Stem Neurons*. New York, Elsevier, 1977, pp 207–222.
59. Cannon SC, Robinson DA: Loss of neural integrator of the oculomotor

system from brain stem lesions in monkey. *J. Neurophysiol* 1987; 57:1383–1409.

60. Noda H, Suzuki DA: The role of the flocculus of the monkey in fixation and smooth pursuit eye movements. *J Physiol* 1979; 294:335–348.
61. King WM, Fuchs AF, Magnin M: Vertical eye movement-related responses of neurons in the midbrain near the interstitial nucleus of Cajal. *J Neurophysiol* 1981; 46:549–562.
62. Maekawa K, Simpson JI: Climbing fiber responses evoked in vestibulocerebellum of rabbit from visual system. *J Neurophysiol* 1973; 36:649–666.
63. Maekawa K, Takeda T: Mossy fiber responses evoked in the cerebellar flocculus of rabbits by stimulation of the optic pathway. *Brain Res* 1975; 98:590–595.
64. Shimazu H, Precht W: Inhibition of central vestibular neurons from the contralateral labyrinth and its mediating pathway. *J Neurophysiol* 1966; 29:467–492.
65. Galiana HL, Outerbridge JS: A bilateral model for central neural pathways in vestibuloocular reflex. *J Neurophysiol* 1984; 51:210–241.
66. Baker R, Gresty M, Berthoz A: Neuronal activity in the prepositus hypoglossi nucleus correlated with vertical and horizontal eye movement in the cat. *Brain Res* 1976; 101:366–371.
67. Precht W: Vestibular mechanisms. *Annu Rev Neurosci* 1979; 2:265–289.
68. Yoshida K, McCrea R, Berthoz A, et al: Properties of immediate premotor inhibitory burst neurons controlling horizontal rapid eye movements in the cat, in Fuchs AF, Becker W (eds): *Progress in Oculomotor Research*. New York, Elsevier, 1981, pp 71–80.
69. Chubb MC, Fuchs AF, Scudder CA: Neuron activity in monkey vestibular nuclei during vertical vestibular stimulation and eye movements. *J Neurophysiol* 1984; 52:724–742.
70. Lisberger SG, Miles FA: Role of primate medial vestibular nucleus in long-term adaptive plasticity of vestibulo-ocular reflex. *J Neurophysiol* 1980; 43:1725–1745.
71. Tomlinson RD, Robinson DA: Signals in vestibular nucleus mediating vertical eye movements in the monkey. *J Neurophysiol* 1984; 51:1121–1136.
72. Guedry FE, Benson AJ: Tracking performance during sinusoidal stimulation of the vertical and horizontal semicircular canals, in Busby DE (ed): *Recent Advances in Aerospace Medicine*. Dordrecht, the Netherlands, Reidel, 1970, pp 276–288.
73. Barnes GR, Benson AJ, Prior ARJ: Visual-vestibular interaction in the control of eye movement. *Aviat Space Environ Med* 1978; 49:557–564.
74. Collewijn H, Conijn P, Tamminga EP: Eye-head coordination in man during the pursuit of moving targets, in Lennerstrand G, Zee DS, Keller EL (eds): *Functional Basis of Ocular Motility Disorders*. Oxford, Pergamon Press, 1982, pp 369–378.

75. Lisberger SG, Evinger C, Johanson GW, et al: Relation between eye acceleration and retinal image velocity during foveal smooth pursuit in man and monkey. *J Neurophysiol* 1981; 46:229–249.
76. Halmagyi GM, Gresty MA: Clinical signs of the visual-vestibular interaction. *J Neurol Neurosurg Psychiatry* 1979; 42:934–939.
77. McKinley PA, Peterson BW: Voluntary modulation of the vestibulo-ocular reflex in humans and its relation to smooth pursuit. *Exp Brain Res* 1985; 60:454–464.
78. Evinger LC, Fuchs AF, Baker R: Bilateral lesions of the median longitudinal fasciculus in monkeys: Effects on the horizontal and vertical components of voluntary and vestibular induced eye movements. *Exp Brain Res* 1977; 28:1–20.
79. Anderson JH, Precht W, Pappas C: Changes in the vertical vestibulo-ocular reflex due to kainic acid lesions of the interstitial nucleus of Cajal. *Neurosci Lett* 1979; 14:259–264.
80. Westheimer G, Blair SM: The ocular tilt reaction—a brain stem oculomotor routine. *Invest Ophthalmol* 1979; 14:833–839.
81. Halmagyi GM, Gresty MA, Gibson WPR: Ocular tilt reaction with peripheral vestibular lesion. *Ann Neurol* 1979; 6:80–83.
82. Hedges TR, Hoyt WF: Ocular tilt reaction due to an upper brainstem lesion: Paroxysmal skew deviation, torsion, and oscillation of the eyes with head tilt. *Ann Neurol* 1982; 11:537–540.
83. Rabinovitch HE, Sharpe JA, Sylvester TO: The ocular tilt reaction: A paroxysmal dyskinesia associated with elliptical nystagmus. *Arch Ophthalmol* 1977; 95:1395–1398.
84. Auerbach SH, De Piero TJ, Romanul F: Sylvian aqueduct syndrome caused by unilateral midbrain lesion. *Ann Neurol* 1982; 11:91–94.
85. Ranalli PJ, Sharpe JA, Fletcher WA: Palsy of upward and downward saccadic pursuit and vestibular movements with a unilateral midbrain lesion: Pathophysiological correlations. *Neurology* 1988; 38:114–122.
86. Cohen B, Raphan T, Waespe W: Vestibulo-cerebellar control of the vestibulo-ocular reflex, in Keller EL, Zee DS (eds): *Adaptive Processes in Visual and Oculomotor Systems*. Oxford, Pergamon Press, 1986, pp 277–283.
87. Darlot C, Lopez-Barneo J, Tracy D: Asymmetries of vertical vestibular nystagmus in the cat. *Exp Brain Res* 1981; 41:420–426.
88. King WM, Leigh RJ: Physiology of vertical gaze, in Lennerstrand G, Zee DS, Keller EL (eds): *Functional Basis of Ocular Motility Disorders*. Oxford, Pergamon Press, 1982, pp 267–276.
89. King WM, Maxwell J: The vertical vestibulo-ocular reflex (VOR) in the cat: I. Responses to head velocity steps and sinusoids. *J Neurophysiol* In press.
90. Snyder LH, King WM: Vertical vestibulo-ocular reflex in cat: Asymmetry and adaptation, in preparation.
91. Matsuo V, Cohen B: Vertical optokinetic nystagmus and vestibular nys-

tagmus in the monkey: Up-down asymmetry and effects of gravity. *Exp Brain Res* 1984; 53:197–216.

92. Bohmer A, Henn V: Horizontal and vertical vestibulo-ocular and cervico-ocular reflexes in the monkey during high frequency rotation. *Brain Res* 1983; 277:241–248.
93. Correia MJ, Perachio AA, Eden AR: The monkey vertical vestibulo-ocular response: A frequency domain study. *J Neurophysiol* 1985; 54:532–548.
94. Miles FA, Lisberger SG: Plasticity in the vestibulo-ocular reflex: A new hypothesis. *Annu Rev Neurosci* 1979; 4:273–299.
95. Ito M, Jasterboff PJ, Miyashita Y: Adaptive modification of the rabbit's horizontal vestibulo-ocular reflex during sustained vestibular and optokinetic stimulation. *Exp Brain Res* 1979; 37:17–30.
96. Gonshor A, Melvill Jones G: Short-term adaptive changes in the human vestibulo-ocular reflex arc. *J Physiol (Lond)* 1976; 256:361–379.
97. Gonshor A, Melvill Jones G: Extreme vestibulo-ocular adaptation induced by prolonged optical reversal of vision. *J Physiol (Lond)* 1976; 256:381–414.
98. Duffose M, Ito M, Jasterboff PJ, et al: A neuronal correlate in rabbit's cerebellum to adaptive modification of the vestibulo-ocular reflex. *Brain Res* 1978; 150:611–616.
99. Lisberger SG: Role of the cerebellum during motor learning in the vestibulo-ocular reflex: Different mechanisms in different species? *Trends Neurosci* 1982; 5:437–441.
100. Melvill Jones G, Barry W, Kowalsky N: Dynamics of the semicircular canals compared in yaw, pitch, and roll. *Aerospace Med* 1964; 35:984–989.
101. Baloh RW, Richman L, Yee RD, et al: The dynamics of vertical eye movements in normal human subjects. *Aviat Space Environ Med* 1983; 54:32–38.
102. Collins WE, Guedry FE: Duration of angular acceleration and ocular nystagmus from cat and man: I. Responses from the lateral and vertical canals to two stimulus durations. *Acta Otolaryngol (Stockh)* 1967; 64:373–387.
103. Berthoz A, Brandt T, Dichgans J, et al: European vestibular experiments on the Spacelab-1 mission: 5. Contribution of the otoliths to the vertical vestibulo-ocular reflex. *Exp Brain Res* 1986; 64:272–278.
104. Ranalli PJ, Sharpe JA: Vertical vestibulo-ocular reflex, smooth pursuit and eye-head tracking in normal subjects. *Inv Ophthalmol Vis Sci* 1987; 28(ARVO suppl):315.
105. Viire E, Tweed D, Milner K, et al: A reexamination of the gain of the vestibuloocular reflex. *J Neurophysiol* 1986; 56:439–450.
106. Buttner-Ennever JA, Buttner U, Cohen B, et al: Vertical gaze paralysis and the rostral interstitial nucleus of the medial longitudinal fasciculus. *Brain* 1982; 105:125–149.

107. Pierrot-Deseillingy C, Chain F, Gray F, et al: Parinaud's syndrome: Electrooculographic and anatomic analyses of six vascular cases with deductions about vertical gaze organization in the premotor structures. *Brain* 1982; 105:667–696.
108. Baloh RW, Furman JM, Yee RD: Dorsal midbrain syndrome: Clinical and oculographic findings. *Neurology* 1985; 35:54–60.
109. Bannister R: *Brain's Clinical Neurology*. London, Oxford University Press, 1975, pp 30–32.
110. Adams RD, Victor M: *Principles of Neurology*. New York, McGraw-Hill, 1981, pp 178–179.
111. Baloh RW, Yee RD, Honrubia V: Internuclear ophthalmoplegia: II. Pursuit, optokinetic nystagmus, and vestibulo-ocular reflex. *Arch Neurol* 1978; 35:490–493.
112. Leigh RJ, Newman SA, King WM: Vertical gaze disorders, in Lennerstrand G, Zee DS, Keller EL (eds): *Functional Basis of Ocular Motility Disorders*. Oxford, Pergamon Press, 1982, pp 257–266.
113. Larmande P, Henin D, Jan M, et al: Abnormal vertical eye movements in the locked-in syndrome. *Ann Neurol* 1982; 11:100–102.
114. Ranalli PJ, Sharpe JA: Vertical vestibulo-ocular reflex, smooth pursuit, and combined eye-head tracking dysfunction in internuclear ophthalmoplegia. *Neurology* 1987; 37(suppl 1):140.
115. Zee DS, Friendlich AR, Robinson DA: The mechanism of downbeat nystagmus. *Arch Neurol* 1974; 30:227–237.
116. Gresty MA, Barratt H, Rudge P, et al: Analysis of downbeat nystagmus: Otolithic vs semicircular canal influences. *Arch Neurol* 1986; 43:52–55.
117. Baloh RW, Spooner JW: Downbeat nystagmus: A type of central vestibular nystagmus. *Neurology* 1981; 31:304–310.
118. Halmagyi GM, Rudge P, Gresty MA, et al: Downbeating nystagmus: A review of 62 cases. *Arch Neurol* 1983; 40:777–784.
119. Cogan DG: Down-beat nystagmus. *Arch Ophthalmol* 1968; 80:757.
120. Phadke JG, Hern JEC, Blaiklock CT: Downbeat nystagmus—a false localising sign due to communicating hydrocephalus. *J Neurol Neurosurg Psychiatry* 1981; 44:459.
121. Donat JR, Auger R: Familial periodic ataxia. *Arch Neurol* 1979; 36:568–569.
122. Saul R, Selhorst JB: Downbeat nystagmus with magnesium depletion. *Arch Neurol* 1981; 38:650–652.
123. Coppeto JR, Monteiro MLR, Lessel S, et al: Downbeat nystagmus: Long term therapy with moderate-dose lithium carbonate. *Arch Neurol* 1983; 40:754–755.
124. Chrousos GA, Cowdry R, Schulein M, et al: Two cases of downbeat nystagmus and oscillopsia associated with carbemazepine. *Am J Ophthalmol* 1987; 103:221–224.
125. Alpert JN: Downbeat nystagmus due to anticonvulsant toxicity. *Ann Neurol* 1978; 4:471–473.

126. Dejong JMBV, Cohen B, Matsuo V, et al: Midsaggital pontomedullary brainstem section: Effects on ocular adduction and nystagmus. *Exp Neurol* 1980; 68:420.
127. Zee DS, Yamazaki A, Butler PH, et al: Effects of ablation of flocculus and paraflocculus on eye movements in primate. *J Neurophysiol* 1981; 46:878–899.
128. Fernandez C, Alzate R, Lindsay JR: Experimental observations on postural nystagmus: II. Lesions of the nodulus. *Ann Otol Rhinol Laryngol* 1960; 69:94–114.
129. Precht W, Volkind R, Maeda M, et al: The effects of stimulating the cerebellar nodulus in the cat on the response of vestibular neurons. *Neuroscience* 1976; 1:301–312.
130. Zee DS, Leigh RJ, Mathieu-Millaire F: Cerebellar control of ocular gaze stability. *Ann Neurol* 1980; 7:37–40.
131. Keane JR, Itabashi HH: Upbeat nystagmus: Clinicopathologic study of two patients. *Neurology* 1987; 37:491–494.
132. Fisher A, Gresty M, Chambers B, et al: Primary position upbeat nystagmus: A variety of central positional nystagmus. *Brain* 1983; 106:949–964.
133. Gilman N, Baloh RW, Tomiyasu U: Primary position upbeat nystagmus. *Neurology* 1977; 27:294–298.
134. Troost BT, Martinez J, Abel LA, et al: Upbeat nystagmus and internuclear ophthalmoplegia with brainstem glioma. *Arch Neurol* 1980; 37:453–456.
135. Cox TA, Corbett JJ, Thompson HS, et al: Upbeat nystagmus changing to downbeat nystagmus with convergence. *Neurology* 1981; 31:891.
136. Holmes GL, Hafford J, Zimmerman AW: Primary position upbeat nystagmus following meningitis. *Ann Ophthalmol* 1981; 13:935.
137. Sibony PA, Evinger C, Manning KA: Tobacco induced primary-position upbeat nystagmus. *Ann Neurol* 1987; 21:53–58.
138. Daroff RB, Troost BT: Upbeat nystagmus. *JAMA* 1973; 225:312.
139. Nakada T, Remler MP: Primary position upbeat nystagmus: Another central vestibular nystagmus? *J Clin Neuro-ophthalmol* 1981; 1:185.
140. Leigh RJ, Zee DS: *The Neurology of Eye Movement*. Philadelphia, FA Davis, 1983, pp 197–198.
141. Keane JR: Sustained upgaze in coma. *Ann Neurol* 1981; 9:409–412.
142. Keane JR, Rawlinson DG, Lu AT: Sustained downgaze deviation: Two cases without structural pretectal lesions. *Neurology* 1976; 26:594–595.
143. Simon RP: Forced downward ocular deviation: Occurrence during oculo-vestibular testing in sedative drug-induced coma. *Arch Neurol* 1978; 35:456–458.

12

New Concepts of Vestibular Nystagmus

David S. Zee, M.D.

This chapter emphasizes the new concepts of nystagmus that are particularly relevant to the clinical diagnosis of vestibular disorders. I will concentrate on three areas: (1) The so-called velocity storage mechanism; the central neural network that improves the inherently limited ability of the semicircular canals to respond to the low-frequency components of head rotation. (2) The analysis of the VOR as a three-dimensional geometrical problem. Much can be gleaned by considering the relationships among the planes in the head in which the semicircular canals lie, the planes in the orbit in which the muscles pull, and the planes in space in which the head is rotating. The analysis of this type of problem has become considerably simplified by the use of the tools of matrices and vectors.[1] But even without a rigorous mathematical analysis, one can appreciate many of the practical implications of these approaches. (3) Otolith influences on the generation and the characteristics of vestibular nystagmus. There are important new perspectives to the perennial question: Is there an otolith-induced nystagmus?

VELOCITY STORAGE AND THE FREQUENCY RESPONSE OF THE VOR

The concept of velocity storage was introduced by Raphan and Cohen.[2] The velocity storage mechanism refers to a central neural network that is probably located in the medulla in the region of the vestibular nuclei and the perihypoglossal nuclei. An important function of this network is to improve the ability of the vestibular system to respond accurately to the low-frequency components of head rotation. Because of the mechanical properties of the endolymph-cupula system, the labyrinth can reliably transmit a signal proportional to the velocity of the head only when the frequency of rotation is above about 0.02 Hz. Any head rotation that is comprised of lower frequencies would not be adequately compensated.

Consider the response to an impulsive (constant-velocity) head rotation. At the onset of rotation, when head velocity is rapidly changing, high-frequency components predominate, and the vestibular periphery transmits a faithful rendition of head velocity. As the rotation continues at a constant velocity, the frequency content of the stimulus shifts toward the lower end of the spectrum. The cupula then gradually returns toward the neutral position and the discharge rate of primary vestibular afferents, which is proportional to the angle of deviation of the cupula, signals (incorrectly) a progressively lower head velocity. The rate of decline of the response can be described by a time constant. The higher the value of the time constant, the longer the duration of the response and, correspondingly, the better the response to the low-frequency components of the stimulus. This dichotomy between the response to high- and low-frequency components of a stimulus can readily be appreciated with sinusoidal stimuli. The amplitude of the response is lower when the frequency of stimulation is low.

Because of the intrinsic limitations of the labyrinthine transducers, the nervous system has evolved a central mechanism—velocity storage—to improve the low-frequency response of the VOR. This mechanism can take the peripheral labyrinthine signal and, by the process of a mathematical integration, increase the range of frequency response of the VOR threefold. Accordingly, the time constant of decay of vestibular nystagmus (about 20 seconds) is three times that of the actual signal recorded on vestibular afferents coming from the semicircular canals (about 7 seconds). Exactly how this integration is accomplished is not settled, but one hypothesis[3] uses a central positive feedback loop, which carries the peripheral vestibular signal away from the secondary vestibular neurons and then, after appropriate processing, feeds a lagged version of head velocity back onto those same secondary vestibular neurons for transmission to the ocular motoneurons.*

The velocity storage mechanism uses every source of sensory information available to it. It has access to signals that discharge in relation to slip of images on the retina, so that during rotation in the light, labyrinthine signals can be supplemented by vision. When vision becomes the only input—as is the case after the cupula has returned to its neutral position during a prolonged constant-velocity rotation—the sustained "vestibular" response is called optokinetic nystagmus (OKN).

Otolith signals can also be used by the velocity storage mechanism. If one rotates at a constant velocity in darkness, but with the body tilted away from the upright position—so-called off-axis rotation—a nystagmus continues to be produced even after the cupula has returned to its neutral position. In the extreme case, with a 90° tilt away from vertical, the sustained response is called "barbeque nystagmus." With off-axis rotation the head continuously changes its orientation with respect to gravity, so that the otolith organs, which detect linear accelerations (e.g., gravity), continue to modulate their discharge even though there is no angular acceleration to excite the semicircular canals. Apparently the velocity storage mechanism can use otolith inputs to abstract the velocity of angular rotation of the head and generate a compensatory nystagmus.[4]

Clinically it is important to keep in mind this division of labor between the semicircular canals, which transmit signals that are used to compensate for high frequencies of rotation, and the velocity storage mechanism, which uses afferent information from a variety of sources (including the semicircular canal inputs themselves, otolith inputs, visual inputs, and even somatosensory inputs) to generate nystagmus that compensates for the low-frequency components of head rotation. A caloric stimulus, for example, is composed of predominantly low frequencies. A constant-velocity rotation of the head contains all frequencies; the high end of the spectrum is represented at the initiation of movement, the low end of the spectrum during the later, sustained portion of the rotation. Thus, one can have absent or markedly attenuated caloric responses (both in duration and in amplitude) in the presence of a normal response to the high-frequency components of a head rotation. The initial amplitude of response to a con-

*The velocity storage integrator must be distinguished from the eye position, gaze-holding integrator that takes eye velocity commands of all types (vestibular, saccades, pursuit) and produces the position-coded information necessary for holding the eyes steady. The medial vestibular nucleus and nucleus prepositus hypoglossi are important in this process.[18]

stant-velocity rotation would be normal but its duration considerably shortened.*

It is important to remember that patients may not experience any symptoms when only the response to the low-frequency components of a stimulus is lost. Even with absent caloric responses, patients need not experience oscillopsia during head movements, since the high-frequency response can be intact. The inability of their labyrinths to respond to low frequencies can be compensated for by visual (optokinetic) inputs. To epitomize, oscillopsia with head motion, when due to a symmetric loss of vestibular function, usually signifies an inadequate response to the high-frequency components of head rotation.

ABNORMALITIES OF VELOCITY STORAGE

A decrease in velocity storage, as shown by a low VOR time constant, is commonly found with peripheral (unilateral or bilateral) lesions. Some patients may have too much velocity storage. An example is periodic alternating nystagmus (PAN).[6] This is a form of central vestibular nystagmus in which the direction of a spontaneous horizontal nystagmus changes every few minutes. Theoretical analysis suggests that PAN arises from an increased "gain" in the central velocity storage mechanism, so that vestibular responses are excessively prolonged to the point of instability. An adaptation mechanism, probably akin to that which produces the reversal phases of caloric and of post-rotatory nystagmus, helps stop the runaway response of the velocity storage mechanism, but when the nystagmus slows down and changes direction, it runs away in the other direction. This sequence of events incessantly repeats itself, leading to PAN. Fortunately, we have a medication, baclofen, with its gamma-aminobutyric acid (GABA)-like action, that disengages velocity storage.[7] Consequently, one can effectively stop periodic alternating nystagmus with relatively low doses of baclofen.

In some patients velocity storage may attenuate rather than perseverate peripheral vestibular responses. Patients who have been deprived of normal visual experience during development of their nervous systems with, for example, congenital blindness or congenital

*This pattern of a dissociated vestibular response to caloric and impulsive stimuli is commonly the case with severe degrees of bilateral vestibular paresis such as that due to ototoxic medication.[5] On rare occasions central lesions may also cause a similar dissociation.

nystagmus may have absent caloric responses and exceedingly low time constants during constant-velocity rotations, even smaller than the 7 seconds that one would predict from cupula-endolymph mechanics.[8, 9] These patients may have a selective defect in one population of vestibular afferents, so that the only fibers that are functional are those with low time constants of discharge. Alternatively, the change in their VOR may be of central origin, since, because of the visual defect, the VOR becomes superfluous. The CNS is unable to calibrate the reflex properly, or it simply attempts to eliminate the VOR completely. One way to dampen the VOR would be to use negative feedback to attenuate the peripheral vestibular signal rather than the positive feedback which is normally used to perseverate the VOR.

The clinician should keep in mind the distinction between the response to the high- and low-frequency components of a vestibular stimulus; the role of the peripheral labyrinth in transducing the former, of central mechanisms in extracting the latter; and the complementary nature of caloric and impulsive rotational testing in defining the full range of responses of the VOR.

THREE-DIMENSIONAL ANALYSIS OF VESTIBULAR NYSTAGMUS

Head-Shaking-Induced Nystagmus

When we rotate our heads, compensatory eye movements must be not only of the correct size and timing but also of the appropriate direction. If the head rotates horizontally, so should the eyes. We became particularly interested in the problem of inappropriate "cross-coupling" of vestibular nystagmus, also known as "perverted nystagmus," as part of an investigation of head-shaking-induced nystagmus (HSN).[10]

Head-shaking-induced nystagmus has been recognized for many years. It refers to the observation that patients with vestibular lesions, of either peripheral or central origin, may show a transient increase in or emergence of a spontaneous nystagmus after a period of vigorous head shaking.[11] This nystagmus has traditionally been ascribed to the activation of a latent vestibular imbalance. We have studied HSN in a group of normal subjects and in a group of patients with a complete unilateral loss of peripheral vestibular function. We found a highly characteristic pattern of HSN in all of our patients. The appearance of this particular pattern might allow the prediction that the caloric response will be markedly depressed on one side.

We elicited HSN by encouraging vigorous, approximately sinusoidal, head shaking for 15–20 seconds. We then asked the patient to stop shaking his head and observed the patient's eyes under Frenzel lenses. Invariably, we found a transient (5–20 sec) but relatively brisk nystagmus with slow phases initially directed toward the impaired ear. This nystagmus was followed by a much longer but lower-amplitude nystagmus with slow phases directed away from the impaired ear. With vertical head shaking we also induced a horizontal nystagmus, but in this case the primary phase was directed away from the impaired ear. The reversal phase was small or absent.

How do we explain this particular pattern of nystagmus? We will invoke three processes to explain the presence and the direction of the two phases of HSN. Of primary importance is Ewald's second law, which states that for high velocities of head rotation, excitation is a more effective stimulus than is inhibition. This asymmetric response occurs because vestibular afferents are silenced—driven into inhibitory cutoff—at a velocity of head rotation that is lower than that which leads to saturation during excitation. The effect of Ewald's law is most apparent when the head is positioned so that the plane of the particular semicircular canal being tested is parallel to the plane in which the head is rotating. In the case of an absent labyrinth, for high speeds of rotation the increase in peripheral vestibular activity that is relayed centrally with rotation toward the good ear (the excitatory direction) is greater than the decrease in vestibular activity that is relayed centrally with rotation toward the bad ear (the inhibitory direction). This nonlinear property of the labyrinthine response forms the basis for using high-speed rotational stimuli to detect unilateral peripheral vestibular lesions. Furthermore, to probe the function of a particular pair of semicircular canals, the head should be positioned with the plane of the canals parallel to the plane in which the head is rotating.

With rapid head shaking, the nonlinearity described by Ewald's second law leads to a continual, asymmetric, increase and decrease in activity that is relayed to the central velocity storage mechanism. Consequently, there is an accumulation of activity for slow phases directed toward the impaired ear. When the head stops shaking, the velocity storage mechanism gradually discharges, leading to a slowly decaying nystagmus with slow phases directed toward the bad ear. To account for the reversal phase of HSN, we invoked a short-term adaptive mechanism, comparable to that which produces the reversal phase of caloric or of post-rotatory nystagmus in normal individuals.

The combination of Ewald's second law, asymmetric velocity storage and adaptation nicely explains the pattern of horizontal nystagmus that occurs after head shaking in patients with a unilateral peripheral vestibular loss. Note that this hypothesis predicts that head rotations of low velocities should not lead to HSN, because Ewald's law should only become apparent when the speed of rotation is high. HSN due to more central lesions, for example, due to asymmetries in the velocity storage mechanism itself, might appear when the speed of head rotation is low. Finally, if velocity storage is relatively ineffective, as indicated by a low VOR time constant, the primary phase of HSN will be shorter and the reversal phase will emerge sooner.

Cross-Coupling Effects in HSN

What is the origin of the horizontally directed component of the nystagmus induced by vertical head shaking? The most likely explanation relates to the fact that in normal individuals excitation of the vertical semicircular canals also contributes to the generation of horizontal slow phases of nystagmus. This "cross-coupling" between activities in the vertical semicircular canals and horizontal nystagmus arises from the geometrical arrangement of the semicircular canals within the head. The lateral canals are pitched up about 30° and the vertical canals are correspondingly tilted backward. Consequently, with certain orientations of the head with respect to the axis of rotation, the vertical canals contribute to the generation of horizontal nystagmus and the lateral canals to the generation of torsional nystagmus. In fact, when the head is pitched up 60°, and the body is rotated around an earth-vertical axis, a significant horizontal component of the VOR (about 50% of that with the head upright) is still generated—as it should be—even though with this head orientation the peripheral vestibular activity arises almost exclusively from the vertical semicircular canals.[12]*

One must also remember that excitation of the vertical semicircular canals leads to ipsilaterally directed horizontal slow phases and that rotation around an earth-vertical axis with the head upright leads to inhibition of activity from the vertical canals in the same labyrinth in which the lateral canal is being excited. Accordingly, during vertical head shaking by a patient with only one functioning labyrinth,

*During rotation of the body around an Earth-vertical axis, one can use measurements of the *horizontal VOR* with the head in different positions of pitch to assay the relative abilities of the vertical and of the lateral semicircular canals to transduce head velocity.

activity for horizontal nystagmus accumulates in central velocity storage. After vertical head shaking, there is a transient horizontal component of nystagmus with slow phases directed toward the intact ear.

OTOLITH-INDUCED NYSTAGMUS

There are several mechanisms by which the otoliths can influence vestibular nystagmus. We are just beginning to develop ways of using this information to assay otolith function in patients. We have already mentioned the use of off-axis, or barbeque, rotation as an example of an otolith-induced nystagmus. Hain et al.[13] have investigated another way to test otolith function, and I will update the results of this study.

Tilt-Suppression of Post-Rotatory Nystagmus

After several minutes of rotation around an earth-vertical axis at a constant velocity in darkness, the vestibular nystagmus dies away. Then, if rotation is abruptly stopped, a post-rotatory nystagmus ensues that decays with a time constant of about 20 sec. If, however, one tilts the head forward, just as the post-rotatory phase of nystagmus begins, a horizontal nystagmus still appears, but its time constant drops to a value close to that of the cupula itself (7 sec). Because of the change in otolith activity due to the reorientation of the head with respect to gravity, the velocity storage mechanism is disengaged; only the decaying peripheral vestibular activity remains. This attenuation of the post-rotatory VOR response has been attributed to "dumping" of velocity storage, or so-called tilt suppression of vestibular nystagmus.[2, 14] In the monkey such tilt suppression is abolished by ablation of the uvula and nodulus of the posterior cerebellar vermis.[15] We have studied several human patients with lesions in the posterior fossa and found that in human beings, too, a loss of tilt suppression is a reliable sign of lesions of the posterior cerebellar vermis.

One can envision a function for the tilt-suppression mechanism, since repositioning of the head during post-rotatory nystagmus leads to incongruous otolith and semicircular canal inputs. When the head is actually rotating around an axis oriented away from the vertical upright, the otoliths should modulate their discharge with respect to the change in position of the head with respect to gravity. In the case of post-rotatory nystagmus, when the head is actually still, the otoliths do not signal a rotation, while the semicircular canals signals do. With the head positioned away from upright the absence of a modulation of otolith activity during post-rotatory nystagmus—which is an intra-vestibular conflict—is presumably interpreted by the CNS as a malfunction. Accordingly the CNS does not "know" what signal to believe. Velocity storage is "dumped," and the vestibular time constant is (appropriately) shortened.

Tilt suppression is a test of the ability of the otoliths to transduce the position of the head with respect to gravity, of the integrity of the pathways that relay otolith information to the uvula and nodulus, and of the ability of the uvula and nodulus to transmit a message to the brain stem to disengage velocity storage. If velocity storage is impaired to begin with —i.e., the time constant of the VOR is low during rotation with the head upright—one can not use tilt-suppression to assay otolith or posterior cerebellar vermal function.

Otolith Modulation of the VOR During Eccentric Head Rotation

It has also been suggested that the otoliths may be able to modulate semicircular canal-induced responses independent of any effect on velocity storage. In other words, there may be an otolith-induced change of the gain of the VOR at high frequencies of rotation. Viirre and co-workers[16] in monkeys and Gresty et al.[17] in human patients investigated this possibility during eccentric head rotation. The head is positioned away from the center of the axis of rotation but not reoriented with respect to gravity. In this circumstance, the gain of the VOR must be adjusted to account for the superimposed linear components of acceleration, if one needs to maintain gaze at any location that is closer than infinity.

Even in natural circumstances, consider fixating on a stationary target located 1 m in front of the head during either horizontal or vertical head oscillation. Because the eyes are being translated with every rotation (the eyes are about 10 cm in front of the axis around which the head naturally rotates), the VOR gain must be adjusted upward, by about 10% in this case, to allow fixation of the target during head rotation. How is this accomplished? In the light, of course, the pursuit system might help, provided the frequency and velocity of rotation are within its range. The angle of vergence or the state of accommodation might also be used as cues for the needed VOR adjustment. Finally, the otolith organs, which relay information about the linear components of head movement, might be the critical sensor.

Both Viirre et al.[16] and Gresty et al.[17] have shown that during rotation in darkness the gain of the VOR can be adjusted appropriately, up or down, according to the relationship between the position of the head and the axis of the rotation. This adjustment, though, is critically dependent on the percept of where gaze is to be directed; i.e., how close the target is to the eyes. Any angular rotation of the globe that is used to compensate for a linear motion of the head requires a trigonometric conversion factor, based on the distance between the eyes and the target. The otoliths may supply one component of the necessary information for adjustment of the VOR as a function of viewing distance. Hence, the ability to adjust the VOR gain during eccentric head rotations in patients is a potential way to assess the integrity of otolith inputs as well as of central canal-otolith interactions. What has not yet been adequately addressed is whether higher-level, cognitive factors play the same type of role in this type of adjustment as they do in other on-line adjustments of the VOR during, for example, imagination of targets rotating with the head.

There are now three relatively new ways to assay otolith function: generation of a sustained nystagmus during off-axis, constant-velocity rotations, tilt suppression of post-rotatory nystagmus, and modulation of VOR gain during combined linear-angular accelerations. Demonstrating the practical usefulness of these tests remains the challenge to the clinician.

Conclusions

I would like to reemphasize the following organizational features of the VOR and analytical approaches to accurate vestibular diagnosis. Vestibular stimuli must be analyzed in terms of both their complement of frequencies and range of velocities. There is a division of labor among labyrinthine, visual, and proprioceptive receptors as to which component of a vestibular stimulus they respond and under what circumstances that particular sensor is best suited to transduce the speed of rotation of the head. A central velocity storage mechanism combines information from all of these sensors to widen the range of frequencies over which the VOR performs properly. The nonlinear properties of the peripheral labyrinthine transducers at high speeds of head rotation lead to Ewald's second law, which makes it possible to diagnose unilateral peripheral labyrinthine lesions using rotational testing. An appreciation of the geometrical relationships of the semicircular canals in the head is crucial to interpreting the directions of both normal and pathologic nystagmus. Finally, the evaluation of the influences of otolith stimulation on nystagmus induced by stimulation of the semicircular canals may become an important clinical tool in our assessment of vestibular disorders.

REFERENCES

1. Robinson DA: The coordinates of neurons in the vestibulo-ocular reflex, in Berthoz A, Melvill Jones G (eds): *Adaptive Mechanisms in Gaze Control.* Amsterdam, Elsevier, 1985, pp 297–311.
2. Raphan T, Cohen B: Velocity storage and the ocular response to multidimensional vestibular stimuli, in Berthoz A, Melvill Jones G (eds): *Adaptive Mechanisms in Gaze Control.* Amsterdam, Elsevier, 1985, pp 123–143.
3. Robinson DA: Linear addition of optokinetic and vestibular signals in the vestibular nucleus. *Exp Brain Res* 1977; 30:447–450.
4. Hain TC: A model of the nystagmus induced by off vertical axis rotation. *Biol Cybern* 1986; 54:337–350.
5. Baloh RW, Honrubia V, Yee RD, et al: Changes in the human vestibulo-ocular reflex after loss of peripheral sensitivity. *Ann Neurol* 1984; 16:222–228.
6. Leigh RJ, Robinson DA, Zee DS: A hypothetical explanation of periodic alternating nystagmus: Instability in the optokinetic-vestibular system. *Ann NY Acad Sci* 1981; 374:619–635.
7. Halmagyi G, Rudge P, Gresty M, et al: Treatment of periodic alternating nystagmus. *Ann Neurol* 1980; 8:609–611.
8. Demer J, Zee DS: Vestibulo-ocular and optokinetic deficits in albinos with congenital nystagmus. *Invest Ophthalmol Vis Sci* 1984; 25:739–745.
9. Sherman KR, Keller EL: Vestibulo-ocular reflexes of adventitiously and congenitally blind adults. *Invest Ophthalmol Vis Sci* 1986; 27:1154–1159.
10. Hain TC, Fetter M, Zee DS: Head shaking nystagmus in unilateral peripheral vestibular lesion. *Am J Otolaryngol* 1987; 8:30–41.
11. Kamei T, Kornhuber HH: Spontaneous and head-shaking nystagmus in normals and in patients with central lesions. *Can J Otolaryngol* 1979; 3:372–380.
12. Fetter M, Hain TC, Zee DS: Influence of eye and head position on the vestibulo-ocular reflex. *Exp Brain Res* 1986; 64:208–216.
13. Hain TC, Zee DS, Maria B: Modification of the dynamics of the vestibulo-ocular reflex by head tilt in patients with cerebellar lesions, in Graham MD, Kemink JL (eds): *The Vestibular System: Neurophysiologic and Clinical Research.* New York, Raven Press, 1987, pp 217–223.
14. Schrader V, Koenig E, Dichgans J: The effect of lateral head tilt on horizontal postrotatory nystagmus I and II and the Purkinje effect. *Acta Otolaryngol (Stockh)* 1985; 100:98–105.

15. Waespe W, Cohen B, Raphan T: Dynamic modification of the vestibulo-ocular reflex by the nodulus and uvula. *Science* 1985; 228:199–202.
16. Viirre E, Tweed D, Milner K, et al: A reexamination of the gain of the vestibuloocular reflex. *J Neurophysiol* 1986; 56:439–450.
17. Gresty M, Barratt H, Bronstein A, et al: Clinical aspects of otolith-oculomotor relationships, in Keller EL, Zee DS (eds): *Adaptive Processes in Visual and Oculomotor Systems.* Oxford, Pergamon Press, 1986, pp 357–365.
18. Cannon SC, Robinson DA: Loss of neural integrator of the oculomotor system from brain stem lesions in monkey. *J Neurophysiol* 1987; 57:1383–1409.

13

*Management of Oscillopsia**

R. John Leigh, M.D.

Oscillopsia[1, 2]—an illusion of movement of the seen world—may be caused by a variety of disorders (Table 13–1). A feature common to all (except "central oscillopsia"*) is excessive slip of images of stationary objects upon the retina. Excessive retinal slip not only causes oscillopsia but also impairs visual acuity. The relationship between retinal image velocity (RIV) and visual acuity is direct: RIV greater than about 4°/second degrades vision.[3, 4] The relationship between RIV and oscillopsia is less well established. What is known is that since the VOR works imperfectly, RIV may reach 4°/second during rotational perturbations of the head; nevertheless, there is no oscillopsia, and visual acuity is unimpaired.[5] How much retinal slip is required to produce oscillopsia has not been determined; however, there is obviously considerable variation among individuals. For example, subjects with congenital nystagmus seldom complain of oscil-

*Supported by Public Health Service grant R01-EY06717, the Veterans Administration, and the Evenor Armington Fund.

* "Central oscillopsia"[2]—in which there is no evidence of excessive image slip—is a rare condition presumably due to disorders of those central mechanisms that normally maintain visual constancy. Although its existence has been questioned, recent experimental studies[6] have shown that transcutaneous electrical stimulation with electrodes on the scalp may produce oscillopsia. Thus, the question of "central oscillopsia" remains open but will not be discussed further here. Our focus will be on disorders that cause oscillopsia by producing excessive retinal image slip.

TABLE 13–1.
Causes of Oscillopsia

Inappropriate vestibulo-ocular reflex
Hypoactive
Hyperactive
Spontaneous oscillations of the eyes
"Central oscillopsia"

lopsia despite large values of RIV. Mechanisms that may contribute to the variable threshold for oscillopsia are discussed below.

OSCILLOPSIA DUE TO ABNORMALITIES OF THE VOR

Loss or deficiency of the VOR is a well-known cause of oscillopsia occurring with head movements (Fig 13–1). Natural perturbations of the head such as those that occur during locomotion are predominantly of much higher frequency than can be coped with by visual following mechanisms.[7] Consequently, individuals with a deficient VOR mainly complain of oscillopsia when they get up and walk, as was described so well by the anonymous physician J.C.[8] Such individuals usually experience spontaneous improvement in their symptoms, however. This improvement may be due to a variety of factors that vary idiosyncratically from patient to patient[9, 10]; they include (1) potentiation of the cervico-ocular reflex, (2) preprogramming of compensatory slow eye movements in anticipation of head movement, (3) improvement of visual following reflexes, (4) perceptual adaptation, so that oscillopsia can be ignored, (5) restriction of head movements, and (6) changes in planning of saccades and quick phases.

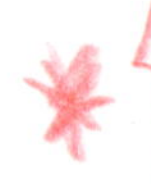

A hyperactive VOR can also cause oscillopsia, since compensatory eye movements that are inappropriately large will lead to slip of retinal images during head movements. Such a state is fairly unusual, except for the hyperactive vertical VOR that is a common accompaniment of downbeat nystagmus due to the Arnold-Chiari malformation.[11, 12]

We have studied a patient with cerebellar degeneration whose VOR gain ranged between 2 and 3.[13] We are aware of only one report of such large values for VOR gain, an experimental study in cats by Demer and Robinson,[14] in which lidocaine was injected into the com-

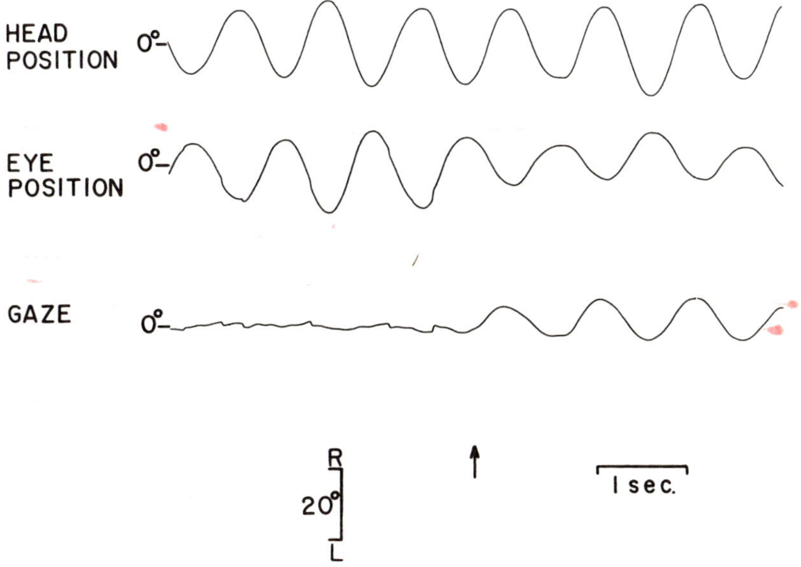

FIG 13–1.
Measurement of horizontal head rotation, eye-in-orbit, and gaze (eye in space) in patient with deficient labyrinthine function (magnetic search coil record). While room lights are on (initial part of record), he uses residual VOR, saccades, and visual following mechanisms to try to hold gaze steady. As soon as room lights are turned off (after arrow), his inadequate VOR is evident. Since the head movements are active, a cervico-ocular reflex may also be contributing.

missure of the inferior olive. We reasoned that if the climbing fiber pathway from the inferior olive to the cerebellar Purkinje cells was cholinergic, a cholinergic agent such as physostigmine might reduce the gain of the VOR. Intravenous physostigmine did indeed reduce the gain of the VOR in our patient, and he currently takes an oral preparation of this medication which he feels improves his vision. Whether such an approach is vindicated in similar patients, however, remains to be seen.

Recent work has stressed the importance of the proximity of the visual scene in modulating VOR gain so that the latter is appropriate to hold images steady on the retina.[15] The otolithic organs appear to be important in this modulation of VOR gain. It therefore seems possible that therapeutic manipulations of visual or otolithic inputs may, in the future, be used to correctly adjust VOR gain so that retinal image slip is not excessive.

OSCILLOPSIA DUE TO SPONTANEOUS OCULAR OSCILLATIONS

Spontaneous ocular oscillations—nystagmus—often cause oscillopsia. To date, the form of nystagmus that has been best studied with respect to its relationship to attendant oscillopsia is downbeat nystagmus. Wist and colleagues[16] showed that the magnitude of the oscillopsia in such patients was, on average, only 37% of the magnitude of the nystagmus. This finding implies that treatment measures may not need to stop the nystagmus to abolish oscillopsia. Wist's finding may reflect changes in perceptual threshold for motion detection[17] or partial use of an extraretinal signal to maintain some visual constancy.[18] The relationship between oscillopsia and other forms of nystagmus, such as acquired pendular nystagmus, has not been systematically investigated.

A variety of treatment measures has been reported to stop acquired nystagmus and so abolish oscillopsia and improve vision; these are listed in Table 13–2. Of the variety of drug treatments, only one, baclofen, can be regarded as a reliable specific treatment for one condition, acquired periodic alternating nystagmus.[19] Other drug successes have mainly concerned individual case reports of a variety of nystagmus types.[20–23] Recently, Currie and Matuso[24] found that a single 1–2-mg dose of clonazepam reduced or abolished nystagmus and

TABLE 13–2.
Treatments for Oscillopsia Due To Acquired Nystagmus

Treatments
Drugs
Baclofen (Lioresal)
Trihexyphenidyl (Artane)/other anticholinergics
Valproic acid (Depakene)
Clonazepam (Clonopin)
Carbamazepine (Tegretol)
Lidocaine
Barbiturates
Optical devices
Base-out prisms
Other prism arrangements
Rotational magnification device
Invasive procedures
Kestenbaum operation
Botulinum toxin
Suboccipital craniotomy for Arnold-Chiari malformation

abolished or reduced oscillopsia in all of their 10 patients with downbeat, see-saw, or circular nystagmus. This drug was not evaluated in a double-blind fashion. However, 7 of their patients profited from long-term administration of clonazepam. Both clonazepam and trihexyphenidyl (the latter in high doses) are worth trying in individuals with acquired forms of nystagmus, provided there are no contraindications. Significant side effects can occur with both drugs. Other drugs are less likely to succeed. There is a need for double-blind studies to evaluate the effect of such medications on acquired nystagmus; to date, this has not been done.

A number of optical devices have been tried as treatment measures for nystagmus. The combination of base-out prisms (typically 7 diopters) and −1 diopter spheres are often useful in patients with congenital nystagmus whose oscillations dampen with convergence.[25] Such a combination is only occasionally successful in acquired nystagmus.[26] Forms of acquired nystagmus that obey Alexander's law (nystagmus greatest with gaze in direction of quick phases) sometimes benefit from prisms that put the eyes into a quiet position in the orbit (e.g., upgaze in downbeat nystagmus). Usually, however, patients simply adopt head positions (e.g., chin down in downbeat nystagmus) to reduce their nystagmus to a minimum. More recent methods (rotational magnification device) are described further below.

The Kestenbaum operation aims to move the attachment of the extraocular muscles so that a "null" or quiet zone corresponds to the eyes' new primary position.[25] It is sometimes helpful in congenital nystagmus but seldom helps acquired forms of nystagmus. Attempts to stop the eyes moving—either by detaching the muscles or paralyzing them with botulinum toxin—are extreme measures that have yet to receive systematic evaluation.

Surgery does, however, have a clear role in the treatment of Arnold-Chiari malformation. Suboccipital decompression often causes an improvement of downbeat nystagmus in addition to stabilization of other neurologic deficits.[27, 28]

NEW OPTICAL TREATMENTS FOR OSCILLOPSIA DUE TO ACQUIRED NYSTAGMUS

Recent studies of the effect of wearing a spectacle lens correction on the gain of the VOR[29] led us to focus our attention on the optical phenomenon that Rubin called "rotational magnification."[30] This term describes the prismatic effect of spectacle lenses; an example is shown in Figure 13–2. In Figure 13–2,A, an aphakic subject followed step displacements of a laser spot ("target position") without her glasses. In Figure 13–2,B, she donned +11 diopter glasses, after which she had to make larger eye rotations (an increase of over 30%) to follow the same movements of the target. Theoretically, by progressively increasing the power of the glasses, the eye would eventually be required to make infinite-sized rotations (i.e., 100% stabilization of retinal images would be possible). The latter would occur when the light rays from a distant object of interest were focused close to the center of rotation of the eye. Of course, such an image would not be clearly visible, since it would be focused at the center of the vitreous. Thus, the spectacle lens alone is not an effective way to stabilize images on the retina.

Working independently, Rushton and Rushton[31] realized that this problem could be overcome if the subject wore a highly negative contact lens, which would extend back the focus from the vitreous to the retina (Fig 13–3). Since the contact lens moves with the eye (the spectacles do not), the stabilizing effect of the positive spectacle lens is

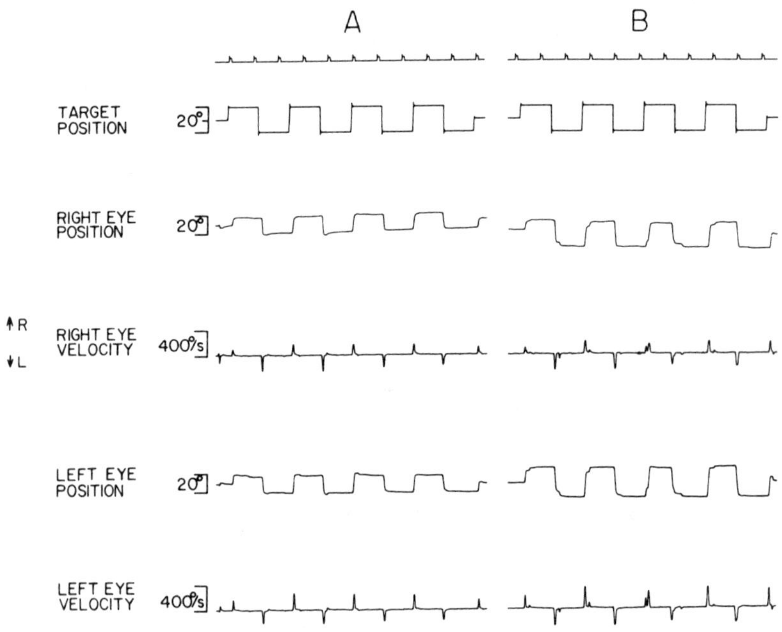

FIG 13–2.
Comparison of saccades made *(A)* without and *(B)* with +11 diopter correction in aphakic subject (EOG record). Time marks are in seconds.

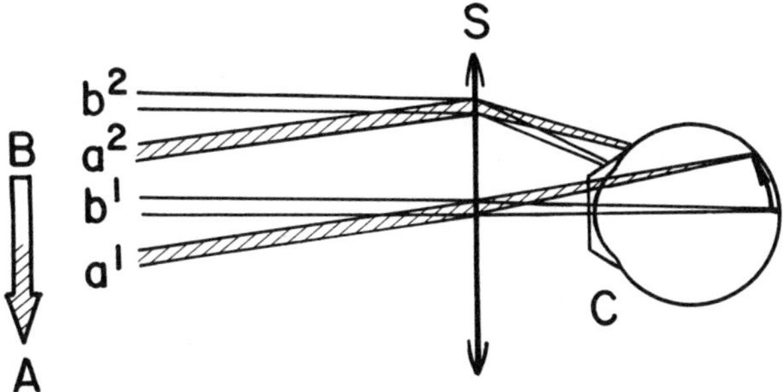

FIG 13–3.
Optical device for stabilizing images on the retina. Rays of light from distant object, *A–B,* are focused by strong spectacle lens at its secondary focal point, which is close to center of rotation of eye. Strongly divergent contact lens, *C,* extends back focus from center of the globe to retina. Since the contact lens moves with the eye, it does not negate the effect of retinal image stabilization produced by the spectacle lens. Rays of light from point *B* remain focused on the foveal region of the retina.

not negated. In practice, the greatest amount of retinal image stabilization (RIS) that can be achieved with this device is determined by the highest power negative contact lens that can be lathed. This is a −58 diopter contact lens made of polymethyl methacrylate* and is shown in Figure 13–4,A. Some features of this contact lens are described by Rushton and Cox.[32] When worn with +32 diopter spectacle lenses (Fig 13–4,B), approximately 90% stabilization of retinal images can be achieved (Fig 13–5). With lower power combinations of contact lenses and spectacle lenses, lower amounts of retinal image stabilization are achieved.

How can we determine how much retinal image stabilization any individual with nystagmus requires to abolish oscillopsia? (We have already noted that the relationship between retinal image velocity and oscillopsia varies from individual to individual and that oscillopsia is usually absent in congenital nystagmus.) One method, used by Rushton and Cox,[32] is (1) to ask the patient to estimate the magnitude of oscillopsia (O) while viewing an Amsler grid; (2) to estimate the magnitude of nystagmus (N) using an ophthalmoscopic method,[33] and then (3) calculate the required retinal image stabilization, as a fraction, from O/N. In practice, patients have difficulty in estimating the amplitude of oscillopsia and the ophthalmoscope method is not reliable for quantitative estimates.

*Jack Allen and Company, London.

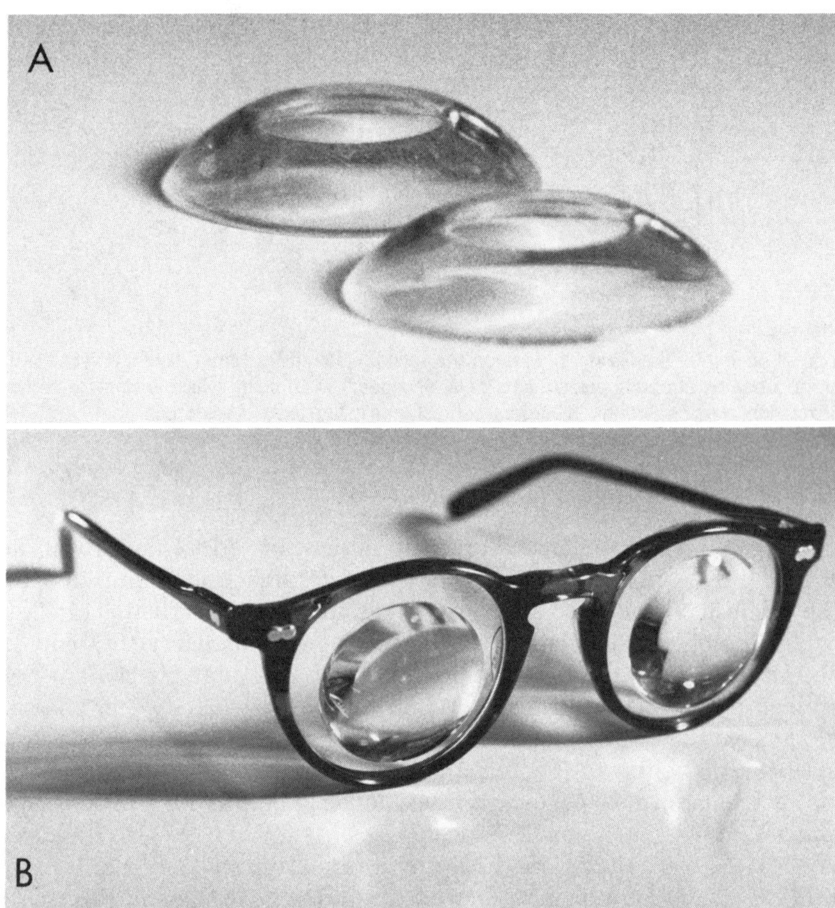

FIG 13–4.
A, −58 diopter contact lenses. **B,** +32 diopter spectacle lenses. When the contact lens and spectacles are worn together, approximately 90% retinal image stabilization is achieved.

We have artificially stabilized images on the retinas of patients with nystagmus using electronic feedback,[34] a method first developed by Drs. David Zee and Michael Harris at Johns Hopkins Hospital. We use the magnetic search coil method to measure horizontal and vertical eye movements with precision and feed these signals through amplifiers to an X-Y mirror galvanometer projection system, which determines the position of a projected Amsler grid on a tangent screen in front of the patient. Thus, the grid is made to move with the patient's

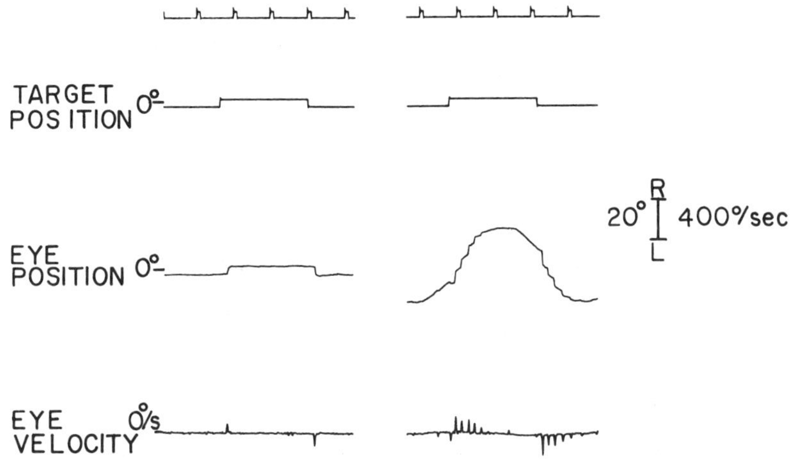

FIG 13–5.
Saccades made by a normal subject as he follows 4° step displacements of a target light. **Left,** eye movements (EOG record) shown while viewing without the optical device. **Right,** the subject wearing −58 diopter contact lens and +32 diopter spectacle lens. Rotation magnification of approximately 10° is evident. Time marks (top) are in seconds.

eyes. By varying the gain of amplifiers, we can vary the amount of retinal image stabilization from 0% to approximately 100%. Our techniques consists of *nulling* the oscillopsia and then directly measuring the amount of retinal image stabilization required. We can then refer to a nomogram[32] to select the appropriate spectacle lens and contact lens power required to achieve the desired amount of stabilization.

Evaluation of the optical device as a treatment for oscillopsia is under way. It suffers from certain limitations: a field of view restricted to approximately 30 × 30°; the need for the head to be stationary (the VOR is negated); and monocular viewing with the higher powers (because vergence movements are rendered ineffective). Nevertheless, certain patients have already benefited from the device and regained the ability to read and watch television.

CONCLUSIONS

Although we still do not clearly understand the pathologic physiology of oscillopsia, a start has been made. Oscillopsia due to an inadequate VOR often spontaneously improves; further study of these compensatory mechanisms may prove fruitful. Oscillopsia due to a hyperactive VOR is uncommon, but of great theoretical interest concerning the normal physiology of the VOR. Study of oscillopsia due to nystagmus offers promise of better understanding of mechanisms that normally maintain visual constancy. New treatments—drugs and optical devices—require careful evaluation in future years.

Acknowledgments

I am grateful to Drs. Stephen Thurston, Richard Hertle, and Stacy Yaiglos for technical help and to Holly Stevens for editorial assistance.

REFERENCES

1. Brickner R: Oscillopsia: A new symptom commonly occurring in multiple sclerosis. *Arch Neurol Psychiatry* 1936; 36:586–589.
2. Bender MB: Oscillopsia. *Arch Neurol* 1965; 13:204–213.
3. Westheimer F, McKee SP: Visual acuity in the presence of retinal-image motion. *J Opt Soc Am* 1975; 65:847–850.
4. Barnes GR, Smith R: The effects on visual discrimination of image movement across the stationary retina. *Aviat Space Environ Med* 1981; 52:466–472.
5. Steinman RM, Collewijn H: Binocular retinal image motion during active head rotation. *Vision Res* 1980; 20:415–429.
6. Katims JJ, Long DM, Ng LKY: Transcutaneous nerve stimulation: Frequency and waveform specificity in humans: *Appl Neurophysiol* 1986; 49:86–91.
7. Grossman GE, Abel LA, Thurston SE, et al: Frequency and velocity ranges of natural head rotations. *Soc Neurosci Abstr* 1986; 12 (pt 1):251.
8. JC: Living without a balancing mechanism. *N Engl J Med* 1952; 246:458.
9. Kasai T, Zee DS: Eye-head coordination in labyrinthine defective human beings. *Brain Res* 1978; 144:123.
10. Chambers BR, Mai M, Barber HO: Bilateral vestibular loss, oscillopsia and the cervico-ocular reflex. *Otolaryngol Head Neck Surg* 1985; 93:403.
11. Zee DS, Frienclich AR, Robinson DA: The mechanism of downbeat nystagmus. *Arch Neurol* 1974; 30:227–237.
12. Gresty M, Barratt H, Rudge P, et al: Analysis of downbeat nystagmus: Otolithic vs semicircular canal influences. *Arch Neurol* 1986; 43:52–55.
13. Thurston SE, Leigh RJ, Abel LA, et al: Hyperactive vestibulo-ocular reflex in cerebellar degeneration: Pathogenesis and treatment. *Neurology* 1987; 37:53–57.
14. Demer JL, Robinson DA: Effects of reversible lesions and stimulation of olivocerebellar system on vestibuloocular plasticity. *J Neurophysiol* 1986; 47:1084–1097.

15. Viire E, Tweed D, Milner K, et al: A reexamination of the gain of the vestibuloocular reflex. *J Neurophysiol* 1986; 56:439–450.
16. Wist ER, Brandt T, Krafczyk S: Oscillopsia and retinal slip. *Brain* 1983; 106:153–168.
17. Brandt T, Dieterich M: Oscillopsia and motion perception, in Rose FC, Kennard C (eds): *Physiological Aspects of Clinical Neuro-ophthalmology*. New York, Springer-Verlag, 1987; In press.
18. Howard IP: *Human Visual Orientation*. New York, John Wiley & Sons, 1982.
19. Halmagyi GM, Rudge P, Gresty MA, et al: Treatment of periodic alternating nystagmus. *Ann Neurol* 1980; 8:609–611.
20. Bender MB, Nathanson M, Gordon GG: Myoclonus of muscles of the eye, face and throat. *Arch Neurol Psychiatry* 1952; 67:44–58.
21. Gresty MA, Ell JJ, Findley LJ: Acquired pendular nystagmus: Its characteristics, localizing value and pathophysiology. *J Neurol Neurosurg Psychiatry* 1982; 45:431–439.
22. Lefkowitz D, Harpold G: Treatment of ocular myoclonus with valproic acid. *Ann Neurol* 1985; 17:103–104.
23. Jabbari B, Rosenberg M, Hosey J: Trihexyphenidyl improves oscillopsia and pendular nystagmus. *Neurology* 1985; 35(suppl):243.
24. Currie JN, Matuso V: The use of clonazepam in the treatment of nystagmus-induced oscillopsia. *Ophthalmology* 1986; 93:924–932.
25. Dell'Osso LF, Flynn JT: Congenital nystagmus surgery: A quantitative evaluation of the effects. *Arch Ophthalmol* 1979; 97:462–469.
26. Lavin PJM, Traccis S, Dell'Osso LF, et al: Downbeat nystagmus with a pseudocycloid waveform: Improvement with base-out prisms. *Ann Neurol* 1983; 13:621–624.
27. Penderson RA, Troost BJ, Abel LA, et al: Intermittent downbeat nystagmus and oscillopsia reversed by suboccipital craniotomy. *Neurology* 1980; 30:1239–1242.
28. Spooner JW, Baloh RW: Arnold-Chiari malformation: Improvement in eye movements after surgical treatment. *Brain* 1981; 104:51–60.
29. Cannon SC, Leigh RJ, Zee DS, et al: The effect of rotational magnification of corrective spectacles on the quantitative evaluation of the VOR. *Acta Otolaryngol (Stockh)* 1985; 100:81–88.
30. Rubin M: *Optics for Clinicians*, ed 2. Gainesville, Fla, Triad Scientific Publishers, 1974.
31. Rushton DN, Rushton RH: An optical method for approximate stabilization of vision of the real world. *J Physiol (Lond)* 1984; 357:3P.
32. Rushton D, Cox N: A new optical treatment for oscillopsia. *J Neurol Neurosurg Psychiatry* 1987; 50:411–415.
33. Zee DS: Ophthalmoscopy in examination of patients with vestibular disorders. *Ann Neurol* 1978; 3:373–374.
34. Leigh RJ, Rushton DN, Thurston SE, et al: Effects of retinal image stabilization in acquired nytagmus due to neurologic disease. *Neurology* 1988; 38:122–127.

PART FOUR

Dizziness: Diagnosis, Treatment

14

Benign (And Not So Benign) Postural Vertigo: Diagnosis and Treatment

Hugh O. Barber, M.D., F.R.C.S.(C.)

*R. John Leigh, M.D.**

Postural vertigo is spinning dizziness that occurs in only one or two of a series of different head positions, and not in all. It may be accompanied by nystagmus, positional nystagmus. It is a common occurrence. Nedzelski et al.[1] made the diagnosis of benign postural vertigo (BPV) in 17% of 2,222 patients attending a Dizziness Unit, and it then represented the third most common diagnosis.

Though interest in the subject goes back at least as far as 1921,[2] it is topical now. At the University of Toronto's Dizziness Up-Date 1986 an experienced panel was asked to rank, in order of importance, six subsets of electronystagmographic (ENG) testing: spontaneous nystagmus, positional nystagmus, ocular motor tests (pursuit, saccades, VOR cancelation), caloric tests, rotation tests, and posturography. The panel placed position tests second only to caloric tests in diagnostic importance.

It is not possible to quantify postural vertigo other than to note its presence or absence, and, if present, its intensity. But positional nys-

*Dr. Leigh is supported by PHS grant EY06717, the Veterans Administration, and the Evenor Armington Fund.

tagmus lends itself readily to classification. Nylén[3] noted that the direction of beat of the nystagmus might change in different (usually opposite) head positions, or retain a constant direction. The first he designated as type I and the second type II. The nystagmus might also be persistent, lasting as long as the provocative head position is maintained, or transitory, ceasing to beat in a relatively short time, perhaps 5–15 seconds. Noting these last features, Aschan[4] proposed a useful modification of Nylén's classification. Thus, Aschan's type I and II were *persistent*, type I direction changing and type II direction fixed, while type III is used to denote all paroxysmal, *transient* forms, of which the Barany-Dix-Hallpike[5] type is the most common.

Types I and II result either from peripheral vestibular or CNS lesions. Type III occurs mainly (but not exclusively) from inner ear abnormality. Vertigo with types I and II is generally absent or minor, with type III prominent and sometimes terrifying. (Thus, in neurotologic physical examination suitable tests for positional nystagmus should be routine, because positional dizziness may not be reported even when specific inquiry for the symptom is made.) Further comments on classification of positional nystagmus are given below.

Dix and Hallpike[5] described postural vertigo, the positional nystagmus that accompanies it, and the maneuvers needed to elicit the nystagmus. They used the term "benign postural vertigo" to denote the symptom, and "positional nystagmus of benign paroxysmal type" to denote the nystagmus; "benign" was used in each instance to emphasize the authors' belief that the causative lesion was always harmless as opposed to dangerous. They considered also that the lesion was peripheral and located in (the utricle of) the ear, which, when undermost, released the nystagmus.

The Barany-Dix-Hallpike nystagmus is distinctive. It occurs when the head is moved into a provocative position (head-hanging right or left, head-hanging sagittal) quickly, but not slowly. There is a latent period of about 1–10 seconds before nystagmus appears. Latency is much more often of the order of 1 or 2 seconds than 8 or 10. When nystagmus appears, it quickly reaches its zenith, then declines more slowly and stops, while a particular head position is maintained, having a typical duration of about 5–10 seconds. To the observer the nystagmus appears to be predominantly rotatory, with the 12 o'clock point of the limbus beating toward the undermost ear, clockwise in head-hanging left position, counterclockwise in head-hanging right. Typically, with each quick rotation there is a visible upward beat of the eye, and, if the observer ignores vertical and rotational movements and concentrates on the horizontal axis, there is often a varying degree of linear horizontal beat, with the quick component directed away from the undermost ear. Vertigo, often severe and at times with nausea, accompanies the nystagmus. On return to a sitting position nystagmus may reappear (again after a short latent period), typically rotating in a direction opposite to that found earlier or directed vertically downward. The nystagmus declines with repetition of the provoking maneuver; it may be absent on the second or third successive test. Typically it occurs mostly in a single (right or left) head-hanging position, infrequently in both.

In most cases, paroxysmal positional nystagmus (PPN) results from a peripheral vestibular disorder. Hence, it is most easily identified when ocular fixation is reduced, as (using ENG recording) with eyes open in dark or closed in light or with the use of Frenzel's goggles in a darkened room. This last test condition is preferred, because it gives the best chance for the observer actually to see the nystagmus. For clinical purposes it is advisable to have the patient maintain the primary position of the eyes while nystagmus is present, because gaze deviations cause eye movements different from those described, including vertical downbeat.[6, 7]

In the great majority of cases, benign postural vertigo (BPV) and its accompanying positional nystagmus result from inner ear abnormality. The majority of these are idiopathic, in the sense that the condition occurs in otherwise normal people. Of the others, a common pathogenesis seems to be any lesion that causes abrupt but subtotal loss of vestibular receptor activity of one ear,[8] as after vestibular neuronitis, stapedectomy, perilymph fistula,[9] head injury, and especially longitudinal fracture of temporal bone.[10] Vitamin B_{12} deficiency has also been connected with the condition.[11]

Schuknecht[12] presented evidence to support his proposal that agglomerations of inner ear debris, perhaps derived from otoconia and with greater specific gravity than the surrounding endolymph, float in the inner ear fluid to contact and displace the cupula of the dependent posterior semicircular canal in a head-hanging lateral position. Alternatively, the debris may be attached (? loosely) to the cupula, making it gravity-sensitive. Schuknecht uses the term "cupulolithiasis" to describe this condition. Probably this explanation is valid for some, or many, of the idiopathic group, and for many of those that follow head injury. There is certainly very good evidence to implicate the posterior semicircular canal as the site responsible for typical positional nystagmus of benign paroxysmal type. Cohen et al.[13] produced rotatory nystagmus in monkeys by stimulation of the ampullary nerve of the posterior canal. There is also anatomical[14] and physiologic[15] evidence that the posterior semicircular canal crista projects to the ipsilateral superior oblique and contralateral inferior rectus muscles, by which both rotatory and vertical eye movements make take place. Finally, singular neurectomy on the affected side eliminates the positional nystagmus.[16]

The natural history of idiopathic BPV is predictable. It occurs most frequently in the middle-aged, in the forties and fifties, and shows no sex preference other than a slightly greater representation of women in the fifth decade (Fig 14–1). It is rare or infrequent in childhood or youth and in old age. Typically the vertigo takes place when the patient lies back supine on a pillow, or on turning in bed so that either right or left ear is on the pillow. (Usually the patient recognizes that the symptom occurs with only one ear down, not both, but this is not invariable.) Vertigo lasts "a minute or two," by which the patient really means about 5–15 seconds—many people judge time poorly. The spinning illusion/sensation recurs on arising from bed in the morning. Often it happens also when the head is extended (as in reaching for an object from the top shelf in the kitchen) and sometimes in the hairdresser's salon when the head is extended for hair washing. Some patients learn that if they move slowly into the provocative position, rather than at their usual pace, the vertigo may be avoided. Nausea may occur with the vertigo, although it usually is not severe.

The vertigo never starts with body erect and head in the neutral position or turned axially (without flexion or extension) to either side, presumably because in each of these positions the same gravity orientation of the vestibular receptors is maintained.

The vertigo persists typically for only a few days or weeks, then declines and stops. The period of remission that follows is usually prolonged, usually a matter of months or even years. Recurrence then takes place. In the group of patients with reasonable antecedent cause, such as head injury or vestibular neuronitis, or in the elderly, the periods of activity may be long, but this is usually not so in the idiopathic group.

The typical positional nystagmus that accompanies typical BPV has been described earlier.

PPN may be *typical*, but it may also be *atypical*, in the sense that it does not conform to the Dix-Hallpike model. The nystagmus may be linear (horizontal, vertical, oblique) rather than predominantly rotatory; latency of onset and/or habituation may be absent; it may occur

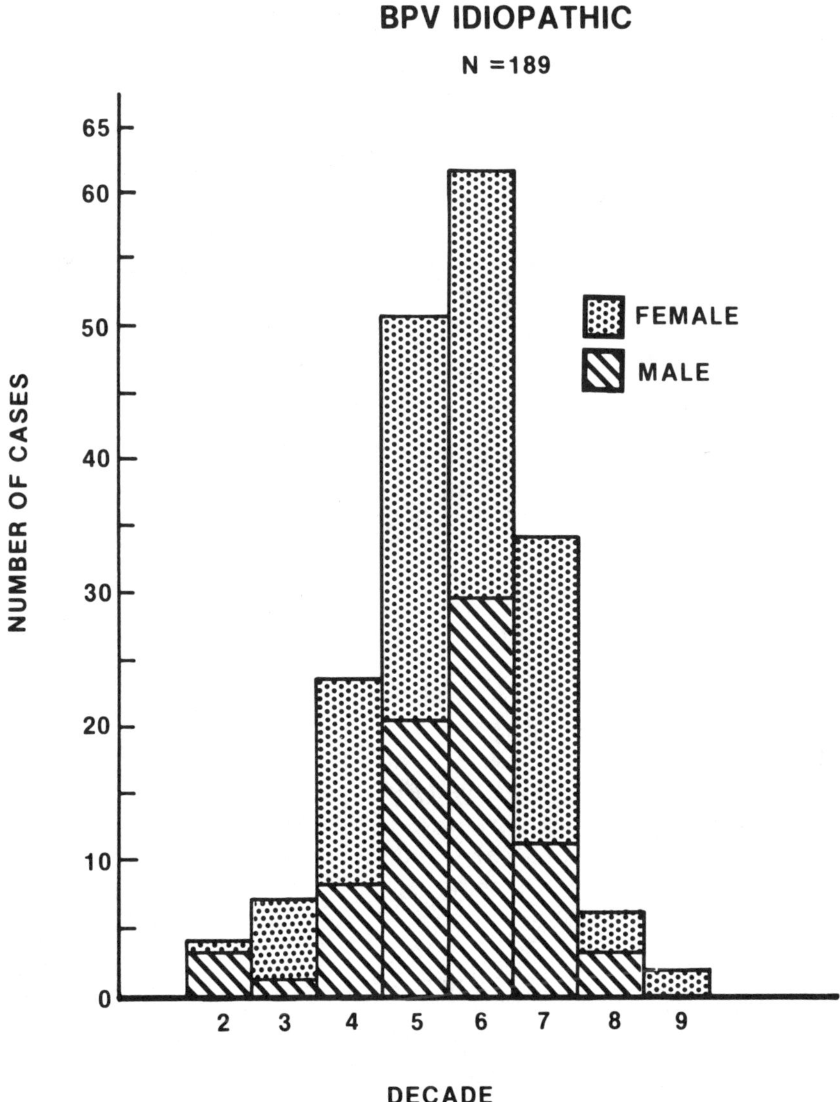

FIG 14–1.
Age and sex distribution of benign postural vertigo where there is no antecedent cause.

with each ear down rather than one. Stahle and Terins[17] noted these and other variations from the typical eye displacements, and Harrison and Ozsahinoglu[18] proposed another classification of positional nystagmus that emphasizes the difference between typical and atypical forms of the paroxysmal type.

Perhaps another word on classification is relevant here.

Persistent forms of positional nystagmus occur from static changes of head position relative to gravity; paroxysmal forms require in addition a certain brisk speed of movement from one position into the provocative position. The first may be described as "static," the second "dynamic." One of us (HOB) suggests the following classification that embodies the main features of current ideas on positional nystagmus:

Type I (Static-Persistent)
- (a) Direction changing
- (b) Direction fixed

Type II (Dynamic-Paroxysmal)
- (a) Typical (Dix-Hallpike)
- (b) Atypical (other)

While PPN is certainly nearly always due to a nonlethal, "benign" inner ear abnormality, this is not always the case. Some examples are due to vertebrobasilar disease,[10, 19] by no means always harmless. Gulati et al.[20] reported an example of PPN which was relieved by surgical restoration of blood flow in the left subclavian and innominate arteries whose lumina had been reduced by occlusive disease. In addition, there has been a steady trickle of reports[18, 21–25] of posterior fossa tumor, of cerebellum (especially vermis) or fourth ventricle, in association with PPN.

No clinician wants to overlook serious disease in a patient. Since typical PPN results from an abnormality of one posterior semicircular canal, it follows that other forms of PPN, the atypical, might arise from other causes. Put another way, when PPN is a physical sign of such serious lesions as neoplastic or ischemic brain disease, the nystagmus is more likely to be atypical than typical. Previous reports support this contention for the most part. Thus, the positional nystagmus reported by Harrison and Ozsahinoglu[18] in their patient with brain stem glioma failed to fatigue on repetition of the testing. Two (one with cerebellar/brain stem astrocytoma, one with hydrocephalus) of three patients described by Watson et al.[23] had atypical paroxysmal positional nystagmus, but the third (fourth ventricle subependymoma) had the typical form, and without other neurologic findings. Watson and Terbrugge[24] also described a patient with headache and dizziness (but not vertigo) who had typical PPN as a single neurologic finding, caused by medulloblastoma of one cerebellar hemisphere and the adjacent vermis. However, the PPN in Barber's[25] case of vermis metastasis was atypical, paroxysmal (linear) downbeat. In the patient with occlusive extracranial vascular disease described by Gulati et al.,[20] in head-hanging right position clockwise rotatory nystagmus appeared, without latency, and lasted 20–30 seconds; it was atypical.

A further case is reported here.

Case Report

A 29-year-old woman complained of dizziness and nausea for about one year. At the beginning she had turned to one side in her sleep when she was awakened by a feeling of something moving in her head for a short time. Quite brief (a few seconds) episodes of postural dizziness persisted, with little or no remission, and later she realized that the dizziness was a sense of movement, and she thought it more likely to occur with the left than right ear undermost (but see below). In the three months before consultation, the vertigo was accompanied by nausea and sometimes vomiting. She was unaware of auditory or focal neurologic symptoms.

On physical examination, tandem gait was unsteady both with eyes open and closed. On position testing there was in head-hanging right paroxysmal, linear, oblique nystagmus beating downward and to the left, lasting 2 or 3 seconds, and accompanied by vertigo. When the erect position was assumed after, a paroxysm of nystagmus appeared for a few seconds, now beating upward and to right. Nystagmus was absent in head-hanging left, in the sagittal-extended position, and on arising from these. The positional nystagmus was found about equally with eyes open in light or behind Frenzel's goggles in dark. No other neurotologic abnormality was found.

Because the positional nystagmus was atypical, computerized tomographic (CT) scanning of the head was requested (Fig 14–2). A 3-cm enhancing mass was found in the midline of the posterior fossa, indenting the fourth ventricle, displacing it upward and forward.

Later, audiometry showed normal pure tone thresholds and speech discrimination but with auditory brain stem response testing both III-V and I-V intervals were prolonged on the right side. ENG recordings then showed no positional nystagmus, whether seen visually or recorded. Caloric activity was normal, and smooth ocular pursuit was normal, but there was slight impairment of visual cancelation of the VOR during sinusoidal rotations at 0.05 Hz.

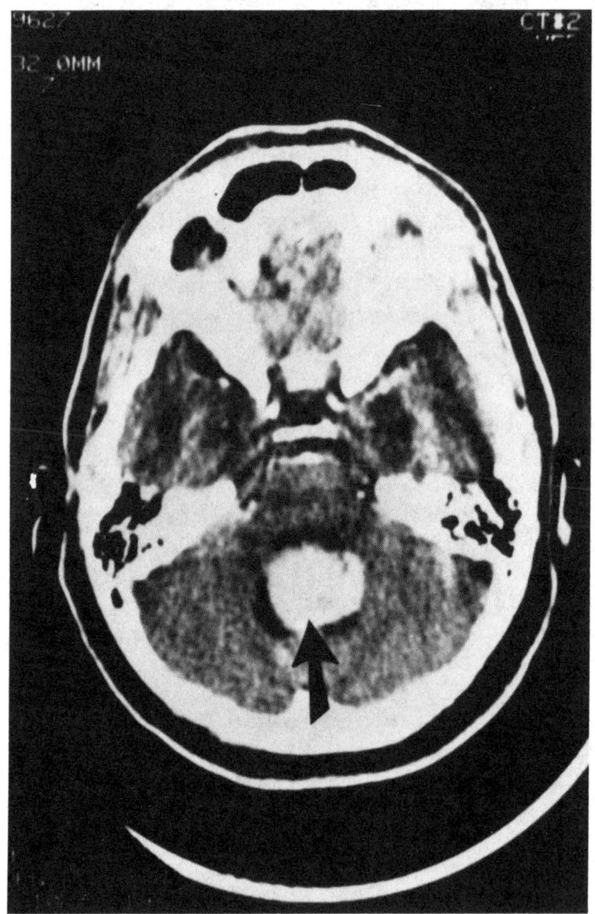

FIG 14–2.
CT scan. *Arrow* points to lesion.

At craniotomy, an encapsulated reddish tumor of the fourth ventricle was found which extended to the cerebellar peduncles and vermis. It was removed. The pathologic diagnosis was choroid plexus papilloma.

Comment

The paroxysmal nystagmus was atypical because it was linear, without rotation, vertical (mainly), and lacked latency.

ENG recording of the eye movements of PPN may also assist in the differentiation between "typical" and "atypical," between our types II(a) and (b).[26, 27] In the great majority of patients with PPN, whether the recordings are made with fixation or without, in the critical dependent position the direction of the horizontal beat (as determined by bitemporal horizontal leads) is *away from* the undermost ear. This is shown in Figure 14–3, and this direction of beat would be typical. On the other hand, horizontal nystagmus beating *toward* the undermost ear, (Fig 14–4) would be atypical. Vertical nystagmus beating *upward* (Fig 14–5) is typical (common), and beating *downward* (Fig 14–6) atypical. In fact, downward beating vertical positional nystagmus, whether paroxysmal or persistent, is always an important physical sign, never to be ignored; it often denotes structural disease of the caudal brain stem or cerebellum, as in our earlier report[25] and in the case reported here.

Probably the great majority of examples of intracranial disease or deformity whose symptoms include "benign" postural vertigo and who have PPN are to be found in the atypical group, II(b) in our classification, rather than the typical group, II(a). This is written with some degree of caution, because, as noted earlier, the occasional brain tumor manifests itself first by history very similar or identical to that of BPV, and Type II(a) positional nystagmus. For clinical purposes, an attempt is made in Table 14–1 to summarize some of the historical, physical, and ENG features that may assist in the differentiation of typical from atypical.

Different features or combinations of the features given in Table 14–1 should guide the clinician to a reasonable diagnostic strategy. In history, postural vertigo that begins at an early age, especially when remissions are inconspicuous, would give rise to suspicion of a CNS cause, perhaps regardless of the eye findings. The development of postural vertigo for the first time in the eighth or ninth decade should have similar meaning. Vertical positional nystagmus in an extended position, especially when vertigo is mild or absent (or on the other hand, with vomiting) would always denote CNS abnormality. When PPN is bilateral, occurring when each ear is undermost, there is a higher incidence of ischemic brain disease than when the finding occurs with only one ear down.[19] One would be alert to the possibility of brain abnormality in a patient whose positional nystagmus lacked latency or fatigability, regardless of age, or where the horizontal nystagmus beat toward the undermost ear on the ENG strip.

But nothing in medicine is 100%; nothing is "always." McClure[28] has described an atypical form of paroxysmal positional nystagmus

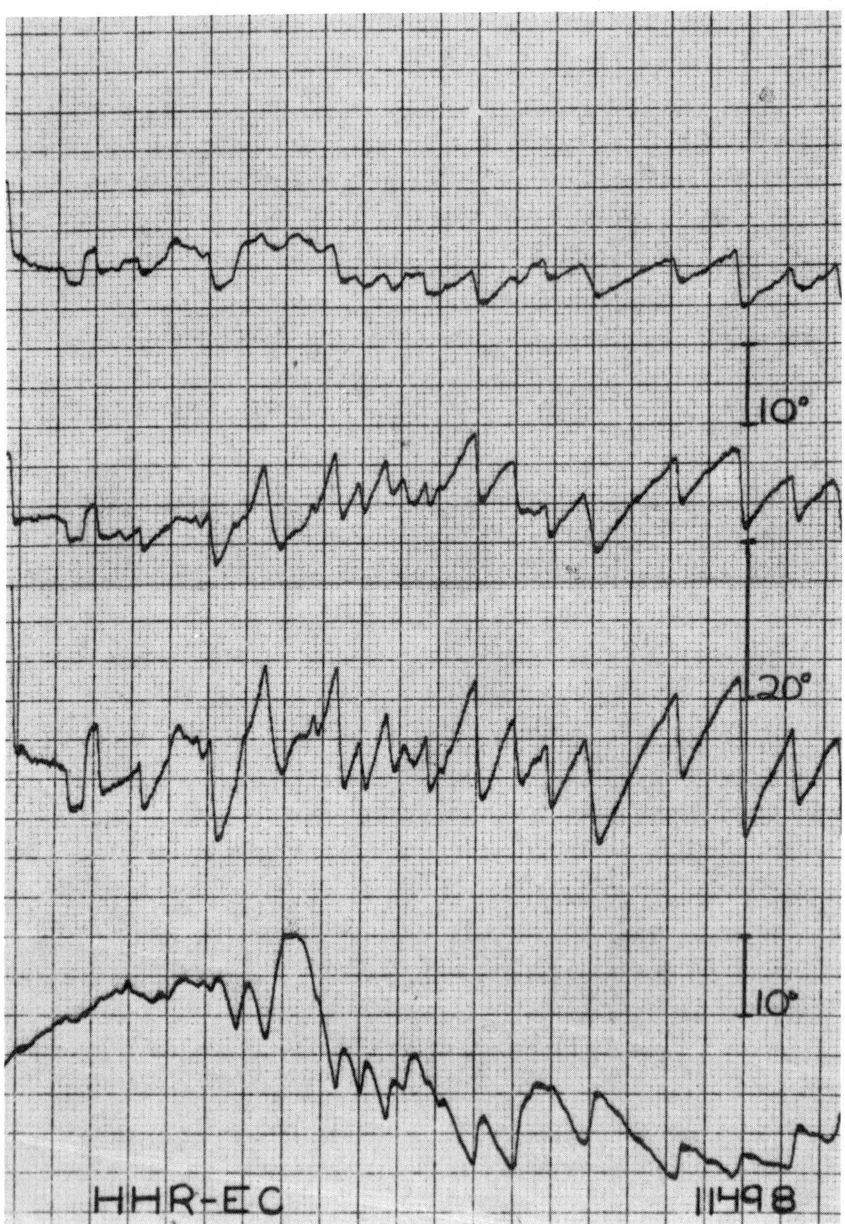

FIG 14–3.
ENG tracing, Hallpike's maneuver, head-hanging-right position, eyes closed. **Top lead,** monocular horizontal right eye; **second lead,** monocular horizontal left eye; **third lead,** bitemporal horizontal; **bottom lead,** vertical left eye. Position is attained at left margin of illustration. (From Barber HO: Positional nystagmus. *Otolaryngol Head Neck Surg* 1984;92:649-655. Used by permission.)

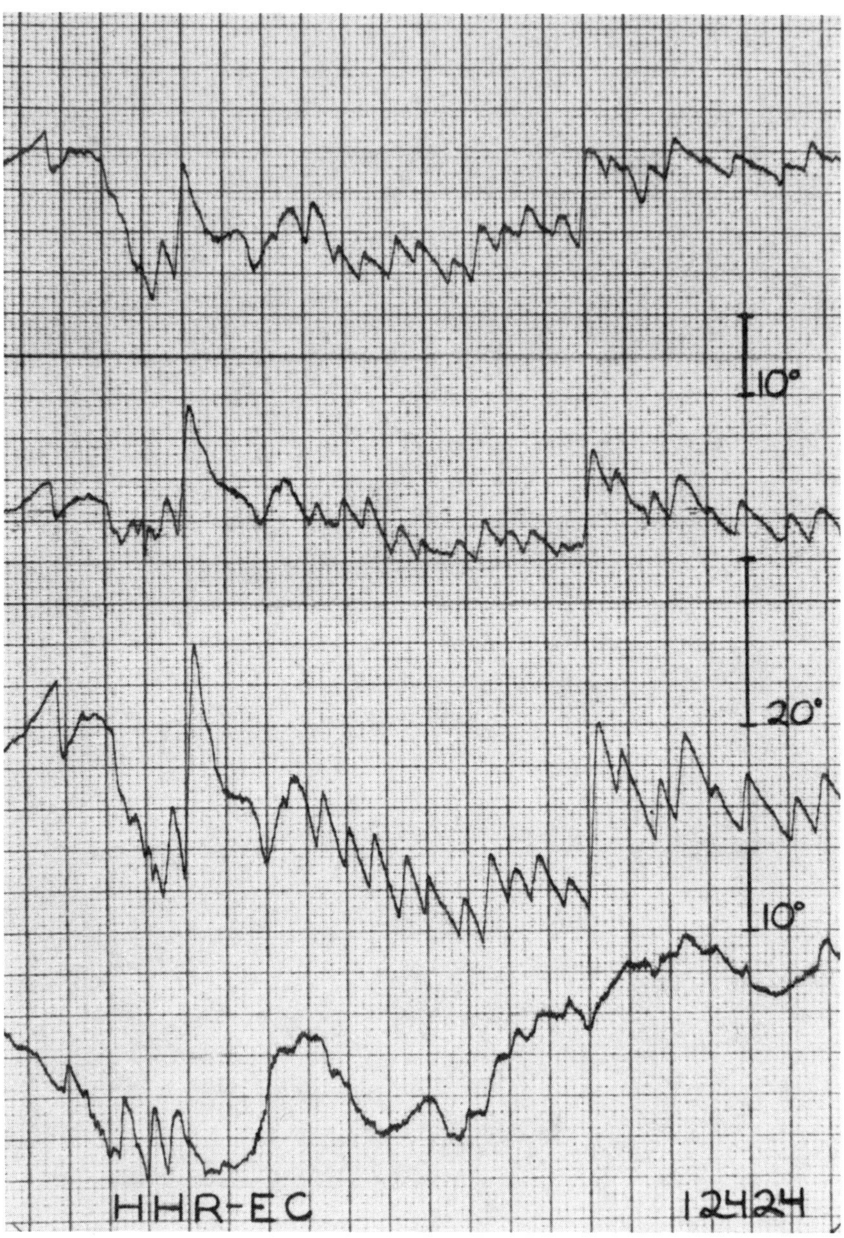

FIG 14–4.
Electrode application, leads, head position, and test conditions identical to Figure 14–3. (From Barber HO: Positional nystagmus. *Otolaryngol Head Neck Surg* 1984;92:649–655. Used by permission.)

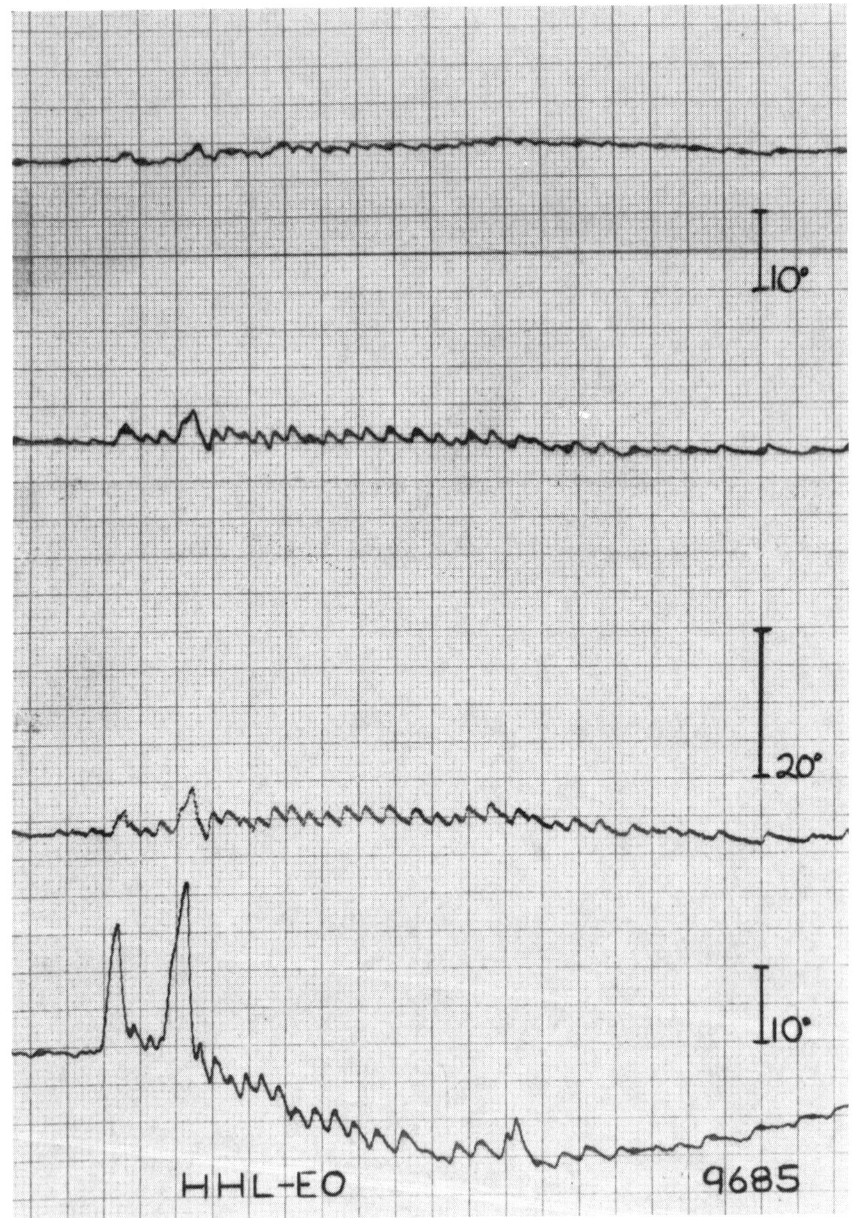

FIG 14–5.
Electrode application, leads as in Figure 14–3, head-hanging-left position, eyes open and fixated in primary position. (From Barber HO: Positional nystagmus. *Otolaryngol Head Neck Surg* 1984;92:649-655. Used by permission.)

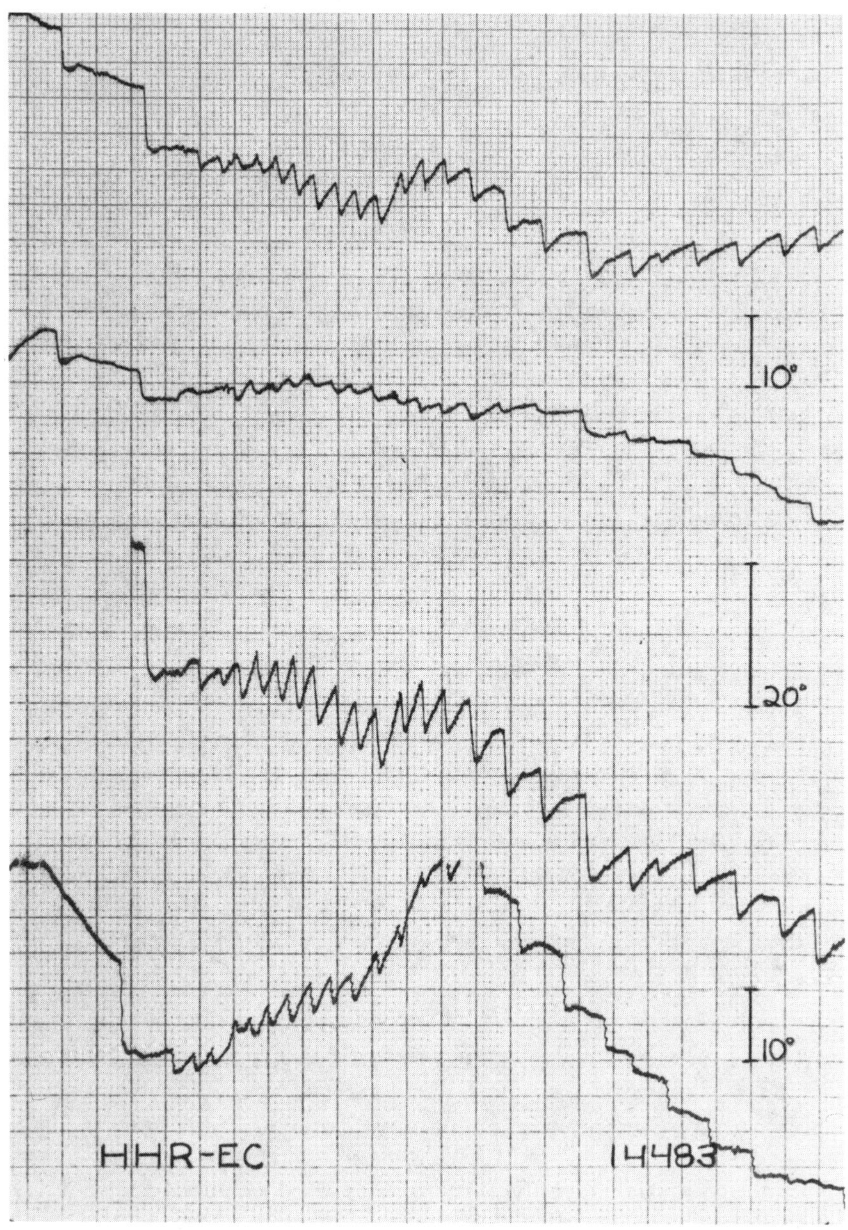

FIG 14–6.
Electrode application, leads, head position, and test conditions identical to those in Figure 14–3. Downward-beating vertical paroxysmal positional nystagmus. (From Barber HO: Positional nystagmus. *Otolaryngol Head Neck Surg* 1984;92:649-655. Used by permission.)

TABLE 14–1.
Differentiation of Typical and Atypical Postural Vertigo

Feature	Variable	Typical	Atypical
History	Age	Middle age	Youth/elderly
	Antecedent cause	Present/absent	Absent
	Periods remission	Prominent/prolonged	Brief/absent
	Vomiting with vertigo	Absent	Absent/present
	Neurologic symptoms	Absent	Absent/present
Positional nystagmus	Latency	Present	Present/absent
	Fatigability	Yes	Yes/no
	Rotational	Prominent	Present/absent
	Downbeat	No	Yes
	Bilateral	No	Yes
	Associated vertigo	Marked	Present/minor absent
ENG	Bitemporal leads	Nystagmus beats away from under ear	Nystagmus beats toward under ear
	Vertical leads	Vertical upbeat	Vertical downbeat

that very likely is due to release of positional nystagmus from a lateral, rather than posterior, semicircular canal. The paroxysmal nystagmus is horizontal rather than rotatory (see chapter 15).

Nevertheless, clinicians should suspect possible CNS origin of paroxysmal positional nystagmus at times, when the history, physical findings, or ENG tracing, or different combinations of these, are inconsistent with the Dix-Hallpike model. Appropriate neurologic investigation is needed for these patients, and, if negative, careful follow-up.

TREATMENT OF BENIGN POSTURAL VERTIGO

Almost all patients who visit a physician because of benign paroxysmal positional vertigo (BPV) are prescribed medications such as meclizine or diazepam. And yet, there is no good evidence that medications are of value in BPV.[29] In many individuals, the symptoms of BPV resolve spontaneously. In others, however, the symptoms persist. On questioning, it is often evident that these latter individuals have studiously avoided head positions that precipitate their symptoms. It is the opinion of one of us (RJL) that almost every patient with BPV can be successfully treated with physical therapy provided that the patient conscientiously carries out the exercises.

A variety of types of physical therapy have been recommended for BPV. It is inevitable that any treatment that is likely to work will cause the patient to have vertigo, nausea, and other discomfort after institution of the exercises. Some physicians recommend that the patient spend time, for example, in the lounge at home, on hands and knees. The philosophy of such an approach is that it provides the brain with strong tactile, proprioceptive and visual cues to enhance any vestibular habituation.

Brandt and Daroff[30] recommended a specific type of physical therapy which they were able to apply to 66 patients with BPV in an inpatient hospital setting (Fig 14–7). Patients sit with their eyes closed and tilt laterally to the precipitating position, with the left lateral aspect of their occiput resting on the bed. They remain in this position until the evoked vertigo subsides and then sit up for 30 seconds before assuming the opposite head-down position for another 30 seconds. This sequence of positionings is repeated at each session until vertigo subsides. The maneuvers are carried out every 3 hours while awake and are terminated after 2 consecutive vertigo-free days. Every one of Brandt and Daroff's patients gained complete relief from their positional vertigo. The number of days required varied from 3 to 14, with most patients requiring about a week.

How do these or other, similar exercises work? One possibility is that habituation of the abnormal vestibular signal is enhanced when the patient is repeatedly put in the offending position. It is a common finding that during clinical examination of patients with BPV, the symptoms become less severe with each positioning, as Barany[2] pointed out. An alternative hypothesis, offered by Brandt and Daroff,[30] is that their exercises shake free otolithic debris from the cupula (hence the positioning shown in Figure 14–7; the right posterior semicircular canal is superior to the utricle when the head is tilted over to the right, and otolithic debris can then detach from the cupula of the posterior semicircular canal).

Whatever the mechanism, these exercises or similar protocols are almost always successful provided the patient adheres to them. When symptoms do not respond to the exercises, it is worthwhile reconsidering the diagnosis and carrying out CT scanning to make sure that a central lesion is not mimicking the BPV. Only very rare cases require singular neurectomy[16]—surgical transection of the pos-

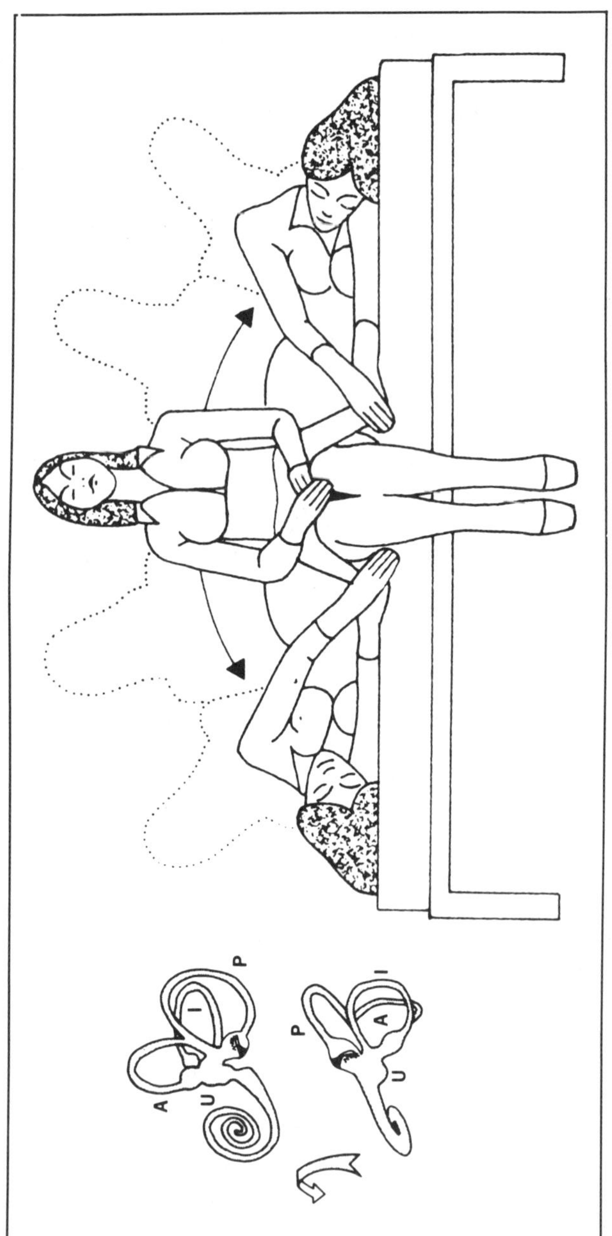

FIG 14–7.
Sequence of repetitive positionings in patients with benign paroxysmal positional vertigo in seated position with eyes closed. Corresponding location of right labyrinth is depicted **(left).** With response to gravity, ampulla of posterior canal *(P)* is situated inferior to utricle *(U)* when head is upright, but superior in precipitating head position. *A* indicates anterior canal; *I*, inferior canal. (From Brandt T, Daroff RB: Physical therapy for benign paroxysmal positional vertigo. *Arch Otolaryngol* 1980; 106:484–485. Used by permission. Copyright 1980, American Medical Association.)

terior ampullary nerve via a middle ear approach—or other surgical procedure.

REFERENCES

1. Nedzelski JM, Barber HO, McIlmoyl L: Diagnoses in a dizziness unit. *J Otolaryngol* 1986; 15:101–104.
2. Barany R: Diagnose von krankheitserscheinungen im bereiche des otolithenapparates. *Acta Otolaryngol (Stockh)* 1921; 2:434–437.
3. Nylén CO: Positional nystagmus: A review and future prospects. *J Laryngol Otol* 1950; 64:295–318.
4. Aschan G: The pathogenesis of positional nystagmus. *Acta Otolaryngol (Stockh)[suppl]* 1961; 159:90–93.
5. Dix MR, Hallpike CS: The pathology, symptomatology and diagnosis of certain common disorders of the vestibular system. *Proc R Soc Med* 1952; 45:341–354.
6. Katsarkas A, Kirkham TH: Paroxysmal positional vertigo—a study of 255 cases. *J Otolaryngol* 1978; 7:320–330.
7. Katsarkas A, Outerbridge JS: Nystagmus of paroxysmal positional vertigo. *Ann Otol Rhinol Laryngol* 1983; 92:146–150.
8. Lindsay JR, Hemenway WG: Postural vertigo due to unilateral sudden partial loss of vestibular function. *Ann Otol Rhinol Laryngol* 1956; 65:692–706.
9. Healy GB, Strong MS, Feldman RG: Ataxia secondary to labyrinthine fistula. *Laryngoscope* 1973; 83:502–507.
10. Barber HO: Positional nystagmus, especially after head injury. *Laryngoscope* 1964; 74:891–944.
11. Mahmud K, Ripley D, Doscherholmen A: Paroxysmal positional vertigo in vitamin B12 deficiency. *Arch Otolaryngol* 1970; 92:278–280.
12. Schuknecht HF: Cupulolithiasis. *Arch Otolaryngol* 1969; 90:113–126.
13. Cohen B, Suzuki J, Bender MB: Nystagmus induced by electric stimulation of ampullary nerves. *Acta Otolaryngol (Stockh)* 1965; 60:422–436.
14. Gacek RR: Anatomical demonstration of the vestibulo-ocular projections in the cat. *Laryngoscope* 1971; 81:1559–1595.
15. Baker R, Precht W, Berthoz A: Synaptic connections to trochlear motoneurons determined by individual vestibular nerve branch stimulation in the cat. *Brain Res* 1973; 64:402–406.
16. Gacek RR: Cupulolithiasis and posterior ampullary nerve transection. *Ann Otol Rhinol Laryngol* 1984; 93(suppl 112):25–29.
17. Stahle J, Terins J: Paroxysmal positional nystagmus. *Ann Otol Rhinol Laryngol* 1965; 74:69–83.
18. Harrison MS, Ozsahinoglu C: Positional vertigo: Aetiology and clinical significance. *Brain* 1972; 95:369–372.
19. Longridge NS, Barber HO: Bilateral paroxysmal positioning nystagmus. *J Otolaryngol* 1978; 7:395–400.

20. Gulati SM, Pugh JE, Whitehouse WM, et al: Paroxysmal positional nystagmus in innominate and subclavian arterial occlusive disease. *J Neurosurg* 1983; 58:443–445.
21. Riesco Mac-Clure JS: Es el vertigo aural de origen exclusivamente periferico? *Rev Otorrinolaryngol* 1957; 17:42–54.
22. Gregorius FK, Crandall PH, Baloh RW: Positional vertigo with cerebellar astrocytoma. *Surg Neurol* 1976; 6:283–286.
23. Watson P, Barber HO, Deck J, et al: Positional vertigo and nystagmus of central origin. *Can J Neurol Sci* 1981; 8:133–137.
24. Watson P, Terbrugge K: Positional nystagmus of the benign paroxysmal type with posterior fossa medulloblastoma (letter to the editor). *Arch Neurol* 1982; 39:601–602.
25. Barber HO: Positional nystagmus. *Otolaryngol Head Neck Surg* 1984; 92:649–655.
26. Barber HO, Stockwell CW: *Manual of Electronystagmography*, ed 2. St Louis, CV Mosby Co, 1980, p 155.
27. Baloh RW, Sakala SM, Honrubia V: Benign paroxysmal positional nystagmus. *Am J Otolaryngol* 1979; 1:1–6.
28. McClure JA: Horizontal canal BPV. *J Otolaryngol* 1985; 14:30–35.
29. McClure JA, Willet JM: Lorazepam and diazepam in the treatment of benign paroxysmal vertigo. *J Otolaryngol* 1980; 9:472–477.
30. Brandt T, Daroff RB: Physical therapy for benign paroxysmal positional vertigo. *Arch Otolaryngol* 1980; 106:484–485.

15

Functional Basis for Horizontal Canal BPV

Joseph A. McClure, M.D.

Benign positional vertigo (BPV) is a syndrome characterized by brief (usually less than 30-sec) episodes of vertigo and nystagmus brought on by certain changes of head position relative to the gravity vector. BPV is suspected on history and is confirmed on physical examination by Dix-Hallpike position testing to elicit the typical rotatory nystagmus that can be observed with eyes open. Since the nystagmus is primarily rotatory, it is not detected by conventional ENG.

The following features of conventional BPV suggest involvement of the posterior semicircular canal:

1. The vertigo and nystagmus are most intense with a change of head position in the plane of one posterior canal.
2. The predominant nystagmus direction is rotatory.
3. Schuknecht[1] has been able to demonstrate a deposit of material on the cupula of one posterior canal in a limited number of patients with the permanent form of BPV (cupulolithiasis).
4. Sectioning the nerve to the involved posterior canal (singular nerve section[2]) relieves the symptoms.

To explain the pathophysiology, Schuknecht and Ruby[3] suggested that loose material in the endolymphatic space will eventually find its way to the most dependent part of the system, which happens to be the ampulla of the posterior semicircular canal. This material, either-loose in the endolymph or attached to the cupula, will move under the influence of gravity when the head changes position in the plane of the affected canal. This theory of differential-density within the posterior canal explains most aspects of conventional BPV.

One might expect on occasion to encounter a similar but modified syndrome if a differential-density condition were to occur in either the superior or horizontal semicircular canals. McClure[4] reported 7 cases with a clinical picture consistent with horizontal canal BPV. These cases were all characterized by intense vertigo and a pure horizontal nystagmus lasting several seconds, with a change of position in the plane of the horizontal canals while recumbent. The horizontal nystagmus could be observed with eyes open and was also recorded with conventional ENG.

With horizontal canal involvement, one would expect detectable changes in canal dynamics as manifested by the frequency response of the VOR with horizontal canal stimulation. To assess canal dynamics, some of the patients with horizontal canal BPV underwent a rotational test that measured the frequency response of the VOR with sinusoidal stimulation (frequency range, 0.04–0.5 Hz) in the plane of the horizontal canals.

CLINICAL PICTURE

Symptoms

As with conventional BPV, patients with horizontal canal BPV complain of a positional vertigo. The history can be somewhat misleading in that the vertigo tends to be more intense than with conventional BPV. In addition, rolling to either side while recumbent is the most provocative position change, whereas getting up and lying down may produce only minimal symptoms. The patient is also sensitive to side-to-side head movements when up and about. With conventional BPV, the symptoms usually persist over several weeks or months, while with horizontal canal BPV, the symptoms persist for relatively short periods of a few days to 3 or 4 weeks, although the patient tends to have multiple recurrences that can have rapid onset and subsidence.

Characteristic Nystagmus

The diagnosis of horizontal canal BPV is confirmed by observing the characteristic nystagmus with eyes open during the physical examination. The characteristic nystagmus is a "pure" horizontal nystagmus lasting up to 60 sec. It is induced by rolling the head to either side while the patient is recumbent. The nystagmus is in the same direction as the direction of the head position change with the initial position of the head not important. The absence of rotatory and/or vertical components of nystagmus strongly suggests that this is a different condition from conventional BPV. Figures 15–1 and 15–2 provide two examples of horizontal canal BPV nystagmus recorded with conventional dc ENG. The nystagmus in Figure 15–1 was induced by whole body position change from the supine to the right and left lateral positions. The nystagmus in Figure 15–2 was obtained by rotating the head into the lateral position while the patient's body remained supine.

CANAL DYNAMICS

Five patients with horizontal canal BPV underwent a sinusoidal rotational test. During this test, the patient was seated in a chair that could rotate about an Earth-vertical axis. The head was fixed in a restraint and tilted 30° forward to bring the horizontal canals into the horizontal plane. Each patient was subjected to sinusoidal rotation in the plane of the horizontal canals at 0.04, 0.1, 0.3, and 0.5 Hz. Horizontal eye movements were recorded using conventional dc ENG. A

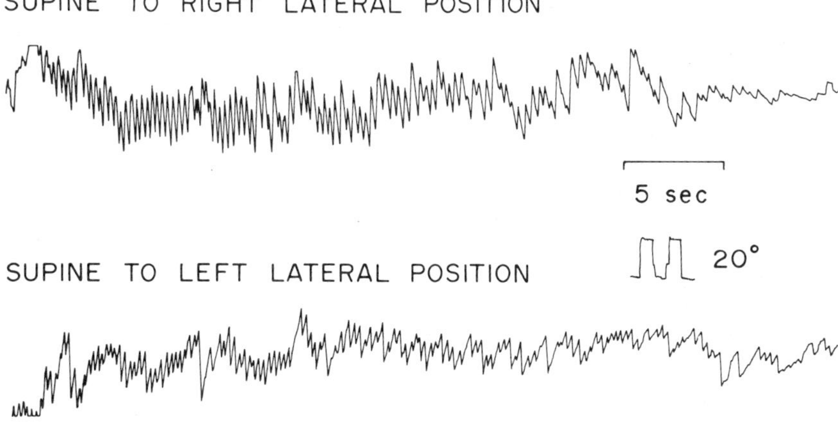

FIG 15–1.
Horizontal nystagmus recording from patient CN with suspected horizontal canal BPV. Nystagmus was induced by whole body position change.

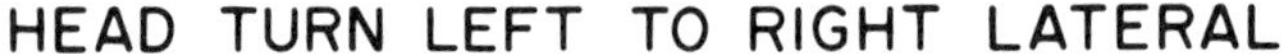

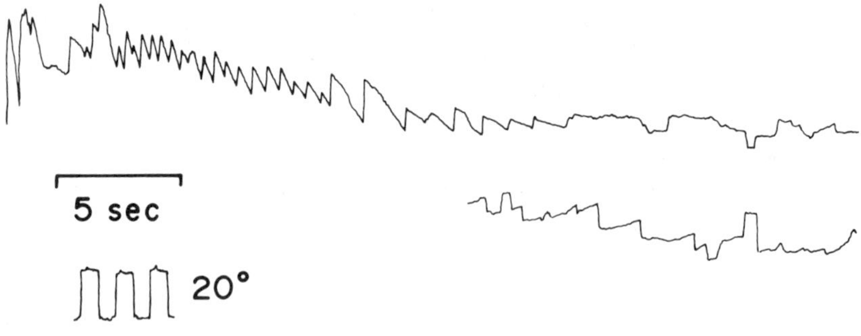

HEAD TURN RIGHT TO LEFT LATERAL

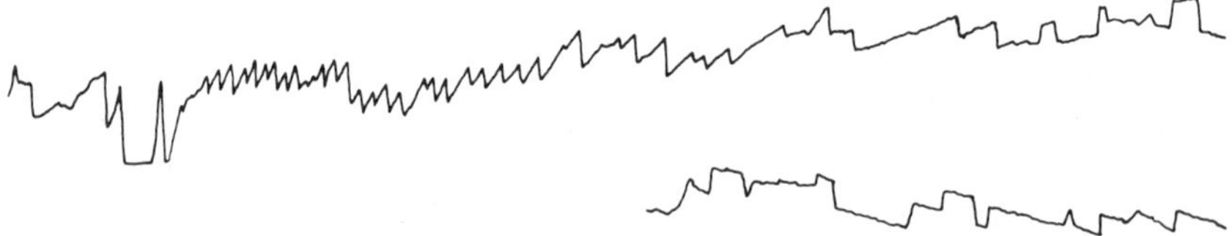

FIG 15–2.
Horizontal nystagmus recording from patient SL with suspected horizontal canal BPV. Nystagmus was induced by turning the head to either side while the patient was supine.

calibration was carried out prior to stimulation at each frequency by having the patient gaze between two points that subtended an angle of 20°. Recordings were made with eyes closed (in a red-lighted room) and with adequate mental alerting. The slow-phase eye velocity was compared to chair velocity (i.e., head velocity) in terms of gain and phase shift. The most obvious finding was a reduced phase shift of eye velocity relative to head velocity at 0.04 Hz compared with normal subjects. This was observed in four of the five patients whose results are illustrated in Figure 15–3.

DISCUSSION

Conventional BPV is attributed to involvement of the posterior semicircular canal mainly on the basis of clinical circumstantial evi-

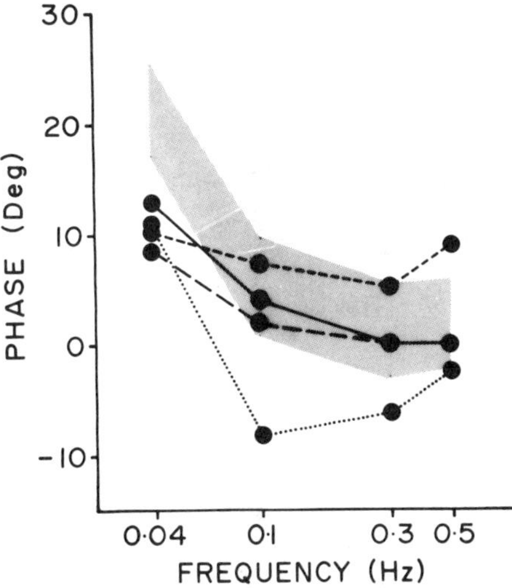

FIG 15–3.
Plot of phase difference (eye velocity relative to head velocity) against frequency of sinusoidal rotation for the four patients with suspected horizontal canal BPV who showed a reduced phase shift at 0.04 Hz. *Shaded area* represents 1 SD for 8 normal control subjects.

dence. Similarly, the horizontal canal is implicated with horizontal canal BPV. However, since horizontal canal dynamics can be measured via the VOR, one is able to look for changes in the system.

One change appears to be the reduced phase shift at frequencies near the lower end of what is considered to be the VOR system's normal frequency range. In effect, the system functions as a velocity sensor (i.e., zero phase shift of eye velocity relative to head velocity) down to a lower frequency. Such a change indicates a lengthening of the system's viscoelastic time constant (often referred to as the "long" time constant of the system). Such a change would result from either reduced elasticity of the cupula or increased viscous friction of the canal fluid.

The concept of loose particles in the fluid of the horizontal canal to explain this condition is not particularly convincing, because the particles are unlikely to remain in the canal and would not necessarily alter friction within the canal. A more attractive theory would be a heavier-than-endolymph "viscous plug" or endolymph "precipitate" caught within the canal. This could be displaced under the influence of gravity and could also alter canal dynamics by increasing resistance to fluid motion. Such a "plug" or "precipitate" could form quickly and be quickly absorbed depending on hormonal, immunologic, or other chemical factors. This would explain the relatively sudden onset and disappearance of the symptoms with this condition.

REFERENCES

1. Schuknecht HF: Cupulolithiasis. *Arch Otolaryngol* 1969; 90:113–126.
2. Gacek RR: Singular neurectomy up-date. *Ann Otol Rhinol Laryngol* 1982; 91:469–473.
3. Schuknecht HF, Ruby RRF: Cupulolithiasis. *Adv Otorhinolaryngol* 1973; 20:434–443.
4. McClure JA: Horizontal canal BPV. *J Otolaryngol* 1985; 14:30–35.

16

Transient Vertigo, Drop Spells and Cerebrovascular Disease

Louis R. Caplan, M.D.

COMMON NONVASCULAR CAUSES OF EPISODIC DIZZINESS

Episodic vertigo or dizziness is one of the most common complaints patients bring to physicians. Dizzy patients are often routinely and falsely diagnosed as having vertebrobasilar occlusive disease, especially if they are within the stroke-prone age group, and warfarin is often prescribed. Attacks of dizziness can be caused by protean disorders ranging from peripheral vestibulopathies to epileptic seizures to psychological disorders such as hysteria and depression.

In my experience, there are four frequent groups of dizzy patients whose clinical features are recognizable. Unfortunately, they are often given the misdiagnosis of cerebrovascular disease and inappropriate investigations are ordered and unnecessary and ineffective treatment is given.

Muscle Contraction Headache

This syndrome is characterized by a cephalic discomfort usually described as a tightness, bandlike feeling, pressure, or sensation as if a tight cap were being worn. Discomfort is maximal on the top and back of the head and may spread to the face and jaws. Some speak of constant "awareness" of their head. Some headache is always present, and, when severe, there often is accompanying episodic dizziness. The neck proprioceptors yield information about the posture and position of the head in space. When the head and neck are gripped tightly by contracted muscles or immobilized by traction, patients report a disorienting, dizzy feeling. Often depressed or anxious, these patients usually describe more how the problem affects them and makes them feel than the specifics of the discomfort and dizziness. They invariably report that the dizziness and cephalic feelings are disconcerting and make them feel depressed and unable to function.

"Multisensory" Dizziness

The principal sensory receptors that tell of the position of the head and body in space are the retina, proprioceptive fibers in the peripheral nerves and posterior columns of the spinal cord, the neck proprioceptors, and the labyrinthine receptors and their vestibular connections.[1] In some older patients all of these systems undergo aging or disease. Presbyopia, cataracts, cataract surgery with the need for new lenses, glaucoma, and macular degeneration affect vision; peripheral neuropathies and cervical osteoarthritis decrease somatosensory input; Meniere's disease, toxic vestibulopathies, and aging alter vestibular function. Dizziness occurs only when these patients move about and walk and is absent when they sit or recline. Examination confirms abnormalities of the optic and vestibular systems and a peripheral neuropathy.

Faintness or Near Syncope

In this condition,[2] episodic decrease in cerebral blood flow is caused by cardiovascular factors not occlusive cerebrovascular disease. Dimming of vision, sweating, pallor, and a sense of "being about to pass out" or "needing more air" accompany the dizziness. Causes vary and include hypovolemia (for example, after diuresis), Addison's disease, postural hypotension, cardiac arrythmias, valvular heart disease, and vasovagal syncope. The dizziness is usually relieved by sitting, lying, or putting the head down; unless the cause is cardiac arrhythmia, attacks rarely begin when patients are supine. Anxious patients with intermittent hyperventilation have similar symptoms.

"Kopfschwindel"

This is an old German term freely translated as "head swimming" or "spinning." It applies to patients whose dizzy feelings are more perceptions of confusion or uncertainty, not a sense of motion or rotation. Intoxication, depression, and dementia can all cause this symptom, which should not be confused with vertigo.

VASCULAR LESIONS CAUSING EPISODIC VERTIGO

Anatomy and Pathophysiology

Cerebrovascular disease does explain some attacks of vertigo. The major anatomical structures subserving vestibular function are the vestibular nuclei and their connections with the flocculonodular lobes of the cerebellum. Information is then relayed centrally to the lateral thalamus and temporal lobes for conscious awareness of motion. All of these CNS structures are supplied by the posterior circulation. The peripheral receptors are fed by branches of the internal auditory arteries which are branches of the anterior-inferior cerebellar artery (AICA) branches of the basilar artery. The vertebral arteries join at the pontomedullary junction to form the basilar artery. Since the vestibular nuclei are primarily located in the lateral tegmentum of the medulla, they are almost entirely irrigated by the vertebral arteries, not the more rostral system, which includes the basilar and posterior cerebral arteries and their branches. The vestibulocerebellum, located far posterior, inferior, and medial in the posterior fossa, is also supplied by the vertebral arteries. More rostral occlusive disease can cause sensations of dizziness, but this symptom is invariably overshadowed by motor, sensory, visual, or cognitive dysfunction. Although ischemia to the labyrinths undoubtedly does occur, it has not been attributable to angiographically visible lesions within the posterior circulation and has not been associated with strokes. For clinical purposes, then, attacks of vertigo, when ischemic, are nearly always due to lesions within the proximal posterior circulation, the subclavian and vertebral arteries in the neck, and the intracranial vertebral arteries. Patients with vertebral artery disease can be conveniently subdivided into two relatively homogeneous but distinct groups, those with proximal lesions (subclavian, innominate, and proximal vertebral arteries), and those with distal disease (terminal portion of the extracranial vertebral arteries and intracranial vertebral arteries). Figure 16–1 depicts the vascular anatomy of this system.

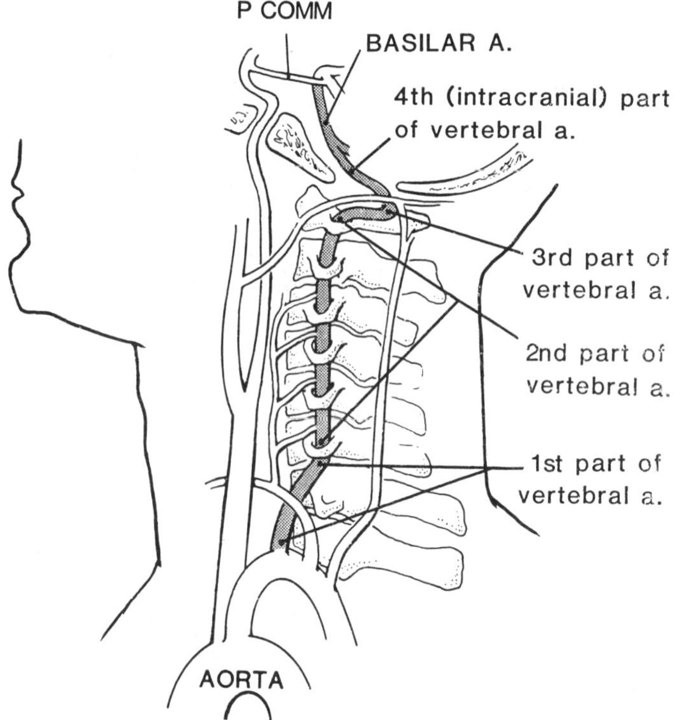

FIG 16–1.
Vertebral artery anatomy.

Subclavian Artery Disease

Subclavian steal was one of the first vascular syndromes described in modern times. Initial reports noted the radiologic findings in patients with occlusion or severe stenosis of one subclavian artery proximal to the vertebral artery origin.[3, 4] Blood flowed from the contralateral vertebral artery to the basilar artery, then down the ipsilateral vertebral artery to supply the ischemic arm (Fig 16–2). We now know more about this syndrome and its recognition, prognosis, and treatment. Routine testing of patients with peripheral vascular and coronary artery disease by noninvasive techniques (Doppler ultrasound and plethysmography) often detects coexistent subclavian artery occlusive disease. Often the patients have no symptoms. When symptomatic, the most common complaints are coldness, cramps, and fatigue in the ischemic arm. CNS symptoms are much less common and include episodic transient spells of dizziness, diplopia, visual blur-

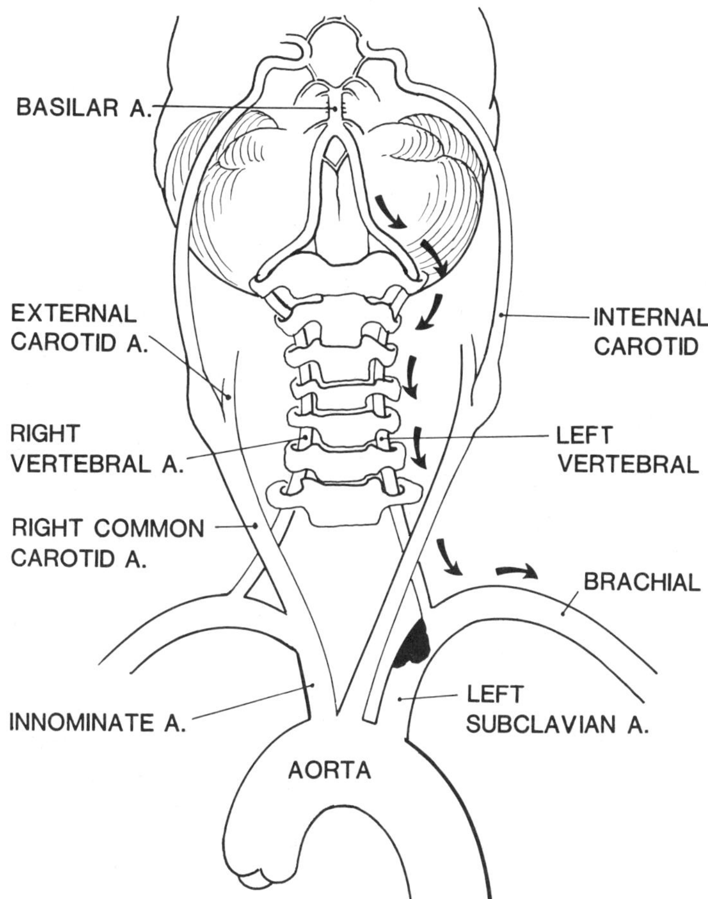

FIG 16–2.
Diagram showing subclavian steal after left subclavian artery occlusion.

ring, and staggering. Neurologic and arm symptoms can be precipitated by exercising the arm, but most often are spontaneous and unprovoked. Although transient attacks are common, strokes are not.[5, 6] The quantity of available collateral circulation usually leads to spontaneous cessation of neurologic symptoms with time. For this reason and because surgery on the proximal intrathoracic subclavian artery is more complex and risky than vascular surgery in the neck, surgical correction of left subclavian steal is seldom warranted for relief of neurologic symptoms. However, in some patients arm symptoms can be disabling and require correction. Subclavian artery occlusive disease is most often caused by atherosclerosis. Serious occlusive disease of the extracranial carotid arteries frequently coexists with and usually explains hemiplegia or other persistent neurologic signs. Physicians are often seduced by the intriguing radiologic display of reversal of vertebral artery flow and ignore the more ordinary but more serious carotid artery occlusive disease.

Disease of the left subclavian artery is much more common than right-sided disease. However, the right subclavian artery is more intimately and directly connected to the carotid system. Clot in the right subclavian artery can enter the parent innominate artery and embolize into intracranial carotid artery branches, causing stroke.[7, 8] For this reason, the risk of right subclavian or innominate artery occlusive disease is much greater than for comparable severity left subclavian disease, and it warrants more aggressive management strategies such as the use of anticoagulants or surgical correction. Subclavian and innominate artery occlusion also occurs in temporal arteritis and Takayasu's disease.

Proximal Vertebral Artery Disease

Atherosclerosis commonly involves the origin of the vertebral arteries. Plaques arise within the subclavian artery and extend into the vertebral artery orifices or originate within the first few millimeters of the vertebral artery. Proximal vertebral artery atherostenosis has a high correlation with disease of the internal carotid artery origin, coronary artery, and peripheral vascular occlusive disease, and hyperlipidemia. Proximal vertebral artery disease is common in white men but is less frequent in women, blacks, and patients of Oriental origin. The symptoms of proximal vertebral artery disease are identical to those found in patients with subclavian steal—episodic dizziness, staggering, diplopia, and blurring of vision. In general, the prognosis of unilateral proximal vertebral artery occlusive disease is benign, with a relatively low incidence of stroke subsequent to known severe occlusive lesions.[9] The good prognosis is probably explained by the availability of rich collateral circulation from branches of the thyrocervical and costocervical branches of the subclavian artery, the occipital branch of the external carotid artery, and many small muscular branches of the vertebral arteries. In contrast, there are no cervical branches of the internal carotid artery. When the vertebral artery is occluded at its origin, nearly always the vessel can be shown to reconstitute in the neck by collateral flow. Chronic hemodynamic insufficiency rarely, if ever, is a problem after proximal vertebral artery occlusion.

Evaluation of patients with sudden onset of symptoms referrable to the more distal vertebrobasilar system sometimes reveals a distal embolus blocking the posterior cerebral artery or one of its branches and a recent occlusion of the proximal vertebral artery. The recently formed clot had served as a source of distal embolization. In some of these patients transient spells of dizziness and diplopia had preceded the stroke and warned of the developing vertebral artery lesion. When a vessel occludes, clot is fresh and loosely adherent to the vertebral artery wall, so it can readily propagate, fragment, or embolize. With time (2–3 weeks), the clot organizes and adheres to the vessel wall. Embolization is rare after organization of the occlusive vascular lesion. A similar situation is well-known in the anterior circulation; evaluation of patients with middle cerebral artery branch occlusion often reveals a source of embolization in the form of recent occlusion in the internal carotid artery in the neck. I currently treat patients who have had recent occlusion of the proximal vertebral artery with heparin, then warfarin for 3–4 weeks. I do not use long-term treatment because of the rarity of chronic hemodynamic insufficiency or late embolization. Even bilateral occlusion of the vertebral artery origins is surprisingly well tolerated.[10]

Vertebral Artery Disease Within the Bony Vertebrae—A Rare Problem

It was once popular to attribute vertebrobasilar insufficiency to compression of the vertebral arteries by bony cervical spine spurs. The vertebral arteries, after their proximal portion, enter C6 and travel within the transverse foramina of C6 – C3. Proponents of the theory of spondylitic vascular insufficiency hypothesized that the arteries were compressed during their intravertebral course, especially when the neck was turned. Some patients had surgery on spondylitic spurs to treat their vertebrobasilar transient ischemic attacks. Time and data have proved this theory a myth. (1) Cervical spondylitis is ubiquitous over the age of 35. (2) In other regions of the body, when arteries or aneurysms are adjacent to bone, the artery, with blood pulsating at systemic blood pressure, erodes bone rather than bone compromising the artery. (3) Spondylic spurs usually form on the posterior aspects of the body of the vertebrae and are not positioned to affect formamen transversara even on turning (Fig 16–3). (4) When large series of patients with vertebral angiography are analyzed, fewer than 1% have occlusive lesions in the vertebral arteries within their intravertebral course in the neck.[11] (5) Autopsy studies document that minor

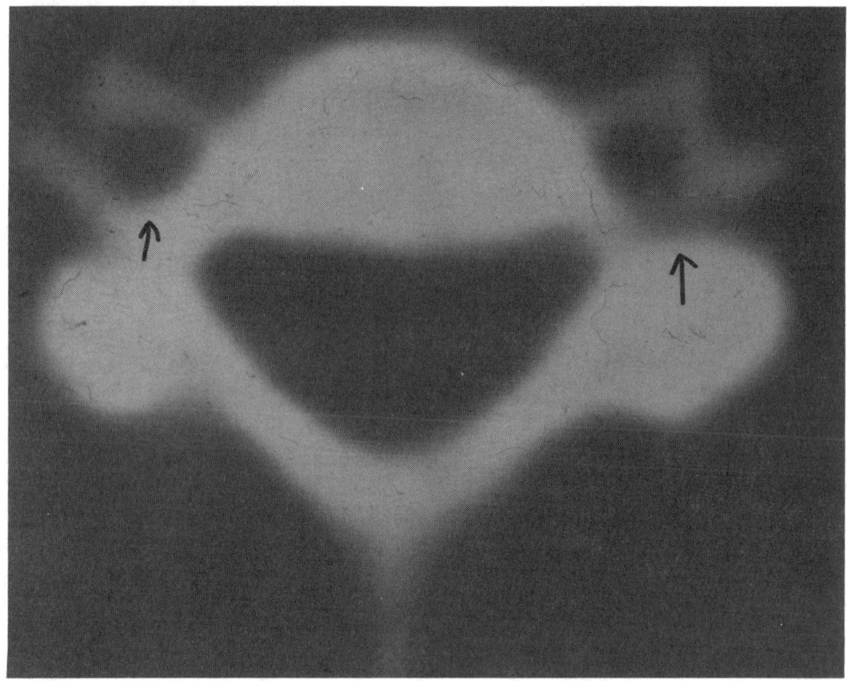

FIG 16–3.
CT cross section of cervical vertebra. *Arrows* point to foramina transversara.

plaques can occur at interspaces, but stenosis is rarely attributable to the adjacent bony disease.[12] Acute neck trauma with vertebral injury can cause occlusion of one or both vertebral arteries with severe posterior circulation infarction.

Distal Extracranial Vertebral Artery Disease

After emerging from the transverse foramina, the vertebral arteries course behind the rostral cervical vertebrae and enter the cranium through the foramen magnum. Anchored caudally within the vertebral column and rostrally within the cranium, this distal free extracranial portion of the vertebral artery is especially vulnerable to injury by sudden motion. Dissection of the distal extracranial vertebral artery can follow neck manipulation or injury during sports activity or neck turning.[13] Spontaneous dissection of the distal extracranial vertebral artery also occurs and is more common than currently recognized.[14] The most frequent symptoms are head, neck, and occipital pain. Elements of the lateral medullary syndrome are also usually present and include vertigo, facial pain or burning, diplopia, hoarseness, difficulty swallowing, and ataxia. Strokes are probably more common than vertebral transient ischemic attacks. When an artery dissects, clot may enter the lumen by an intimal tear or may form spontaneously in the compressed lumen. This fresh clot propagates or embolizes intracranially, causing lateral medullary or cerebellar ischemia. The arterial lesion usually heals over a period of 6 weeks to 6 months. Anticoagulants may control embolization of clot during the period of healing.

Intracranial Vertebral Artery Disease

Intracranial stenosis or occlusion of the vertebral artery is usually caused by atherosclerosis. The lesions favor the proximal intradural segment and region proximal to the vertebrobasilar junctions. Figure 16–4 depicts an intracranial vertebral artery occlusion extending beyond the origin of the posterior inferior cerebellar artery (PICA). Uni-

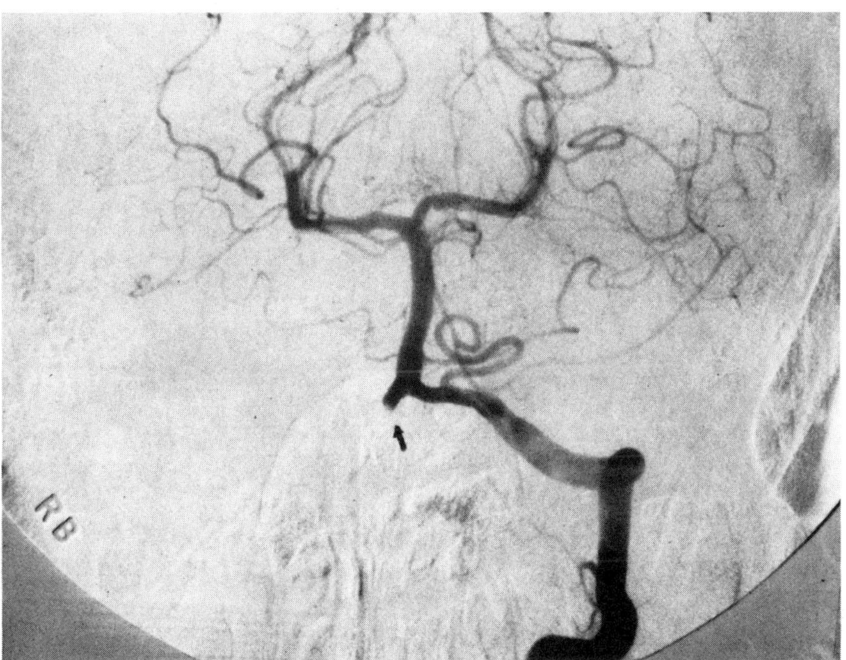

FIG 16–4.
Vertebral angiogram, AP view. Occlusion of right intracranial vertebral artery *(arrow)*.

lateral intracranial vertebral artery occlusive disease causes ischemia of the lateral and medial medulla and the cerebellum. Figure 16–5 diagrams the various syndromes caused by intracranial vertebral artery occlusion. Some patients have transient symptoms that mimic the lateral medullary syndrome which include: (1) headache, mostly in the occiput or neck, (2) spinning dizziness or wavering feelings, (3) sensation of being pulled to one side on sitting or standing, (4) vomiting, (5) pain or jabbing or burning feeling on one side of the face, (6) dysphagia and hoarseness. Table 16–1 lists the most common findings

VERTEBRAL ARTERY OCCLUSION
(INTRACRANIAL)

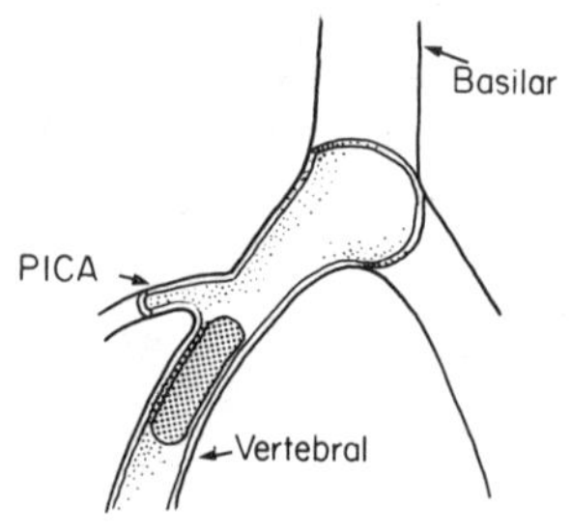

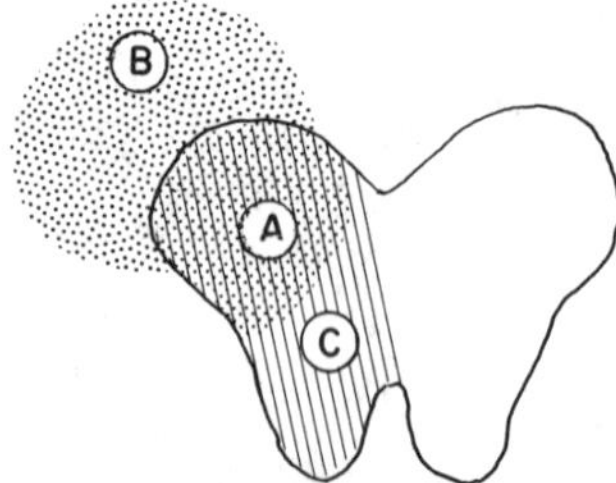

Ⓐ LATERAL MEDULLARY INFARCTION
Ⓑ CEREBELLAR INFARCTION
Ⓒ HEMIMEDULLARY SYNDROME
D TRANSIENT EPISODES ONLY ESPECIALLY DIZZINESS
E EMBOLUS TO MORE DISTAL BASILAR ARTERY
F EXTENSION OF CLOT TO BASILAR ARTERY

FIG 16–5.
Unilateral intracranial vertebral artery occlusion—clinical syndromes.

TABLE 16–1
Lateral Medullary Syndrome

Symptoms and Signs	
Ipsilateral	Contralateral
Limb and gait ataxia	Loss of pain and temperature sensation on the body
Dizziness and nystagmus	
Loss of pain and temperature and corneal reflex	
Horner's syndrome	
Hoarseness; dysphagia; paralysis of pharynx, palate, and vocal cord; hiccups	
Loss of taste	

in patients with lateral medullary infarcts. Hemiplegia indicating medial medullary or lower pontine paramedian basal ischemia is much less common. When ischemia is limited to the cerebellum, patients report occipital or generalized headache, dizziness, inability to walk, and vomiting.

As in most other recent vascular occlusions, the danger of serious or permanent infarction is highest at the time of occlusion. Collateral circulation is not well developed, and the fresh, poorly adherent clot can propagate or embolize. When the contralateral vertebral artery is of normal size and widely patent, the prognosis in patients with lateral medullary or small cerebellar infarcts is good. I often use short-term heparin or warfarin for patients with complete occlusion of the vertebral artery intracranially and continue this treatment for 4–6 weeks. When the vascular lesion is tight stenosis or bilateral intracranial vertebral artery disease, I prescribe longer-term warfarin anticoagulation.[15]

Bilateral severe intracranial vertebral artery stenosis or occlusion is potentially a much more serious vascular lesion than unilateral disease. When symptoms develop, they are often progressive and in my experience are not halted by anticoagulants. Chronic insufficiency to the medulla and cerebellum persist. Some have treated such patients with a surgically created bypass connecting usually the occipital branch of the internal carotid artery with posterior inferior cerebellar artery branches.[16] I have discussed the symptoms, diagnosis, and treatment of ischemic vertebrobasilar disease in more detail elsewhere.[5, 15, 17]

Sometimes the intracranial vertebral artery lesion is an aneurysm. Aneurysms of the intracranial vertebral artery are of three types—saccular (berry), fusiform, and dissecting. Saccular aneurysms are most common at the vertebral-PICA junction[18] and generally produce no symptoms unless they bleed, causing subarachnoid hemorrhage. Fusiform, dolichoectatic aneurysms, on the other hand, frequently cause symptoms by pressure effects on the adjacent lower brain stem and cranial nerves.[19] The most frequent cranial nerve symptoms are vertigo, tinnitus, lancinating pain in the throat ("glossopharyngeal neuralgia"), and hiccoughs. Mass effects on the lateral brain stem can produce signs similar to any other extracranial posterior fossa tumor. Occasionally, clot will form within large saccular or dolichoectatic aneurysms and obliterate the orifices of penetrating arteries, causing ischemia. Clot can also embolize distally to basilar artery branches. Dissection of the intracranial vertebral artery causes subarachnoid hemorrhage when the dissection extends into and through the adventitia. In other patients, the intramural dissection can obliterate the lumen and usually extends into the basilar artery, causing severe brain stem ischemia and headache.[20]

DROP SPELLS

The term "drop spell" has become synonymous in the minds of some with vertebrobasilar disease. No statement, in my opinion, could be farther from the data. Sudden dropping to the ground with loss of consciousness can be caused by myriad conditions; e.g., tripping, near syncope, loss of postural reflexes, loss of balance, spinal cord dysfunction, akinetic seizures. Stepping on a stone often gives a triple flexion reflex that includes leg buckling. Falling among elderly persons is a problem of large proportions, since falls can cause broken hips, a common cause of fatality in the old and infirm. Some patients with posterior circulation vascular disease do fall, but invariably in my experience there are other signs and symptoms that point to a vascular etiology. Meissner et al.[21] reviewed the Mayo Clinic experience with patients who had drop attacks, and the authors could not identify a single instance of drop attacks as an isolated sign in vertebrobasilar disease. Causes of drop spells in their series were quite varied, and prognosis depended on cause. The etiology in many instances escapes definition. (Editor's note: Drop attacks are also a rare manifestation of endolymphatic hydrops, attributed to abrupt disturbances of otolith receptor control of postural tone against gravity, and known as Tumarkin's otolithic crises.[26])

DIAGNOSIS

Diagnosis of patients with episodic vertigo depends on the background medical history of the patient, the duration, nature, and timing of the spells, and their precipitants and accompanying symptoms and signs. CT occasionally helps by identifying cerebellar infarction. MRI is superior to CT in detecting brain stem and cerebellar infarction.[22] "Dynamic CT" (sequential CT films of the posterior structures after dye injection), ENG, caloric testing, and auditory brain stem-evoked responses (BAER) have not helped in the problem case. Noninvasive testing of the vertebral arteries is in widespread use in Germany and will undoubtedly spread. Pulsed Doppler and plethysmography are very accurate in detecting significant subclavian artery occlusive disease.[23, 24] Continuous wave (CW) Doppler has proved very useful in evaluating severe obstructive lesions of the vertebral arteries, even when the lesion involves the distal vertebral or proximal basilar arteries.[25] Transcranial Doppler is a very promising technique for imaging the intracranial vertebral and basilar arteries. Definitive diagnosis of the location of vascular lesions is by angiography. Digital subtraction angiography can opacify the intracranial system. The dye load is high, films are often suboptimal, and intracranial opacification is seldom ideal. For these reasons intra-arterial digital subtraction angiography has become the method of choice for posterior circulation opacification. The dye load is small, and visualization is excellent. The complication rate in patients with vertebral angiography is lower than in carotid disease. It is far better in problem cases to define the vascular lesion than to guess or to use warfarin empirically. I do not use long-term warfarin therapy in patients with occlusive vertebrobasilar disease without angiographic confirmation of the lesion.

REFERENCES

1. Drachman D, Hart C: An approach to the dizzy patient. *Neurology* 1980; 22:323–334.
2. Caplan LR, Kelly JJ: Syncope, in *Consultations in Neurology*. Toronto, BC Decker, Inc, 1988, pp 41–44.
3. Reivich M, Holling E, Roberts B, et al: Reversal of blood flow through the vertebral artery and its effect on cerebral circulation. *N Engl J Med* 1961; 265:878–885.
4. Fisher CM: A new vascular syndrome—"the subclavian steal" (editorial) *N Engl J Med* 1961; 265:912–913.

5. Caplan LR: Vertebrobasilar occlusive disease, in Barnett HJ, Mohr JP, Stein BM, et al (eds): *Stroke, Pathophysiology, Diagnosis, and Management.* New York, Churchill Livingstone, 1986, pp 549–619.
6. Baker R, Rosenbaum A, Caplan LR: Subclavian steal syndrome. *Contemp Surg* 1974; 4:96–104.
7. Symonds C: Two cases of thrombosis of subclavian artery with contralateral hemiplegia of sudden onset, probably embolic. *Brain* 1927; 50:259–260.
8. Fields WS, Lemak N, Ben-Menachem Y: Thoracic outlet syndrome, review and reference to stroke in a major league pitcher. *Am J Neuroradiol* 1986; 7:73–78.
9. Moufarrij N, Little JR, Furlan AJ, et al: Vertebral artery stenosis: Long term follow-up. *Stroke* 1986; 15:260–263.
10. Fisher CM: Occlusion of the vertebral arteries. *Arch Neurol* 1970; 22:13–19.
11. Radner S: Vertebral angiography by catheterization. *Acta Radiol* 1951(Suppl 87), 1–134.
12. Moosy J: Morphology, sites, and epidemiology of cerebral atherosclerosis. *Proceedings Assoc Res Nerv Ment Dis Cerebrovascular Disease* 1966; vol 51, pp 1–22.
13. Easton JD, Sherman DG: Cervical manipulation and stroke. *Stroke* 1977; 8:594–597.
14. Caplan LR, Zarins C, Hemmatti M: Spontaneous dissection of the extracranial vertebral arteries. *Stroke* 1985; 16:1030–1036.
15. Caplan LR: Treatment of patients with vertebrobasilar occlusive disease. *Compr Ther* 1986; 12:23–28.
16. Ausman J, Caplan LR, Diaz F: Surgically created posterior circulation vascular shunts. *Clin Neurosurg* 1986; 33:327–330.
17. Caplan LR: Vertebro-basilar artery system, in Vinken PJ, Bruyn GW, Klawans H (eds): *Handbook of Clinical Neurology*: Revised series, vol II: Toole J (ed): Vascular diseases. Amsterdam, Elsevier Biomedical Publishers, 1988, in press.
18. Bull J: Contribution of radiology to the study of intracranial aneurysms. *Br Med J* 1962; 2:1701–1708.
19. Caplan LR: Miscellaneous cerebrovascular disorders, in Yatsu F, Grotta J, Pettigrew L (eds):*Seminars in Neurology, Stroke.* New York, Thieme Medical Publishers, 1986, 6:267–276.
20. Caplan LR, Baquis GD, Pessin MS, et al: Dissection of the intracranial vertebral artery. *Neurology* 1988, in press.
21. Meissner I, Wiebers D, Swanson J, et al: The natural history of drop attacks. *Neurology* 1986; 36:1029–1034.
22. Kistler JP, Buonanno FS, DeWitt LD, et al: Vertebral-basilar posterior cerebral artery territory stroke—delineation by proton nuclear magnetic resonance imaging. *Stroke* 1984; 15:417–426.
23. Berguer R, Higgins R, Nelson R: Non-invasive diagnosis of reversal of vertebral artery blood flow. *N Engl J Med* 1980; 302:1349–1351.

24. White DN, Ketelaars E, Cledgett PR: Non-invasive techniques for the recording of vertebral artery flow and their limitations. *Ultrasound Med Biol* 1980; 6:315–327.
25. Ringelstein E, Zeumer H, Poeck K: Non-invasive diagnosis of intracranial lesion in the vertebrobasilar system: A comparison of doppler sonographic and angiographic findings. *Stroke* 1985; 16:848–855.
26. Black FO, Effrom MZ, Burns DS: Diagnosis and management of drop attacks of vestibular origin: Tumarkin's otolithic crises. *Otolaryngol Head Neck Surg* 1982; 90:256–262.

17

The Management of Patients With Vestibular Disorders

David S. Zee, M.D.

Management of a vestibular disorder is frequently vexing for both patient and physician. In many instances the cause is uncertain, the treatment empirical, and the outcome less than satisfactory. Furthermore, despite a burgeoning scientific knowledge about basic vestibular physiology,[3, 85] the standard therapeutic regimen for vestibular disorders has undergone little modification, and effective treatment strategies remain elusive. This chapter presents a critique of the current approach to management and provides a theoretical framework on which diagnosis and treatment can be based.*

GENERAL PROBLEMS IN MANAGING PATIENTS WITH VESTIBULAR DISORDERS

Difficulty of Diagnosis: Vestibular Function Tests

One major problem in diagnosing vestibular disturbances is the limited information provided by routine laboratory vestibular function tests. There are five vestibular sensory organs within each labyrinth—three semicircular canals and two otolith organs—and each

*The reader is also referred to several recent related articles.[2, 16, 19, 91, 92]

contributes to two types of postural reflexes: vestibulo-ocular and vestibulospinal. Yet routine vestibular function studies, with either caloric or rotational stimuli, probe only the lateral semicircular canals, and even then just the vestibulo-ocular response.

Vestibular function studies have other shortcomings. Caloric stimulation is imprecise; the thermal gradient delivered to the cupula and endolymph cannot be accurately quantified. Furthermore, caloric stimuli only mimic head motions comprised of low-frequency components. Patients who have no response to caloric stimuli may show a nearly normal rotational response if the frequency of head rotation is sufficiently high.[4] In other words, an absent caloric response does not preclude some function of the lateral semicircular canal. Finally, the usual explanation for the caloric response—induction of convection currents within the endolymph—may not be entirely correct. Caloric stimulation of astronauts in the microgravity environment of the Space Shuttle still elicited a nystagmus response.[7] This finding suggests that at least some component of the caloric response is due to direct thermal activation of the labyrinthine hair cells or their primary vestibular neurons.

Rotational tests have advantages over caloric tests: the stimulus can be controlled precisely, a wide range of frequencies can be tested, and the response is little affected by anatomical variations within the temporal bone. But since rotational tests must always stimulate both labyrinths simultaneously, they are unable to detect unilateral peripheral vestibular lesions reliably. Furthermore, although rotational-testing responses are easy to quantify, there is still a wide range of normal values.[3] Here, as for caloric tests, many factors—age, level of alertness, mental set, use of a variety of medications (sedatives, hypnotics, anticonvulsants, etc.), and even whether the patient wears glasses—may influence the results and confound their interpretation.[3, 23, 57, 83, 89]

Impaired Adaptive (Compensatory) Mechanisms

The CNS has a variety of mechanisms to cope with vestibular disturbances. They include the ability to adjust VOR and vestibulospinal reflexes directly and the flexibility to substitute reflexes mediated by other sensory modalities. The former mechanism is exemplified by the elimination of spontaneous vestibular nystagmus by rebalancing the tone between the vestibular nuclei centrally.[49] Another example is the modulation of VOR and vestibulospinal reflexes in response to wearing glasses with a new prescription.[23, 42] Substitution of reflexes mediated by other sensory modalities is illustrated by patients with complete loss of labyrinthine function. They rely on proprioception—from both the neck and the limbs—and upon vision, to provide the stimuli for generating compensatory eye movements during head and body motion.[14, 38, 58] If there is some impairment of the patient's ability, either to adaptively modulate vestibular responses or to substitute other sensory inputs for those from the labyrinth, it becomes more difficult to overcome a superimposed vestibular disturbance.

Several structures within the CNS are important in vestibular compensation. These include the cerebellum, vestibular commissure, reticular formation, spinal cord, and cerebral hemispheres.[35, 40, 55, 65, 72, 78] Patients with a vestibular disorder due to or associated with a lesion within one of these structures may have incapacitating and unremitting imbalance, dizziness, or vertigo.[69, 76] Lesions that eliminate or distort the sensory feedback needed by adaptive networks to monitor vestibular performance may retard or forestall appropriate vestibular compensation or even result in decompensation in a previously compensated patient.[29, 72, 78] Disabling dizziness and imbalance are common symptoms of elderly patients with failing vision (e.g., cataracts) or blunted proprioception (e.g., cervical osteoarthritis or peripheral neuropathy). In such patients, multiple sensory deficits prevent adequate signaling of, or appropriate sensory substitution for, incorrect vestibular responses.[33]

These considerations suggest an obvious, practical course: improving the quality of inputs from the visual and proprioceptive senses—for example, a cataract extraction followed by an intraocular lens implant—helps patients to develop more accurate postural readjustments in response to movements of the head and body.

Lack of Coherent Treatment Strategies

"Vestibular Suppressants" and Sedation

Symptomatic treatment of vertigo and imbalance with medications is largely trial and error. Often drugs are prescribed without regard to the effects they may have on the natural processes by which compensation takes place. Before prescribing "vestibular suppressants," one must remember that the CNS must be made aware that something is wrong so that it can calculate the necessary adjustments to restore vestibular balance. Much of the required information only becomes available through sensory feedback, when the patient attempts to use his vestibular reflexes. In other words, sensory conflicts, either intravestibular (e.g., between the otolith organs and the semicircular canals) or intersensory (between vision, proprioception and the labyrinths), are necessary to help signal the need for and direction of adaptive change. Unfortunately, such conflicts provoke the severe vegetative symptoms that can incapacitate and immobilize patients. The paradox then seems to be that we have to encourage a patient to feel even more sick before he can become well.

Work in experimental animals provides compelling evidence that a period of immobilization after an acute unilateral loss of labyrinthine function not only retards but actually limits the ultimate degree of vestibular compensation that is reached.[35, 49, 50, 61, 62, 70, 78] Conversely, it has been shown that enforced activity that appropriately challenges the vestibular system enhances the rate of compensation.[35, 49, 70]

It has been suggested that there is a "critical period" immediately after a vestibular insult during which the potential capacity of the CNS to adapt to a lesion is greatest. This interval may coincide with an inhibition of activity within the vestibular nuclei; the initial mechanism used by the CNS to reduce the imbalance of tonic activity between the vestibular nuclei.[66]

One important caution in interpreting the results of these studies of immobilization and activity is that the standard measure of recovery was restoration of vestibulospinal balance. Immobilization may not retard vestibulo-ocular as much as vestibulospinal compensation,[56, 78] since information from the somatosensory system may be more important for the latter. Furthermore, some rebalancing between the vestibular nuclei, which diminishes spontaneous nystagmus, can occur in complete darkness without any visual feedback.[29, 44] But dynamic compensation—restoration of appropriate amplitude and symmetry during head movements—can only take place if the CNS is apprised of a need for it.[93, 99, 100] It is the error signal associated with the use of an inappropriate vestibular reflex that serves as the necessary stimulus for adaptive change. Therefore, patients with an acute vestibular disorder must be encouraged to become active early.

Thus, we are left with the potentially paradoxical effects of vestibular suppressants on patients with an acute vestibular disorder. Suppressing their vestibular imbalance and its consequent distressing symptoms may not be in the best interests of the patient. The optimal therapeutic strategy is to use medications to relieve the vegetative symptoms (nausea, vomiting, headache, etc.) but not the vestibular imbalance, the sensory conflicts it creates, or the adaptive mechanisms that remove it. Obviously, when deciding what medications to prescribe, the prudent physician must adroitly balance the patient's needs for comfort and for rehabilitation.

A possible exception to this approach is the management of an acute but transient and self-limiting vestibular imbalance such as that posed by Meniere's disease. In such cases the vestibular imbalance usually resolves itself promptly. Therefore, it is reasonable to prescribe immobilization and sedation for the acute attack. Chronic vestibular imbalance due to permanent damage should be treated as described above, by encouraging vestibular rehabilitation based on natural compensatory mechanisms.

The Neuropharmacology of Medications Used to Treat Vestibular Disturbances

Motion Sickness Versus Pathologic Vestibular Disorders.—Another important gap in our knowledge of the pharmacotherapy of vertigo is the lack of reliable data on the effectiveness of the many drugs used in treatment. There is much information about the use of various drugs in the prevention of symptoms of motion sickness.[18, 73, 88] These findings often do not apply to the treatment of the symptoms of a patient with a pathologic vestibular imbalance. While the symptoms of normal subjects with motion sickness and patients with vestibular lesions are similar, the vestibular imbalance in each case proceeds from a different cause. The vestibular stimuli that produce motion sickness, while excessively prolonged and/or in conflict with other sensory stimuli, nevertheless are appropriate. They provoke a normal, reciprocal (push-pull) change in peripheral activity: the discharge of afferents from one labyrinth increases while that from the other decreases. In contrast, when the function of one labyrinth is reduced (e.g., acute vestibular neuritis), the CNS does not receive a reciprocally balanced input. The tonic level of afferent input from the affected side is decreased because of the lesion but the normal side does not change. Likewise, during head rotations only the activity of the intact labyrinth is modulated. Thus, there is a barrage of incongruous labyrinthine inputs on the CNS whether the head is still or moving. This unnatural pattern of sensory input may incite the severe vegetative symptoms commonly associated wtih peripheral labyrinthine lesions.

Furthermore, central vestibular lesions, while also producing an acute vestibular imbalance, usually involve structures where afferent information from both labyrinths already has been combined. Asymmetry in vestibular activity then may be perceived as a naturally induced imbalance likely to cause relatively milder symptoms, similar to those associated with motion sickness in normal individuals. Consequently, vegetative symptoms may be less severe with central than with peripheral vestibular lesions (unless, of course, the medullary vomiting centers are directly involved).

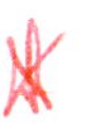

Effects of Drugs on Activity Within Vestibular Neurons.—Several experimental studies have reported the effects of drugs on activity within vestibular neurons. Many medications—anticholinergics, monoaminergics, diazepam, GABA and glycine antagonists, antihistaminics, and narcotics—alter and usually suppress the level of tonic activity within vestibular neurons.[21, 34, 43, 48, 60, 71, 77] Some drugs affect vestibular neurons (primary or secondary) directly; others alter vestibular activity secondarily by changing the activity of neurons within the reticular formation or cerebellum. Autoradiographic studies have demonstrated a high density of histamine and muscarinic (acetylcholine) receptors within the medial vestibular nucleus.[68, 84] But these studies probably have little relevence to the more important question: Will a particular drug be effective for patients? The many ways that drugs can modulate activity within the vestibular nuclei make it that much more difficult to predict the mechanisms of action of medications proposed for patients. Most such drugs have more than one type of action, and which one predominates may depend on the dose. For example, the phenothiazines frequently have antidopaminergic, anticholinergic, and antihistaminic activity, and each may have some effect on activity within the vestibular system.

Effects of Drugs on Vestibular Responses.—Similar considerations apply to the measurement of the effects of various drugs on vestibular responses in normal human and animal subjects. Knowing the effects of any drug on, for example, the amplitude of response to a rotational vestibular stimulus does not enable one to predict whether that drug will have any symptomatic benefit for patients. For example, in normal monkeys subjected to rotational stimuli, diazepam increases the time constant, decreases the amplitude, and abolishes any inherent asymmetries of the response.[12] Despite these effects, it has not been established that diazepam facilitates the ultimate level of recovery in primates.[95] In normal human subjects, drugs used to prevent motion sickness, such as scopolamine, promethazine, and dimenhydrinate, decrease the amplitude of the vestibular response.[28, 74, 97] Sedatives, however, such as alcohol and secobarbital, do the same but are not known to prevent motion sickness.[27] Yet the combination of promethazine plus amphetamine, which does not affect the vestibular response, produces one of the most effective antimotion sickness medications. Thus, while quantifying the effects of medications on normal

vestibular responses is of interest, it certainly does not answer the crucial question: Does the drug have any effect—good or bad—on the state of recovery eventually reached by a patient with a vestibular lesion?

Effects of Drugs on Vestibular Adaptation.—Recent experimental work suggests a basis for trials of various drugs in human patients with vestibular disorders (Table 17–1). In animals that have undergone a unilateral labyrinthectomy and given time to compensate, cholinomimetic, adrenergic, or GABA agents and even alcohol produce a reversible decompensation.[1, 8, 9, 37, 78] Conversely, anticholinergic agents and adrenergic and GABA blockers result in reversible overcompensation. Furthermore, if during compensation a drug is given that causes transient decompensation, the final state of compensation is achieved more rapidly.[35] This last finding reinforces the idea that for vestibular compensation to be most successful intense signals of a vestibular imbalance must be available to central structures.

Studies in guinea pigs have shown that sedatives (e.g., barbitu-

TABLE 17–1.

Drugs That May Affect Vestibular Compensation[37, 49, 78, 94, 96, 97, 98]

Retard compensation
Alcohol
Phenobarbital
Chlorpromazine
Diazepam*
ACTH antagonists
Accelerate compensation
Caffeine
Amphetamines
ACTH
Diazepam*
Produce decompensation
Cholinomimetics, cholinesterase inhibitors
Adrenergic agents
GABA agonists
Alcohol
Produce overcompensation
Anticholinergics
α-Adrenergic blockers
GABA blockers

*There is conflicting evidence about the effects of diazepam on vestibular adaptation.

rates, alcohol, chlorpromazine, diazepam) retard vestibular compensation while stimulants (caffeine, amphetamines) accelerate it.[78] A peptide fragment of ACTH ($ACTH_{4-10}$) also increases the rate of compensation; a specific ACTH antagonist or hypophysectomy slows it.[36, 96] But when the ACTH is stopped, the animal's state of compensation reverts to the level reached by control animals. In the few studies performed in primates, cholinomimetic agents produce decompensation in monkeys that had compensated to a unilateral labyrinthectomy,[49] while depletion of catecholamines with 6-hydroxydopamine inhibited adaptive responses that adjust the amplitude of the VOR.[59, 95] Both $ATCH_{4-10}$ and thyrotropin-releasing hormone promote vestibular compensation in monkeys.[96, 101]

Finally, there is evidence that increases in metabolic activity are necessary to maintain compensation. In unilaterally labyrinthectomized rats, metabolism of 2-deoxyglucose within the vestibular nuclei and cerebellum is increased even after complete compensation is achieved.[65]

These pharmacologic and metabolic studies all suggest that the state of compensation for a vestibular lesion is both dynamic and fragile. Achieving and maintaining compensation probably require continuous metabolic activity. The state of compensation is influenced by exogenous factors (e.g., medications) as well as by fluctuations in the endogenous neurohumoral milieu. The "spontaneous" fluctuations in intensity of symptoms that patients so frequently report probably reflect the tenuous state of vestibular compensation and its susceptibility to pharmacologic manipulation.

There are caveats, of course, in attempting to apply the results of these experimental studies to patients. There seem to be inconsistencies between studies. For example, there are discrepancies in the reported effects of adrenergic agents and of diazepam on adaptation.[9, 78, 98] Experimental results are based for the most part on studies in lower animals, and the compensatory mechanisms for human beings may be different. Furthermore, in most work vestibulospinal, not vestibulo-ocular, compensation was examined. This is important because the adaptive mechanisms for each are, at least partially, under separate control.[56, 78] Finally, the processes underlying the restoration of static vestibular balance (with the head stationary) and of dynamic vestibular balance (with the head moving) and the readjustment of the amplitude of the vestibular response may be mediated by different structures and may have different biochemical bases. Nevertheless, taken together, these experimental studies suggest that a variety of centrally acting drugs may influence the rate of acquisition and the maintenance of compensation after a vestibular lesion. However, the effectiveness of any specific medication regimen for patients remains to be demonstrated convincingly.

Physical Therapy for Symptoms of a Vestibular Disorder

In addition to prescribing drugs for a patient with a vestibular disorder, the physician must designate a level of activity and set forth a plan for physical rehabilitation. As discussed above, there is experimental evidence that inactivity retards the rate and possibly the ultimate degree of compensation reached after a vestibular lesion; enforced activity accelerates compensation. Even prolonged bed rest in normal subjects degrades subsequent performance on balance tests, possibly because there is some degree of vestibular decompensation associated with inactivity.[45] Therefore, the therapeutic strategy for acute vestibular imbalance is to encourage the patient to actively engage his vestibular system. Again, a possible exception is the patient with a transient self-limiting vestibular imbalance, such as that brought on by an attack of Meniere's disease. In such cases one might not attempt to stimulate compensation until the acute attack has ended.

When a patient has recovered sufficiently from an acute vestibular insult, or in a patient with chronic symptoms of vestibular dysfunction, a formal program of rehabilitative therapy should be instituted. Although there are no controlled studies conclusively demonstrating that vestibular exercise programs are of long-term benefit to these patients, abundant experimental evidence and compelling theoretical considerations point to their efficacy.[20, 22]

Several principles should govern the program of vestibular training exercises.[91]

1. Training tasks should exceed the level of capability of the patient, and difficulty should be increased progressively as improvement is achieved.

2. Stimuli should be designed to mimic those body movements and environmental conditions that produce symptoms during natural behavior. This often means abrupt, rapid movements in a high-contrast visual environment that fills the entire field of view. Stimulation of large portions of the visual field, including the periphery, seems to have the strongest effects on vestibular responses.[32]

3. Both self-generated and passively induced head movements should be practiced. Still unsettled is what proportions of each result in optimal compensation. Different frequencies of head motion should be attempted; there is experimental evidence that vestibular adapta-

tion is frequency specific. When experimental animals wear magnification spectacles, adaptation is greatest for the frequency of head rotation used during the training periods.[64]

4. Training tasks should be chosen that not only tax the capabilities of labyrinthine receptors but also promote the development of alternative patterns of motor behavior based on nonlabyrinthine sensory inputs (e.g., visual and somatosensory afferents). Patients should attempt to selectively stimulate each sensory modality while eliminating the effect of the others. For example, the patient is instructed to balance on one foot with the eyes closed to eliminate visual inputs; while standing on foam rubber to blunt somatosensory inputs; or with the head tilted forward or backward to elicit different combinations of otolith inputs.[20] There is also evidence that repetitive exposures to purely visual (optokinetic) stimuli may hasten restoration of vestibular balance.[69]

5. Vestibular training should also be used to develop higher levels of volitional control over vestibular compensatory responses. The patient should practice creating an internal model of the outside world that can be used when sensory stimuli are lacking.[5, 57]

TREATMENT OF SPECIFIC DISORDERS

Acute Peripheral Vestibular Imbalance

As indicated above, the strategy for treating patients with acute vestibular imbalance depends on the specific cause and whether the episode is expected to be short-lived and spontaneously reversible. Therapy can be specific or symptomatic. Specific therapy depends on the diagnosis. Epilepsy, migraine, neurosyphilis,[86] thyroid disease, collagen vascular disease, pyogenic infections, blood dyscrasias, etc., should be treated with appropriate specific medications. Surgically remediable conditions (e.g., tumors, congenital malformations, perilymph fistulae[80]) also must be diagnosed appropriately and treated.

Symptomatic therapy for acute vestibular imbalance includes medications, a plan of physical activity, and a careful explanation to the patient of the nature of the illness.[2, 19, 91] The last, in particular, is essential. The ideal medication for treating patients with vertigo should suppress the vegetative symptoms but not the vestibular imbalance. The latter must be allowed to correct itself naturally. Thus, except in conditions such as Meniere's disease, sedation and immobilization should be avoided. Antiemetics with as little sedative effect as possible, or combined with ephedrine, should be used. At the same time the patient should be encouraged to keep his eyes open and move about as soon and as much as possible to stimulate rebalancing and recalibration of VOR and vestibulospinal reflexes. Naturally, some patients with severe symptoms are so anxious and vertiginous that they refuse to open their eyes or move their heads at all. With these individuals an explanation of the nature of the problem and plan of treatment usually obviates sedatives or tranquilizers.

When the initial severe symptoms have been controlled, physical therapy must be forcefully encouraged and the patient started on an exercise program based on the principles enumerated above. One must prod the patient to move about to accelerate adaptation, but the initial movements must not provoke such severe symptoms that the physician loses the patient's confidence and cooperation.

Meniere's Disease

Meniere's disease is a particularly challenging therapeutic problem. Attacks are unpredictable in occurrence, duration, and intensity; even the direction of vestibular asymmetry may spontaneously fluctuate. Thus, adaptive recalibration is difficult, sometimes impossible. Acute attacks can be treated with antiemetics. When necessary, strong sedation is reasonable, since the vestibular imbalance usually resolves promptly of its own accord. To prevent attacks, strict adherence to a low-salt diet in association with a diuretic frequently is helpful.[41] An antimotion sickness agent also may be of value. It must be remembered, though, that the rate of spontaneous remission in Meniere's disease is so high that all therapies appear effective.

Surgical therapy can give enduring relief to patients with Meniere's disease.[47, 81] Drainage procedures, such as cochleosacculotomy,[79] sometimes help; labyrinthectomy (when hearing is already lost) or selective vestibular nerve section may be indicated. Both local (within the middle ear) and systemic streptomycin have been used to induce a chemical labyrinthectomy.[87] One problem with such destructive procedures is that in many patients with Meniere's disease both labyrinths eventually become involved. It should be emphasized that symptoms similar to those in Meniere's disease appear in patients with a variety of other conditions, including thyroid disease, neurosyphilis, collagen vascular disease, perilymph fistula, and otosclerosis. The last condition, which commonly runs in families, usually is associated with hearing loss (typically conductive but sometimes sensorineural). Calcium carbonate, vitamin D, and sodium fluoride are reported to relieve symptoms, but carefully controlled studies are lacking.[24]

Chronic Vestibular Imbalance

Many patients with chronic symptoms of vestibular dysfunction have lost adaptive capabilities and/or have coincident defects in other sensory systems. Diminished vision or dulled proprioception interferes with vestibular rehabilitation. Even disordered inputs from neck afferents probably exacerbate symptoms of vestibular dysfunction, by virtue of the important role neck proprioception plays in the perception of head relative to body motion.[13]

For all patients with enduring symptoms vestibular training exercises should be instituted. If appropriate, an empirical trial of one of the many different medications used to treat vertigo can be attempted. Acetazolamide, β-blockers, tricyclic antidepressants, dopaminergic agents, anticholinergics, and antihistaminics seem to benefit some patients.[2, 19, 91] Well-designed controlled trials of these drugs have not been performed, and there is no way at present to confidently predict which patients will be helped by what medications.

One drug that has a specific therapeutic effect on a type of central vestibular imbalance is baclofen.[46] Baclofen abolishes the acquired form of periodic alternating nystagmus, a central vestibular disorder usually due to posterior fossa lesions. It has been proposed that periodic alternating nystagmus arises from instability within the central vestibular connections that normally act to perseverate vestibular responses beyond what one would expect from the activity of peripheral afferents alone.[63] Baclofen presumably acts by potentiating inhibition within this circuit and thereby stopping the nystagmus.[102] (See chapter 12 for further discussion of baclofen and periodic alternating nystagmus.) There is no information, however, about the clinical effectiveness of baclofen in vestibular disorders other than periodic alternating nystagmus.

Treatment of Positional Vertigo

Vestibular exercises are most helpful in the treatment of benign paroxysmal positional vertigo (BPPV).[17] The exact mechanism by which such exercises work is not known, although it seems likely that the recovery is achieved by restoring the normal mechanical relationships of the cupula and endolymph within the posterior semicircular canal. In severe cases it is often helpful to medicate the patient with an antimotion sickness agent, for example, about 1 hour before each exercise period. Occasionally, the patient must be admitted to the hospital to be helped to perform the exercises. The major drawback to such a physical therapy program is the extreme reluctance of some patients to precipitate their symptoms voluntarily.

A rare patient with BPPV has such intractable symptoms that section of the ampullary nerve that supplies the offending posterior semicircular canal is undertaken.[39] This surgical procedure is reported to completely relieve the symptoms but carries a risk of loss of hearing.

Finally, a recent report suggests that some patients with intractable vestibular symptoms, often exacerbated by changes in position, benefit from microvascular decompression of the vestibular portion of the 8th cranial nerve where it courses through the cerebellopontine angle.[54] The ultimate effectiveness of this procedure in well-categorized groups of patients remains to be proved. It should be remembered also that almost all patients reported to have benefited from this procedure also had symptoms and signs of involvement of the auditory portion of the 8th cranial nerve, thus removing them from the diagnostic category of BPPV.

PERSPECTIVES

How can we improve our approach to the management of patients with vestibular disorders? An important step will be to develop more reliable ways of testing the vertical semicircular canals and the otolith organs. The vertical VOR can be measured by rotating a patient with his head tilted to one side or, in the appropriate type of stimulator, with the head upright.[6] Otolith function can be assessed by measuring the amount of counter-rolling (cyclotorsion) of the eyes during a sustained lateral head tilt,[30, 31] by measuring the nystagmus response during constant-velocity rotation of the head (and body) around an axis tilted away from the vertical,[25] and by measuring the effect of head tilt on the time course of decay of post-rotatory nystagmus.[25] (See chapter 12 for further discussion of otolith function tests.) The clinical efficacy of such tests remains to be proved.

Perhaps what is more important in developing better ways to test vestibulo-ocular responses is to choose stimuli unfettered by the limitations of current vestibular tests. In particular, one wants a stimulus to which the CNS is either unable to adapt or to which it has not had the exposure that make adaptive modifications necessary. One can choose patterns of head rotation rarely encountered in natural behavior, such as rotations of high velocities,[53] or with the head placed so as to be able to stimulate specific pairs of semicircular canals selectively. Recent theoretical formulations suggest that a mathematical analysis (using matrices) of the contributions of the various pairs of semicircular canals enables one to predict how particular lesions of specific canals might alter slow-phase amplitude and direction during vestibular stimulation.[75]

Another potential diagnostic tool is full-field optokinetic responses. Optokinetic afternystagmus—the response when the lights are turned off during optokinetic stimulation—is another index of activity within the vestibular nuclei altered by both peripheral and central vestibular lesions.[51, 52, 90]

A promising approach is the application to clinical problems of quantitative measures of vestibulospinal reflexes using posturography. This is especially important, since a large proportion, perhaps even a majority, of patients with chronic vestibular disorders complain of imbalance, not vertigo or oscillopsia.

Visual-proprioceptive-labyrinthine interactions can be tested easily with posturography by selectively eliminating proprioceptive or visual stimuli.[11, 67] For example, a specific pattern of abnormal postural control has been identified in patients with BPPV. Such patients rely more heavily on visual cues for postural stability than do normal subjects. If during posturography visual feedback is eliminated by experimentally causing the visual scene to move in exact register with the motion of the body (opening the feedback loop), patients with BPPV are more unstable than if they simply close their eyes.[10] Likewise, patients who have recently lost labyrinthine function also rely more on visual than somatosensory inputs to compensate for postural disequilibrium.[15] Patients with more chronic lesions show an increased reliance on both vision and proprioception.[67] Thus, one can monitor postural control quantitatively during the various stages of compensation that follow a labyrinthine lesion. A battery of vestibular function tests combining measurements of both VOR and vestibulospinal reflexes will improve the capability to detect vestibular disturbances and to monitor the effects of treatment.[82]

An important potential tool for evaluation of a patient with a vestibular disorder is measurement of adaptive capabilities. Can the patient promptly change the amplitude of the VOR, measured in darkness, after briefly wearing magnifying spectacles?[26] Can the patient promptly learn to decrease postural sway during a brief period of training exercises.[22] Does he show a normal pattern of habituation to multiple repetitions of the same vestibular stimulus? If so the time course of adaptation and habituation can be measured and compared with those of the normal range of responses.

The pharmacologic manipulation of adaptive capabilities is a potential strategy for management of patients with vestibular disorders. Evidence indicates that a variety of drugs alter the rate of vestibular compensation. Ultimately we should be able to optimize the pharmacotherapy of vestibular patients so that we can selectively diminish symptoms without retarding and perhaps even enhancing compensation. Likewise, as we learn more about adaptation and motor learning in general, we can plan more effective physical therapy programs to speed recovery, to encourage appropriate sensory substitution, and to optimize vestibular performance. All such therapeutic innovations—with both drugs and physical therapy—must be critically evaluated in patients using carefully controlled studies with objective measurements of vestibulo-ocular and vestibulospinal function.

Acknowledgments

Tim Hain and Leonard Proctor made helpful suggestions. Vendetta Matthews provided editorial assistance.

REFERENCES

1. Abeln W, Bienhold H, Flohr H: Influence of cholinomimetics and cholinolytics on vestibular compensation. *Brain Res* 1981; 222:458–462.
2. Baloh RW: The dizzy patient: Symptomatic treatment of vertigo. *Postgrad Med* 1983; 73:317–324.
3. Baloh RW, Honrubia V: *Clinical Neurophysiology of the Vestibular System*. Philadelphia, FA Davis Co, 1979.
4. Baloh RW, Honrubia V, Yee RD, et al: Changes in the human vestibulo-ocular reflex after loss of peripheral sensitivity. *Ann Neurol* 1984; 16:222–228.
5. Baloh RW, Lyerly K, Yee RD, et al: Voluntary control of the human vestibulo-ocular reflex. *Acta Otolaryngol (Stockh)* 1984; 97:1–6.
6. Baloh RW, Richman L, Yee RD, et al: The dynamics of vertical eye movements in normal human subjects. *Aviat Space Environ Med* 1983; 54:32–38.
7. Baumgarten R von, Benson A, Berthoz A, et al: Effects of rectilinear acceleration and optokinetic and caloric stimulations in space. *Science* 1984; 225:208–212.
8. Berthoz, A, Young L, Oliveras F: Action of alcohol on vestibular compensation and habituation in the cat. *Acta Otolaryngol (Stockh)* 1977; 84:317–327.

9. Bienhold H, Abeln W, Flohr H: Drug effects on vestibular compensation, in Flohr H, Precht W (eds): *Lesion-Induced Neuronal Plasticity in Sensorimotor Systems.* Amsterdam, Springer-Verlag, 1981, pp 265–273.
10. Black FO, Nashner LM: Postural disturbance in patients with benign paroxysmal positional nystagmus. *Ann Otol Rhinol Laryngol* 1984; 93:595–599.
11. Black FO, Wall C, Nashner LM: Effects of visual and support surface orientation references upon postural control in vestibular deficient subjects. *Acta Otolaryngol (Stockh)* 1983; 95:199–210.
12. Blair SM, Gavin M: Modifications of vestibulo-ocular reflex induced by diazepam: Experiments in the macaque. *Arch Otolaryngol* 1979; 105:698–701.
13. Bles W, Vianney de Jong JMB: Cervico-vestibular and visuo-vestibular interaction. *Acta Otolaryngol (Stockh)* 1982; 94:61–72.
14. Bles W, Vianney De Jong JMB, De Wit G: Somatosensory compensation for loss of labyrinthine function. *Acta Otolaryngol (Stockh)* 1984; 97:213–221.
15. Bles W, Vianney de Jong JMB, de Wit G: Compensation for labyrinthine defects examined by use of a tilting room. *Acta Otolaryngol (Stockh)* 1983; 95:576–579.
16. Brandt Th, Daroff RB: The multisensory physiological and pathological vertigo syndromes. *Ann Neurol* 1980; 7:195–203.
17. Brandt Th, Daroff RB: Physical therapy for benign paroxysmal positional vertigo. *Arch Otolaryngol* 1980; 106:484–485.
18. Brandt Th, Dichgans J, Wagner W: Drug effectiveness on experimental optokinetic and vestibular motion sickness. *Aerospace Med* 1974; 45:1291–1297.
19. Brandt Th: Medikamentose und physikalische therapie des schwindels und der ataxie. *Fortschr Neurol Psychiatr* 1981; 49:88–100.
20. Brandt Th, Krafczyk S, Malsbenden I: Postural imbalance with head extension: Improvement by training as a model for ataxia therapy. *Ann NY Acad Sci* 1981; 374:636–649.
21. Brown RD, Wood CD: Vestibular pharmacology. *Trends Pharmacol Sci* 1980; 1:150–153.
22. Buchele W, Knaup H, Brandt Th: Time course of training effects on balancing on one foot. *Acta Otolaryngol (Stockh) [Suppl]* 1984; 406:140–142.
23. Cannon SC, Leigh RJ, Zee DS, et al: The effect of the rotational magnification of corrective spectacles on the quantitative evaluation of the VOR. *Acta Otolaryngol (Stockh)* 1985; 100:81–88.
24. Cody DTR, Baker HL: Otosclerosis: Vestibular symptoms and sensorineural hearing loss. *Ann Otol Rhinol Laryngol* 1978; 87:778–796.
25. Cohen B, Suzuki J, Raphan T: Role of the otolith organs in generation of horizontal nystagmus: Effects of selective labyrinthine lesions. *Brain Res* 1983; 276:159–164.
26. Collewijn H, Martins AJ, Steinman RM: Compensatory eye movements

during active and passive head movements: Fast adaptation to changes in visual magnification. *J Physiol* 1983; 340:259–286.

27. Collins WE, Schroeder DJ, Elam GW: Effects of D-amphetamine and of secobarbital on optokinetic and rotation-induced nystagmus. *Aviat Space Environ Med* 1975; 46:357–364.
28. Collins WE, Schroeder DJ, Elam GW: A comparison of some effects of three antimotion sickness drugs on nystagmic responses to angular accelerations and to optokinetic stimuli. *Aviat Space Environ Med* 1982; 53:1182–1189.
29. Courjon JH, Jeannerod M, Ossuzio I, et al: The role of vision in compensation of vestibulo-ocular reflex after hemilabyrinthectomy in the cat. *Exp Brain Res* 1977; 28:235–248.
30. Diamond SG, Markham CH: Ocular counterrolling as an indicator of vestibular otolith function. *Neurology* 1983; 33:1460–1469.
31. Diamond SG, Markham CH, Furuya N: Binocular counterrolling during sustained body tilt in normal humans and in a patient with unilateral vestibular nerve section. *Ann Otol Rhinol Laryngol* 1982; 91:225–229.
32. Dichgans J, Brandt Th: Visual-vestibular interaction: Effects on self-motion perception and postural control, in Teuber H-L, Held R, Leibowitz H (eds): *Handbook of Sensory Physiology*. Berlin-Heidelberg-New York, Springer, 1978, Vol III, pp 753–804.
33. Drachman DA, Hart CW: An approach to the dizzy patient. *Neurology (Minneap)* 1972; 22:323–334.
34. Ehrenberger K, Benkoe E, Feln D: Suppressive action of picrotoxin—a GABA antagonist—on labyrinthine spontaneous nystagmus and vertigo in man. *Acta Otolaryngol (Stockh)* 1982; 93:269–273.
35. Flohr H, Bienhold H, Abeln W, et al: Concepts of vestibular compensations, in Flohr H, Precht W (eds): *Lesion-induced Neuronal Plasticity in Sensorimotor Systems*, Amsterdam, Springer-Verlag, 1981, pp 153–172.
36. Flohr H, Luneburg U: Effects of $ACTH_{4-10}$ on vestibular compensation. *Brain Res* 1982; 248:169–173.
37. Flohr H, Abeln W, Luneburg U: Neurotransmitter and neuromodulator systems involved in vestibular compensation, in Berthoz A, Melvill Jones G (eds): *Reviews of Oculomotor Research, Adaptive Mechanisms in Gaze Control*. New York, Elsevier, 1985, pp 269–277.
38. Furuya K, Takemori S: Visual compensation after unilateral sudden loss of vestibular function. *Adv Otorhinolaryngol* 1983; 30:338–340.
39. Gacek RR: Singular neurectomy update. *Ann Otol Rhinol Laryngol* 1982; 91:469–473.
40. Galiana HL, Flohr H, Jones GM: A reevaluation of intervestibular nuclear coupling: Its role in vestibular compensation. *J Neurophysiol* 1984; 51:242–259.
41. Glasscock ME, Davis WE, Hughes GB, et al: Medical management of Meniere's disease. *Ann Otol Rhinol Laryngol* 1981; 90:142–147.
42. Gonshor A, Jones GM: Postural adaptation to prolonged optic reversal of vision in man. *Brain Res* 1980; 192:239–248.

43. Guth SL, Norris CH: Pharmacology of the isolated semicircular canal: Effects of GABA and picrotoxin. *Exp Brain Res* 1984; 56:72–78.
44. Haddad GM,Friendlich AR, Robinson DA: Compensation of nystagmus after VIIIth nerve lesions in vestibulo-cerebellectomized cats. *Brain Res* 1977; 135:192.
45. Haines RF: Effect of bed rest and exercise on body balance. *J Appl Physiol* 1974; 36:323–327.
46. Halmagyi G, Rudge P, Gresty M, et al: Treatment of periodic alternating nystagmus. *Ann Neurol* 1980; 8:609–611.
47. Hammerschlag PE, Schuknecht HF: Transcanal labyrinthectomy for intractable vertigo. *Arch Otolaryngol* 1981; 107:152–156.
48. Harris T, Eviatar A, Goodhill V: Droperidol and fentanyl citrate compound as a vestibular depressant. *Arch Otolaryngol* 1969; 89:482–487.
49. Igarashi M: Vestibular compensation: An overview. *Acta Otolaryngol (Stockh) [Suppl]* 1984; 406:78–82.
50. Igarashi M, Levy JK, O-Uchi T, et al: Further study of physical exercise and locomotor balance compensation after unilateral labyrinthectomy in squirrel monkeys. *Acta Otolaryngol (Stockh)* 1981; 92:101–105.
51. Ireland DJ, Jell RM: Optokinetic after-nystagmus in man after loss or reduction of labyrinthine function—a preliminary report. *J Otolaryngol* 1982; 11:86–90.
52. Ireland DJ, Jell RM: Symmetrical optokinetic after-nystagmus loss in Wallenberg's syndrome and multiple sclerosis. *Acta Otolaryngol (Stockh) [Suppl]* 1984; 406:235–238.
53. Istl YE, Hyden D, Schwarz DWF: Quantification and localization of vestibular loss in unilaterally labyrinthectomized patients using a precise rotatory test. *Acta Otolaryngol (Stockh)* 1983; 96:437–445.
54. Jannetta PJ, Moller MB, Moller AR: Disabling positional vertigo. *N Engl J Med* 1984; 310:1700–1705.
55. Jeannerod M, Courjon JH, Flandrin JM, et al: Supravestibular control of vestibular compensation after hemilabyrinthetomy in the cats, in Flohr H, Precht W (eds): *Lesion-Induced Neuronal Plasticity in Sensorimotor Systems*. Amsterdam, Springer-Verlag, 1981, pp 208–220.
56. Jensen DW: Reflex control of acute postural asymmetry and compensatory symmetry after a unilateral vestibular lesion. *Neuroscience* 1979; 4:1059–1073.
57. Jones GM, Berthoz A, Segal B: Adaptive modification of the vestibulo-ocular reflex by mental effort in darkness. *Exp Brain Res* 1984; 56:149–154.
58. Kasai T, Zee DS: Eye-head coordination in labyrinthine-defective human beings. *Brain Res* 1978; 144:123–141.
59. Keller EL, Smith MJ: Suppressed visual adaptation of the vestibuloocular reflex in catecholamine-depleted cats. *Brain Res* 1983; 258:323–327.
60. Kirsten EB, Schoener EP, Wang SC: Effects of d-amphetamine on single vestibular neurons. *J Pharmacol Exp Ther* 1974; 191:377–383.
61. Lacour M, Roll JP, Appaix M: Modifications and development of spinal

reflexes in the alert baboon *(Papio papio)* following an unilateral vestibular neurotomy. *Brain Res* 1976; 113:255–269.
62. Lacour M, Xerri C: Vestibular compensation: New perspectives, in Flohr H, Precht W (eds): *Lesion-Induced Neuronal Plasticity in Sensorimotor Systems*. Amsterdam, Springer-Verlag, 1981, pp 240–253.
63. Leigh RJ, Robinson DA, Zee DS: A hypothetical explanation of periodic alternating nystagmus: Instability in the optokinetic-vestibular system. *Ann NY Acad Sci* 1981; 374:619–635.
64. Lisberger SG, Miles FA, Optican LM: Frequency selective adaptation: Evidence for channels in the vestibular reflex? *J Neurosci* 1983; 3:1234–1244.
65. Llinas R, Walton K: Vestibular compensation: A distributed property of the central nervous system, in Asanuma H, Wilson VJ (eds): *Integration in the Nervous System*. Tokyo, Igaku-Shoin, 1979, pp 145–146.
66. McCabe BF, Ryu JH, Sekitani T: Further experiments on vestibular compensation. *Laryngoscope* 1972; 82:381–396.
67. Nashner LM, Black FO, Wall C: Adaptation to altered support and visual conditions during stance: Patients with vestibular deficits. *J Neurosci* 1982; 2:536–544.
68. Palacios JM, Wamsley JK, Kuhar MJ: The distribution of histamine H1-receptors in the rat brain: An autoradiographic study. *Neuroscience* 1981; 6:15–37.
69. Pfaltz CR: Vestibular compensation: Physiological and clinical aspects. *Acta Otolaryngol (Stockh)* 1983; 95:402–406.
70. Precht W: Neurophysiological and diagnostic aspects of vestibular compensation. *Adv Otorhinolaryngol* 1983; 30:319–329.
71. Precht W, Schwindt PC, Baker R: Removal of vestibular commissural inhibition by antagonists of GABA and glycine. *Brain Res* 1973; 62:222–226.
72. Putkonen PTS, Courjon JH, Jeannerod M: Compensation of postural effects of hemilabyrinthectomy in the cat: A sensory substitution process? *Exp Brain Res* 1977; 28:249–257.
73. Pyykko I, Schalen L, Jantti V: Transdermally administered scopolamine vs. dimenhydrinate: 1. Effect on nausea and vertigo in experimentally induced motion sickness. *Acta Otolaryngol (Stockh)* 1985; 99:588–596.
74. Pyykko I, Schalen L, Matsuoka I: Transdermally administered scopolamine vs. dimenhydrinate: II. Effect on different types of nystagmus. *Acta Otolaryngol (Stockh)* 1985; 99:597–604.
75. Robinson DA: The use of matrices in analyzing the three-dimensional behavior of the vestibulo-ocular reflex. *Biol Cybern* 1982; 46:53–66.
76. Rudge R, Chambers BR: Physiological basis for enduring vestibular symptoms. *J Neurol Neurosurg Psychiatr* 1982; 45:126–130.
77. Ryu JH, McCabe BF: Effects of diazepam and dimenhydrinate on the resting activity of the vestibular neuron. *Aerospace Med* 1974; 45:1177–1179.
78. Schaefer K-P, Meyer DL: Aspects of vestibular compensation in guinea

pigs, in Flohr H, Precht W (eds): *Lesion-Induced Neuronal Plasticity in Sensorimotor Systems.* Amsterdam, Springer-Verlag, 1981; pp 197–207.

79. Schuknecht HF: Cochleosacculotomy for Meniere's disease: Theory, technique and results. *Laryngoscope* 1982; 92:853–858.
80. Singleton GT, Post KN, Karlan MS, et al: Perilymph fistulas: Diagnostic criteria and therapy. *Ann Otol Rhinol Laryngol* 1978; 87:797–803.
81. Snow JB, Kimmelman CP: Assessment of surgical procedures for Meniere's disease. *Laryngoscope* 1979; 89:737–747.
82. Wall C, Black FO: Postural stability and rotational tests: Their effectiveness for screening dizzy patients. *Acta Otolaryngol (Stockh)* 1983; 95:235–246.
83. Wall C, Black FO, Hunt AE: Effects of age, sex and stimulus parameters upon vestibulo-ocular responses to sinusoidal rotation. *Acta Otolaryngol (Stockh)* 1984; 98:270–278.
84. Wamsley JK, Lewis MS, Young WS, et al: Autoradiographic localization of muscarinic cholinergic receptors in rat brainstem. *J Neurosci* 1981; 2:176–191.
85. Wilson VJ, Jones GM: *Mammalian Vestibular Physiology.* New York, Plenum Press, 1979.
86. Wilson WR, Zoller M: Electronystagmography in congenital and acquired syphilitic otitis. *Ann Otol Rhinol Laryngol* 1981; 90:21–24.
87. Wilson WW, Schuknecht H: Update of use of streptomycin therapy for Meniere's disease. *Am J Otol* 1956; 2:108–111.
88. Wood CD, Graybiel: Evaluation of antimotion sickness drugs: A new effective remedy revealed. *Aerospace Med* 1970; 41:932–933.
89. Yagi T, Sekine S, Shimizu M: Age-dependent changes in the gains of the vestibular-ocular reflex in humans. *Adv Otorhinolaryngol* 1983; 30:9–12.
90. Zasorin NL, Baloh RW, Yee RD, et al: Influence of vestibulo-ocular reflex gain on human optokinetic responses. *Exp Brain Res* 1983; 51:271–274.
91. Zee DS: Treatment of vertigo, in Johnson RT (ed): *Current Therapy in Neurologic Disease.* Philadelphia, BC Decker Inc, 1985, pp 8–13.
92. Zee DS: Perspectives on the pharmacotherapy of vertigo. *Arch Otolaryngol* 1985; 3:609–612.
93. Fetter M, Zee DS, Proctor LP: Vestibular compensation in normal and cortically blind monkeys. *Soc Neurosci Abstr* 1986; 12:255.
94. Ishikawa K, Igarashi M: Effect of diazepam on vestibular compensation in squirrel monkeys. *Arch Otolaryngol* 1984; 240:44–54.
95. McElligott IG, Freedman W: Modification of the vestibulo-ocular reflex during behavioral and amphetamine arousal in cats before and after 6-OHDA induced norepinephrine depletion. *Soc Neurosci Abstr* 1986; 12:1087.
96. Igarashi M, Ishikawa K, Ishii M, et al: Effect of ACTH-(4–10) on equilibrium compensation after unilateral labyrinthectomy in the squirrel monkey. *Eur J Pharmacol* 1985; 119:239–242.

97. Ishikawa K, Igarashi M: Effect of atropine and carbachol on vestibular compensation in squirrel monkeys. *Am J Otolaryngol* 1985; 6:290–296.
98. Bernstein P, McCabe BF, Ryu TH: The effect of diazepam on vestibular compensation. *Laryngoscope* 1974; 84:267–272.
99. Fetter M, Zee DS: Recovery from unilateral labyrinthectomy in the rhesus monkey. *J Neurophysiol*, in press.
100. Fetter M, Zee DS, Proctor LP: Effects of lack of vision and of occipital lobectomy upon recovery from unilateral labyrinthectomy in the rhesus monkey. *J Neurophysiol*, in press.
101. Nasonori I, Igarashi M: Effect of thyrotropin-releasing hormone on vestibular compensation in primates. *Am J Otolaryngol* 1986; 7:177–180.
102. Cohen B, Helwig D, Raphan T: Baclofen and velocity storage: A model of the effects of the drug on the vestibulo-ocular reflex in the rhesus monkey. *J Physiol* 1987; 393:703–725.

Index

R

S